NONINVASIVE
TECHNIQUES
IN CARDIOLOGY
FOR THE NURSE
AND TECHNICIAN

NONINVASIVE TECHNIQUES IN CARDIOLOGY FOR THE NURSE AND TECHNICIAN

A. Benchimol, M.D.

Director, Institute for Cardiovascular Diseases
Good Samaritan Hospital
Phoenix, Arizona

A WILEY MEDICAL PUBLICATION

JOHN WILEY & SONS

New York • Chichester • Brisbane • Toronto

Library of Congress Cataloging in Publication Data:

Benchimol, Alberto.
    Noninvasive techniques in cardiology for the
nurse and technician.

    (A Wiley medical publication)
    Includes index.
    1. Heart—Diseases—Diagnosis. 2. Ultra-
sonic cardiography. 3. Vectorcardiography.
I. Title. [DNLM: 1. Phonocardiography.
2. Vectorcardiography. 3. Echocardiography.
4. Heart diseases—Diagnosis. WG141.5.P4 B457n]

RC683.5.U5B45   616.1'2'0754   78-9047
ISBN 0-471-04440-7

Printed in the United States of America

10 9 8 7 6 5 4 3 2 1

*To my wife Helena, our sons Nelson and Alex, my beloved
father Isaac, my mother Nina, and my sisters and brothers*

Foreword

It is a twofold honor to have been privileged to be a technician for a great clinician and teacher and to have been involved in much of the testing that constitutes the material in this book.

Dr. Benchimol has fulfilled a vast need for a concise text dealing with noninvasive studies in cardiology. He has, through his clinical experience, realized the importance of well-trained nurses and technicians and recognized their need for fundamental and practical knowledge. The time and effort put forth by Dr. Benchimol to provide us with such a useful text is a great compliment. It encourages us to strive continually to keep abreast of technological advances.

Bettie J. Massey
Supervisor, Invasive and Non-Invasive Laboratories
Institute for Cardiovascular Diseases
Good Samaritan Hospital
Phoenix, Arizona

Preface

This book is the result of the author's 15 years of experience in recording and analyzing phonocardiograms, pulse waves such as carotid, jugular venous, and apexcardiograms and other precordial pulsations, echocardiograms, transcutaneous ultrasonic techniques, and vectorcardiograms.

The text is divided into 12 chapters. Chapter 1 describes the anatomy and physiology of the cardiovascular system, which is extremely important in understanding phonocardiographic pulse waves and particularly echocardiography. Chapter 2 is devoted to the description of instrumentation used for phonocardiography, and discusses the basic principles of sound formation, transducers, different types of microphones, amplifiers, and recorders. Emphasis is also placed on the recognition of artifacts. The reader will find basic guidelines for pattern recognition of heart sounds, murmurs, and pulse waves as well as how to measure systolic time intervals and other intervals of the cardiac cycle. In Chapter 3 the field of vectorcardiography is discussed. Instrumentation and lead systems are described in detail. Again emphasis is placed on the importance of recognizing a technically adequate recording as well as artifacts. Comparison is made with the electrocardiogram, although the two techniques differ greatly. Chapter 4 is dedicated to the study of ultrasonic techniques as used in cardiovascular diagnosis. Both echocardiography and the basic Doppler flowmeter techniques are described. The principles of ultrasound, different types of probes, recognition of artifacts, and various types of recorders are described. Chapters 5 through 12 deal with specific disease states. In each of these chapters there is a standard format including recognition of abnormal patterns on phonocardiograms, carotid and jugular venous tracings, apexcardiograms, systolic time intervals, vectorcardiograms, and echocardiograms.

The book is clinically oriented and distinctly dedicated to technicians and nurses working in this field. It may also be useful to medical students and others interested in the technical aspects of noninvasive diagnosis. Areas of major controversy have purposely been avoided. The author does not intend to review all the literature available, but a list of useful references is given at the end of each chapter. A book of this size describing extremely broad issues will suffer in some areas due to the omission of other valuable techniques such as electrocardiography, exercise stress testing, and so forth.

A. B.

Acknowledgments

The author's initial experience that resulted in a lasting interest in cardiovascular diagnosis was obtained under the supervision of Dr. E. Grey Dimond. I am very grateful for his stimulation and support during my training at the University of Kansas School of Medicine, Kansas City, Kansas, and later, as his associate at Scripps Clinic and Research Foundation in La Jolla, California.

Good Samaritan Hospital in Phoenix, Arizona, has provided the necessary support to maintain a research and training program for the past 11 years, and the tracings shown in this book were all recorded there.

The assistance of postgraduate fellows, technicians, nurses, and secretaries who have worked in The Institute for Cardiovascular Diseases at Good Samaritan Hospital, Phoenix, Arizona, has been invaluable. I especially want to thank Bettie J. Massey, Supervisor of the Invasive and Non-Invasive Laboratories, for her outstanding efforts and assistance during the recording of tracings illustrated in this book. Dr. Paul Howard was very helpful during the manuscript preparation. I also want to acknowledge the outstanding efforts of Connie Sheasby, echocardiography technician, and Karen McCullough, phono- and vectorcardiography technician. I am greatly indebted to Sydney Peebles, who prepared all the illustrations and diagrams shown. I want to express my appreciation to Carole Crevier for her outstanding efforts during preparation of the manuscript and for editing and indexing this book and to Frances Maldonado and Bonnie Griner for their great assistance in the transcription, typing, and preparation of each chapter.

A. B.

Contents

NONINVASIVE TECHNIQUES IN CARDIOLOGY FOR THE NURSE AND TECHNICIAN

1
Basic Anatomy and Physiology of the Cardiovascular System

The heart functions as a pump circulating blood to the rest of the body. It performs this job tirelessly 24 hours a day, 7 days a week, and 365 days of the year. The heart continues this process without deterioration of function and will not fail unless disease alters its course.

In order to gain a close understanding of the subsequent chapters of this book, it would be of benefit to go into some detail about the normal anatomy and physiology of the heart at this time. The heart is a muscular structure that serves as a double pump, circulating blood returning from the body to the lungs for oxygenation and subsequently returning it to the heart for further circulation to the body tissues. The size of the heart is approximately 250–350 grams, or the size of a large fist. It lies in the center of the chest behind the sternum, with the greater portion of its muscular mass slightly to the left of the midline and posteriorly. The heart is protected within the chest by the sternum and rib cage anteriorly and the vertebral column and rib cage posteriorly. There are many other structures within the chest cavity that are in close approximation to the heart. These structures include the lungs, which lie on each side of the heart slightly covering it anteriorly, the esophagus, and the descending thoracic aorta, which lies just posterior to the heart (Fig. 1.1).

Other structures in the chest are protected from the heart's constant muscular contractions by a fibrous sac called the pericardium. The outer portion of this protective membrane (pericardium) is very tough and fibrous in nature. The pericardial membrane is attached to the great vessels entering and leaving the heart, to the diaphragm just below the heart, and to the sternum anteriorly. The inner portion of the pericardium folds around the heart and is adherent to the outer surface of the muscular layers. With this protective membrane, the heart is able to beat freely within the chest cavity without producing undue friction between itself and the other structures around it. Also, the pericardial sac protects the heart from all but the most severe infection that may occur in an adjacent thoracic structure.

The heart lies within this pericardial sac tethered by its attachment to the great vessels and its close attachment to the pericardial membrane. The heart is basi-

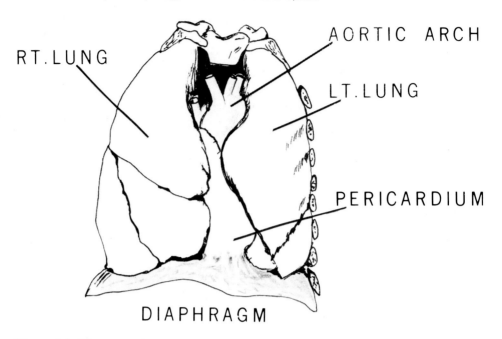

Figure 1.1. Diagrammatic representation of the heart from the frontal view showing the various intracardiac chambers and their relationship to each other.

cally composed of three layers. The outermost layer, the epicardium, is composed of the inner folding of the pericardium, which is in contact with the outer surface of the heart. The second layer, the myocardium, is composed of muscle layers that encompass the heart in a circular fashion. The innermost layer is called the endocardium and it lines the cardiac chambers and covers the valves. The smooth surface of this endocardial layer also extends outside the heart in continuity with the smooth inner surface of the great vessels. The smooth interface of the endocardium is designed to reduce friction on the fragile red blood cells as well as to prevent formation of blood clots within the heart chambers.

Before we look at the heart inside the pericardium, remember that spatial orientation of the heart valves and chambers is important. We talk about the right and left sides of the heart, but their orientation in the chest does not readily compare with that terminology. The heart lies in the center of the chest with the bulk of its muscular mass posterior and to the left. Right heart chambers actually lie anteriorly in the chest, and the left heart chambers lie posteriorly. With this fact in mind, we can look at the heart in detail.

We will now remove the pericardial sac from the heart and view the heart as it is set in the chest from an anterior view (Fig. 1.2). On the outer surface of the heart, or epicardium, one can see small arteries and veins that supply blood to the heart muscle. These vessels, the coronary arteries and veins, are adherent to the outer surface of the heart and have small branches that penetrate the myocardium in order to deliver oxygen and nutrients to the heart muscle. There are two such blood vessels that supply the heart, the right and left coronary arteries, and they have their origin at the very beginning of the ascending aorta. The cardiac veins

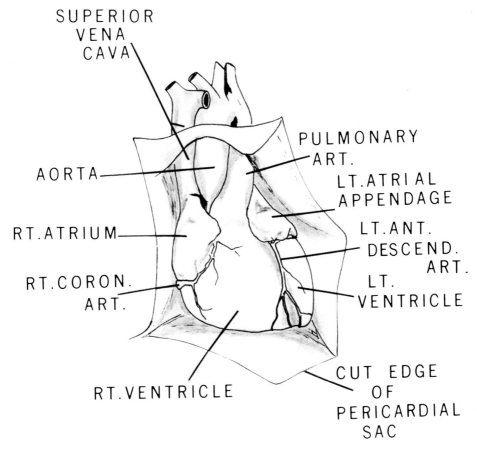

SUPERIOR
VENA
CAVA

PULMONARY
ART.

LT.ATRIAL
APPENDAGE

AORTA

LT.ANT.
DESCEND.
ART.

RT.ATRIUM

RT.CORON.
ART.

LT.
VENTRICLE

RT.VENTRICLE

CUT EDGE
OF
PERICARDIAL
SAC

Figure 1.2. Diagrammatic representation of the heart from the frontal view after the pericardial membrane has been removed. The position of the right and left coronary arteries and veins is shown in the epicardial surface of the heart. In addition, note the relationship of the right ventricle, which is the anterior chamber, and the left ventricle, which is the posterior chamber.

are also on the surface of the heart. They empty into what is known as the great cardiac vein, which lies on the posterior surface of the heart and empties into the right atrium at an entrance called the coronary sinus.

Looking at the heart from the frontal position, one can see that the right atrium lies anteriorly and on the right border of the heart. The right atrium receives blood from the upper and lower body through rather large veins called the superior and inferior vena cava, respectively. This blood is low in oxygen as it returns from the body tissues. The blood enters the right atrium and then is circulated to the right ventricle, which occupies the greater portion of the anterior surface of the heart. The right ventricle subsequently pumps the blood into the pulmonary artery, which immediately branches into a right and left vessel in order to transmit this desaturated blood to the lungs for reoxygenation. Blood returning from the lungs, high in oxygen content, enters the left atrium, which is on the posterior surface of the heart and cannot be seen from the front view. From the left atrium, it is then transmitted to the left ventricle where this oxygenated blood is then pumped to the body tissues through the aorta. From the front of the heart, the left ventricle is barely seen and occupies only a small portion of the left border of the heart.

In order to visualize the left atrium and the left ventricle more thoroughly, one must view the heart from a posterior vantage point (Fig. 1.3). In this view, the left atrium can be seen receiving reoxygenated blood from the four pulmonary veins that are coming from the lungs. This blood is then transmitted to the left ventricle, which occupies the greater portion of the heart's posterior surface.

To understand the anatomical configuration of the heart and why certain chambers lie anteriorly and posteriorly, it is of benefit to look at some of the physiologic functions that these chambers possess. Basically speaking, the right and left atria, as their names suggest, are chambers for receiving blood returning to the heart from the body and lungs, respectively. These receiving chambers hold the blood until the pumping chambers (right and left ventricles) have relaxed from their contractions and are able to accept a new volume for ejection to the lungs and body. The atria, then, do not have thick muscular walls; as a result, they function as receiving and filling chambers for the more powerful ventricles. The ventricles,

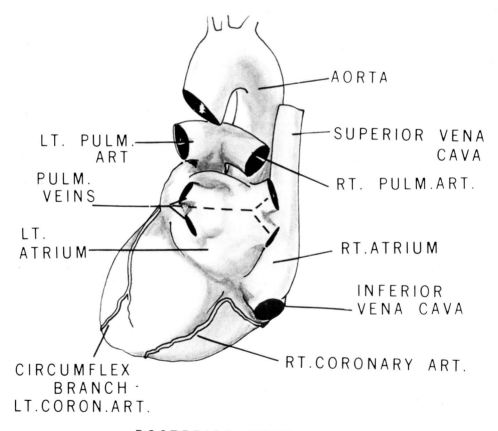

POSTERIOR VEIW

Figure 1.3. Diagrammatic representation of the heart as seen from a posterior view. The left atrium lies posterior to the right atrium and is connected with the pulmonary veins.

on the other hand, have much thicker muscular walls because of their inherent function of pumping blood out of the heart. There are, however, major differences between the right and left ventricles in their size and the amount of muscle mass they possess. The right ventricle is a somewhat larger chamber than the left ventricle but has thinner muscular walls. The left ventricle, on the other hand, has a smaller chamber size but thicker muscular walls. The major difference in the characteristics of the right and left ventricles again resides in their functional needs. The right ventricle receives the desaturated blood returning from the body through the right atrium. This blood in turn is pumped under *low pressure* into the lungs for reoxygenation. The left ventricle receives the oxygenated blood from the lungs, through the left atrium, and must pump this blood out into the aorta to all the tissues of the body. This contraction is done under a *higher pressure*, and more work must be done in order to eject the same amount of blood. Because of these major differences, the size and thickness of the right and left ventricle vary. Despite structural differences, the amount of blood pumped into the lungs is exactly the same as the amount of blood returned from the lungs and pumped out by the left side of the heart. In this manner, a balance between the right and left sides of the heart is maintained and no overloading occurs.

In order to accomplish this complex series of events, there are valves placed between the chambers of the heart and great vessels leading away from the heart to prevent back flow of blood. Thus, the heart basically has two types of heart valves. The atrioventricular valves are located between the atria and the ventricles. These valves permit forward flow of blood into the right and left ventricles during the period of relaxation. At the same time the semilunar valves prevent back flow of blood from the pulmonary artery and aorta. At the time of muscular contraction, the atrioventricular valves form a blood-tight seal to prevent back flow while the ventricles contract and eject the blood out of the heart into the pulmonary artery and aorta.

We will look at the cardiac chambers in more detail and study the different characteristics of these heart valves. In Figure 1.4, we see the right atrium, which occupies the right border of the heart. This cardiac chamber receives desaturated blood returning from the body tissues. The blood is transmitted into the right atrium from the superior and inferior vena cava. The right atrium also receives blood returning from the heart muscle through the great cardiac vein at an opening called the coronary sinus. This blood is then transmitted into the right ventricle at the time of heart relaxation (diastole) through the tricuspid valve. This valve is one of the atrioventricular valves that prevents back flow of blood into the atria at the time of muscular contraction (systole). Located between the right atrium and the right ventricle, the tricuspid valve has three leaflets that are attached to small muscular bundles in the right ventricle by little fibrous strands called chordae tendineae. Looking into the right ventricle, one can see the small papillary muscles with their chordae tendineae attachments connected to the very tips of the tricuspid leaflets. The purpose of the papillary muscles and the chordae tendineae is to prevent the leaflets from bulging back into the right atrium during contraction of the right ventricle. These attachments keep the valve leaflets stationary and prevent blood from leaking across the valve during muscular contraction. The right ventricle is a much more muscular structure than the right atrium. It has many muscular strands crossing over its inner surface (endocardium), which are

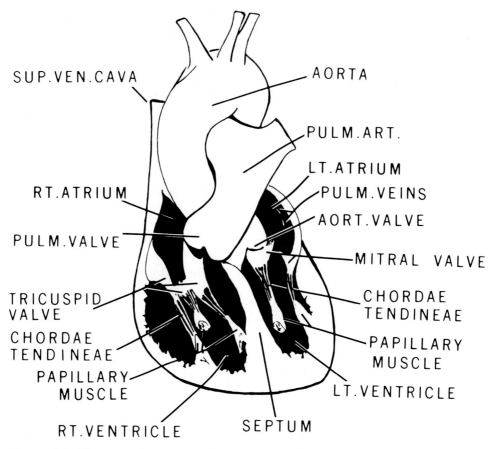

Figure 1.4. Diagrammatic representation of the heart from the frontal view. Note the various relationships of the intracardiac chambers, pulmonary artery and aorta, and the position of the tricuspid valve. Also shown in this figure is the pulmonary valve connecting the right ventricle with the pulmonary artery.

called trabeculae. The muscular wall of the right ventricle is approximately three times as thick as the muscular wall of the right atrium. In the outflow tract of the right ventricle, the pulmonary valve is noted. This is one of the semilunar valves that prevent back flow of blood from the pulmonary artery during the relaxation phase of the heart.

Beyond the pulmonary valve is the main pulmonary artery, which lies anterior to the aorta and subsequently branches into a right and left pulmonary artery to transmit unoxygenated blood to the right and left lungs. The left atrium receives the oxygenated blood from the lungs via four pulmonary veins, two from each lung. This oxygenated blood is then transmitted into the left ventricle during diastole by muscular contraction of the left atrium through the second atrioventricular valve called the mitral valve. The mitral valve has two leaflets, an anterior and a posterior one. As with the tricuspid valve, the mitral valve also has chordae tendineae, which extend from the edge of the leaflets to an anterior and posterior papillary muscle located in the left ventricular cavity. Looking at the left ventricle, one can see that this chamber is slightly smaller than the total size of the right ventricle, and its muscular walls are approximately three times thicker than those of the right ventricle. One can also note the muscular interventricular septum, which separates the right and left ventricles. The aortic valve lies in the outflow tract of the left ventricle, just posterior to the pulmonic valve. The aorta then ascends into the thoracic cavity to form an arch giving off major branches to the head and upper extremities. At the very origin of the aorta just outside of the aortic valve lies a slight dilatation of the aorta called the sinuses of Valsalva. These sinuses are in close relationship with the three cusps of the aortic valve and are called the right, left, and posterior (noncoronary) sinuses.

From the right and left sinuses of Valsalva are the origins of the right and left coronary arteries, respectively. These coronary arteries then course over the outer surface of the heart (epicardium) to supply blood to the myocardial tissue. The right coronary artery, which gains its origin in the right sinus of Valsalva, courses anteriorly in a groove between the right atrium and right ventricle to give off branches to the right atrium and sinus node (in 55% of hearts) and then turns posteriorly and inferiorly to descend in the posterior interventricular groove to supply the blood to this region of the heart. The right coronary artery in 90% of hearts supplies this area of the posterior wall and includes the atrioventricular nodal tissue (Fig. 1.5). The left coronary, on the other hand, originates from the left sinus of Valsalva and courses around the anterior and lateral aspects of the aorta. It immediately divides into two major branches. The first branch, called the left anterior descending, passes downward around the left side of the pulmonary artery in the anterior interventricular groove. This branch gives off smaller branches to the interventricular septum and anterolateral walls of the left ventricle. The other branch of the left coronary artery, called the circumflex branch, runs in the left atrioventricular groove around the left atrium and circles behind the heart. It then supplies branches that course down the posterior wall of the left ventricle as well as branches that supply blood to the posterior and lateral walls of the left ventricle. In 10% of hearts, the circumflex branch is much larger than the posterior branch of the right coronary artery and it is the one that supplies the blood to the atrioventricular nodal tissue.

THE CONDUCTION SYSTEM OF THE HEART

As we have looked into the anatomical aspects of the heart and some of the functional characteristics of specific heart chambers, we have not commented on how the heart actually performs its pumping action. The heart is able to perform this complex pumping action because of a synchronized cycle of contraction. This synchronized contraction pattern is accomplished by electrical stimulation of the muscle. Thus, the heart, just below its endocardial surface, has a complex system of conduction fibers that transmit electrical impulses to the cardiac chambers in order to produce a unified, synchronous muscular contraction (Fig. 1.6).

The location of this initial electrical stimulus, which is the major pacemaker center of the heart, is in the sinus node. This area is in the right atrium at the junction of the superior vena cava. In this region lies a group of specialized myocardial cells that have an inherent rate of electrical discharge. This electrical

POSTERIOR

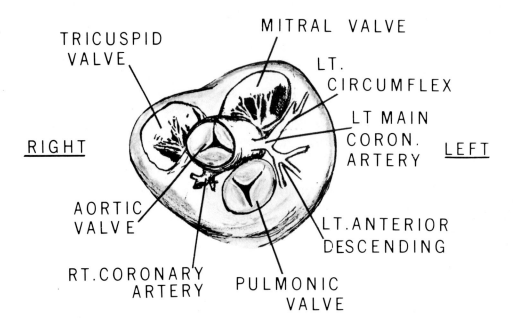

Figure 1.5. Diagrammatic representation of the heart from a posterior view showing the relationship of the right coronary artery to the atrioventricular nodal tissue. Also shown in this figure is the position of the left coronary artery. The left coronary artery provides most of the blood supply to the left ventricle.

discharge is then transmitted by specialized atrial conduction fibers lying just below the endocardial surface of the right atrium. By means of these specialized atrial conduction fibers the electrical impulses are transmitted throughout the right atrium and across the intra-atrial septum to the left atrium. The first chambers to contract are the atria, which discharge their volume of blood into the relaxed right and left ventricles. The electrical charge is then transmitted from the atrial conduction fibers to an area of specialized tissue called the atrioventricular (AV) node. The AV node lies between the atria and the ventricles in the upper portion of the interventricular septum. Delay of the transmission of the electrical impulse from the atria to the ventricle allows for further filling of the right and left ventricles prior to their electrical stimulation. After transmission of the impulse through the AV node, it is transmitted into the ventricular conduction network. The main trunk of the ventricular conduction network is the bundle of His, which

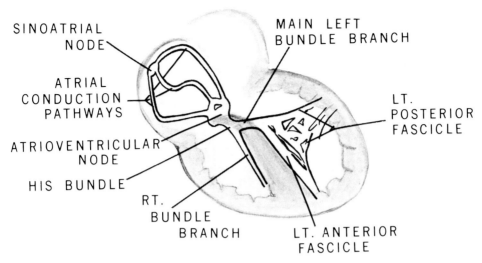

Figure 1.6. Diagrammatic representation of the conduction system of the heart from a frontal view. Note that the main left bundle is of greater width than the right bundle. In addition, the main left bundle has a short proximal segment and is divided into branches, the anterior–superior, which supplies conduction fibers to the anterior and superior aspects of the left ventricular muscle, and the left posterior fascicle, which supplies the posterior and inferior walls of the left ventricle. The right bundle is a single structure until it enters the left ventricular wall and bifurcates into the Purkinje system. The sinoatrial node is shown, as well as the atrioventricular node which is located between the atrium and ventricle in the upper portion of the interventricular septum.

lies below the AV node in the interventricular septum. The bundle of His then divides into two major branches called the right and left bundles. The right bundle then penetrates through the interventricular septum to transmit the electrical stimulus to the endocardial surface of the right ventricle. The left bundle travels for a short distance before dividing into two branches: an anterior–superior branch, which stimulates the anterior and superior wall of the left ventricle; and a posterior–inferior branch, which stimulates the posterior and inferior walls of the left ventricle.

This entire electrical conduction system, which is very complex, lies just under the endocardial surface (inner surface) of the heart. Because of its location, it can be damaged easily by disease.

The heart's function as a circulation pump for the body is quite efficient. This single pumping action of cardiac chambers occurs after a complex series of events that includes electrical activation of first the atria and then the ventricles. This action allows maximum filling of the ventricles for a more efficient pumping action. The complex valves of the heart passively assist in filling the ventricles and ejecting blood from the heart with a minimum of resistance, but at the same time are efficient in preventing any back flow of blood. The heart completes this process over and over again in a tireless effort. It is amazing that these complex events can produce such a single and efficient mode of action.

BIBLIOGRAPHY

Benchimol, A.:   Non-invasive diagnostic techniques in cardiology. Baltimore: Williams & Wilkins, 1977.

Benchimol, A.:   Vectorcardiography. Baltimore: Williams & Wilkins, 1973.

Grant, J.C.B.:   An atlas of anatomy. 6th ed. Baltimore: Williams & Wilkins, 1972.

Guyton, A.C.:   Textbook of medical physiology. Philadelphia: W.B. Saunders, 1975.

Hollinshead, W.H.:   Textbook of anatomy. 2nd ed. New York: Harper and Row, 1967.

Hurst, J.W.:   The heart, arteries, and veins. 3rd ed. New York: McGraw-Hill, 1974.

James, T.N.:   Anatomy of the coronary arteries. New York: Hoeber Medical Division, Harper and Row, 1961.

2
Instrumentation for Phonocardiography and Basic Principles of Sound Formation

Heart sounds originate within the cardiac structures as a result of valve motion and acceleration or deceleration of blood into the cardiac chambers. The heart sounds, as heard with the stethoscope, are recorded on the phonocardiogram, and have a waveform configuration. The strongest vibrations of heart sounds, such as first and second heart sounds, cause large upward and downward deflections of the baseline on the phonocardiogram. The weaker vibrations, such as third and fourth heart sounds, are recorded as upward and downward deflections, i.e., below the baseline, and they are usually 2 to 4 millimeters in amplitude (Figs. 2.1, 2.2). The number of these vibrations per unit of time is defined as wave frequency. Frequency characteristics of heart sounds and murmurs are important in auscultation and phonocardiography because variations in frequency have clinical importance for the physician interpreting the tracings. The number of waves per unit of time (cycles per second or Hertz) represent the number of completed wave cycles (upward and downward deflections) and by definition they determine whether the heart sound or murmur has high or low frequency characteristics.

A murmur is due to turbulent flow of blood across a defective valve or a congenital anomaly in the heart. For example, murmurs in patients with mitral or tricuspid stenosis (atrioventricular murmur) have low frequency characteristics because the flow of blood originates in low pressure chambers such as the left or right atrium and flows through a narrowed or stenotic mitral or tricuspid valve. On the phonocardiogram the vibrations are separated from each other, and that by itself characterizes the low frequency murmur (see Chap. 5). High frequency murmurs of the type seen in patients with aortic or pulmonic narrowing or stenosis have a greater number of vibrations per unit of time (see Chap. 6).

Every heart sound has four major characteristics: (1) time, (2) frequency, (3) amplitude or intensity, and (4) quality. Time and frequency have been described above. Amplitude (loudness or intensity), as defined by the magnitude or size of the vibrations of a sound or murmur, is ordinarily expressed in auscultation by grading it from I to VI (Levine classification)—the higher the amplitude, the higher the grade. Quality is a characteristic derived from the combination of time and the

11

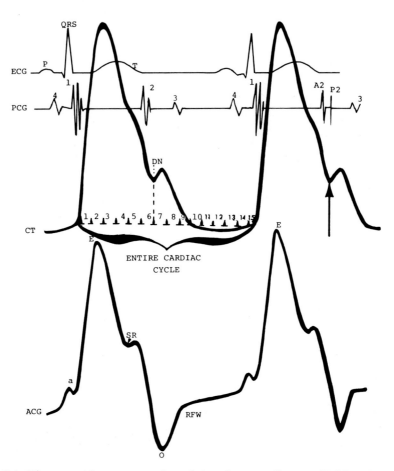

Figure 2.1. Diagrammatic representation of the electrocardiogram (ECG), phonocardiogram (PCG), carotid pulse tracing (CT) showing the four heart sounds that can be recorded on the phonocardiogram. The fourth heart sound, recorded shortly after the P wave of the electrocardiogram, precedes the QRS complex. The first heart sound has a series of vibrations, which are probably due to mitral and tricuspid valve closure. However, the origin of the first heart sound is still controversial. The second heart sound is represented by a single vibration due to aortic valve closure. Note that this sound precedes the dicrotic notch (DN) on the carotid pulse. The next vibration is the third heart sound, which is usually recorded 0.12 to 0.16 sec after the aortic component of the second heart sound. This sound is due to rapid filling of the ventricles in early diastole. A normal carotid pulse tracing shows a sharp rise and reaches its peak in early systole. The downward slope is smooth and terminates with the dicrotic notch. Ejection time is measured from the beginning of the rise at the baseline of the carotid pulse to the dicrotic notch. Each time line interruption represents 0.04 sec. This time multiplied by the number of lines (in this case it is 6 × 0.04 or 0.24 sec) equals the ejection time. Then measure the entire cycle length, which extends from the beginning of the carotid pulse to the next carotid pulse, to get the cardiac cycle. To obtain the ejection time corrected for heart rate you divide the ejection time by the square root of the cycle length.

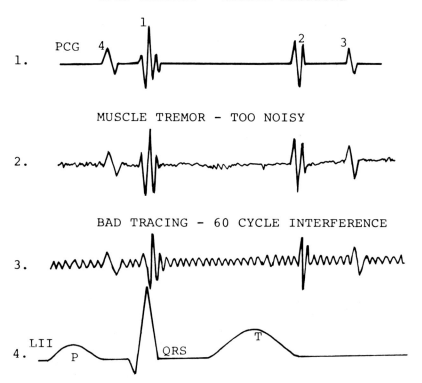

Figure 2.2. Diagrammatic representation of: (1) A normal, technically satisfactory phonocardiogram (PCG) showing a very smooth baseline interrupted by the presence of heart sounds. (2) A tracing illustrating muscle tremor with the baseline oscillating quite a bit. These tracings are usually inadequate for interpretation. Muscle tremor is seen when the patient is shivering or has a condition associated with tremor such as Parkinson's disease, the room is too cold, or the microphone does not have good contact with the skin. This type of tracing is sometimes obtained on a patient with a hairy chest that was not shaved. (3) An illustration of 60 cycle interference, which makes the tracing technically inadequate for the reader to interpret. (4) The bottom tracing shows the electrocardiogram and its relationship to the heart sounds.

number and amplitude of waves. On the basis of quality, heart murmurs are defined as noisy or musical. Noisy murmurs have vibrations or baseline oscillations that vary considerably during the cardiac cycle and are frequently seen in patients with aortic valve narrowing or stenosis without calcification of the valve (see Chap. 6). Musical murmurs are characterized on the phonocardiogram as regular sets of vibrations that have harmonic features.

Propagation of sounds or murmurs originating in the heart and moving toward the chest wall is a function of the various structures that are interposed between them. Air is a poor conductor of sound; therefore, the interposition of large masses of lung tissue causes marked diminution of heart sounds over the precordium. A technically adequate phonocardiogram is difficult to obtain in patients with a large chest, lung disease, or chest wall deformity.

Throughout this book all illustrations indicate settings of the filter system used in phonocardiographic amplifiers, called band pass filters (Fig. 2.3). A band pass filter is an electronic network that allows the technician to control settings of the phonocardiographic amplifier. Fortunately, most heart sounds, clicks, and murmurs are within the theshold of human hearing with vibrations in the range of approximately 30 to 2,000 cycles per second (CPS) or Hertz (Hz).

Heart sounds due to valve motion or rapid acceleration and deceleration of blood within the intracardiac chambers are of short duration. They are also called transients. Heart murmurs have vibratory waves of longer duration and varying frequency. Most phonocardiographic amplifiers record these vibrations within a wide range of frequencies. Since there are several commercial recording units available, technicians must be thoroughly familiar with the filtering systems in their phonocardiographic unit (Fig. 2.3).

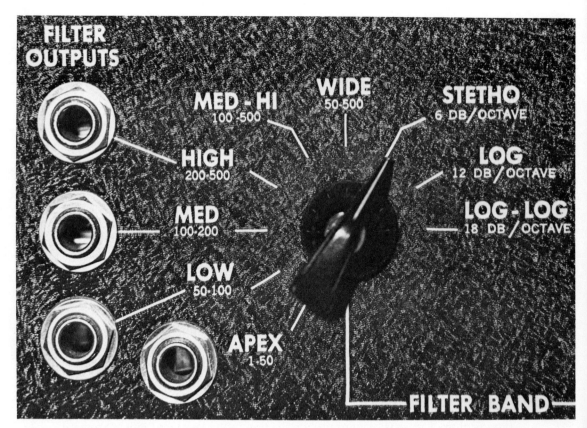

Figure 2.3. Illustration of one type of phonocardiographic amplifier used in our laboratory. It is an Electronics for Medicine unit that has the capability of obtaining stethoscopic (STETHO), log–arithmic (LOG) and log–log recordings. Outputs are shown on the left. (From A. Benchimol: Non-Invasive Diagnostic Techniques in Cardiology. Copyright 1977 by The Williams & Wilkins Company, Baltimore. Used by permission.)

The main purpose of filtering vibrations is to attempt to simulate what is heard with the stethoscope. When the recorder is set for a stethoscope recording, high frequency vibrations are filtered and low frequency waves are amplified. When the filter is set for log or log–log, the low frequency waves are eliminated and the high frequency waves are amplified.

A minimum of four consecutive cardiac cycles should be obtained while recording the phonocardiogram and the configuration, amplitude, and frequency characteristics of heart sounds and murmurs should be identical in all cycles if the patient is in sinus rhythm. In patients with cardiac arrhythmias, a larger number of cardiac cycles (7–10) should be recorded since rhythm abnormalities effect heart sounds and murmurs significantly, depending upon the disease state being analyzed. If a patient has any type of cardiac arrhythmia, be sure to provide the physician with tracings recorded during atrial or ventricular premature contractions as well as tracings for several beats following the arrhythmia. As we will demonstrate in subsequent chapters, very important clinical information can be obtained through careful analysis of the beats recorded during and following premature contractions.

EQUIPMENT FOR PHONOCARDIOGRAPHY
AND PULSE WAVE RECORDINGS

A good phonocardiographic unit should have at least two phonocardiographic amplifiers and be equipped with a band pass filter system to provide the capability for stethoscopic (stetho) and logarithmic (log) recordings (Fig. 2.3). One of the pulse waves (carotid, jugular venous or apexcardiogram) and one lead of the electrocardiogram should be recorded simultaneously with the phonocardiogram (Fig. 2.4). The advantage of this system is that it allows measurements at various times during the cardiac cycle. The unit should also have the capability of multiple speed recordings. Phonocardiograms recorded at a speed of 75 mm/sec or greater are quite satisfactory in the majority of patients to record heart murmurs and abnormal heart sounds. For measurements of systolic and diastolic time intervals, another recording should be made at a paper speed of 100 or 150 mm/sec. Slower paper speed is important in patients with prosthetic cardiac valves for good reproducibility of prosthetic valve sounds in a large number of cardiac cycles. A speed of 25 to 50 mm/sec with a time line interruption of one-tenth second is important to record heart sounds during inspiration, expiration, maneuvers, and administration of drugs.

The most popular microphones for clinical phonocardiography have piezoelectric crystals, which are usually made of barium titanate. Other types used in phonocardiography include condensor, capacitor, contact and electromagnetic or dynamic microphones, which utilize a movable coil located in the range of a magnetic field. Unfortunately, they are not as sensitive to low frequency vibrations as the piezoelectric crystal microphone and are unsuitable for pulse wave recordings. A disadvantage of piezoelectric crystal microphones is that they are sensitive to variations in environmental humidity, which changes their frequency characteristic response, and they are susceptible to fractures if a unit is acciden-

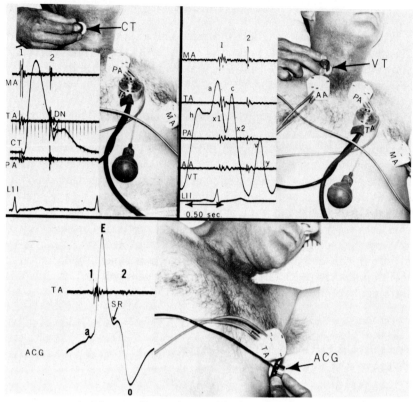

Figure 2.4. *Top Left:* Diagram illustrating positioning of the APT-16 transducer over the right carotid artery with three microphones placed at the mitral (MA), tricuspid (TA), and pulmonic areas (PA). Note that the patient's head is slightly hyperextended. The first (1) and second (2) heart sounds are normal. There are no murmurs. The carotid pulse tracing (CT) is normal. *Top Right:* This illustrates the position of the transducer for recording the jugular venous pulse (VT). It should be held with slight pressure over the anatomical area. The four microphones are located at the mitral, tricuspid, pulmonic, and aortic areas (AA). The first and second heart sounds are normal. The contour of the jugular venous tracing is normal. The normal A wave follows the P wave of the electrocardiogram and precedes the QRS complex. The A wave is due to active atrial contraction. After the A wave there is a downward deflection called X1 descent. The tracing rises again in midsystole reaching a peak called the C wave. The origin of the C wave is not quite clear. Following the peak of the C wave, the tracing moves toward the baseline and this is called X2 descent. The X2 descent terminates near the second heart sound and then the tracing begins to rise again, reaching a peak called the V wave. Near the peak of the V wave, the tricuspid valve opens and this is followed by the Y descent. At the very end of diastole, there is another wave usually noted in patients with a slow heart rate called the H wave. Origin of the H wave is not clear. *Bottom:* Illustrates position of the transducer for recording the apexcardiogram (ACG) with a microphone located near the tricuspid area. The tracing was recorded on a normal subject and shows normal first and second sounds. On a normal apexcardiogram there is an A wave that precedes the first heart sound and is due to ventricular filling secondary to atrial contraction. The tracing then rises rapidly to a sharp point that follows the second vibration of the first heart sound called the E point. The E point represents opening of the aortic valve. From the E point, the tracing begins to return to the baseline reaching a little plateau in midsystole called systolic retraction (SR). This is followed by a continuation of the downslope of the tracing to the O point, which represents opening of the mitral valve. Following the O point, the tracing rises rapidly. This is the rapid filling wave, which is due to rapid filling of the left ventricle.

16

tally damaged. Some advantages of contact microphones are that there are no air conduction delays, air leaks, or movable parts and they have a higher frequency response. Although some microphones have theoretical advantages over the crystal barium titanate microphone, they are more difficult to use for routine clinical evaluation of patients with heart disease. All microphones are very sensitive to artifacts; therefore, great caution must be exercised in the interpretation of phonocardiograms. Crystals should be replaced at fairly frequent intervals (approximately 4–6 months), particularly in geographic areas that have high humidity and atmospheric pressure. For most practical uses piezoelectric crystal microphones are quite suitable, inexpensive, and easy to use. Leatham microphones manufactured by the Cambridge Company were used to record phonocardiograms in most of our tracings (Fig. 2.4). However, many other types of recorders, amplifiers, and microphones available commercially are quite satisfactory for most clinical use.

Transducers are electronic units that change one form of energy to another. For example, strain gauge transducers used in catheterization laboratories transform intracardiac pressures (mechanical pressure) into electrical voltage that can be recorded with a pressure amplifier. A transducer used in phonocardiography for recording a carotid or venous pulse, an apexcardiogram, or any form of pulse wave transforms mechanical displacement caused by motion of these structures to electrical energy. This is recognized by the recording apparatus and displayed on the oscilloscope as a waveform. Transducers should faithfully reproduce vibrations with a long range frequency that is defined as a *time constant*. When purchasing phonocardiographic and pulse wave recording equipment, be sure to ask the manufacturer about the time constant of the instrument. If the time constant of the transducer is less than 3 seconds, it lacks the required electronic characteristics to obtain tracings that are free of artifacts. The time constant of the transducer circuit is defined as the length of time, in seconds, required for the output voltage to reach 63% of the applied input voltage. Therefore, transducers with a long time constant are the most desirable and dependable and this is particularly important in recording apexcardiograms, other precordial motion, carotid or jugular venous tracings. For the past several years, we have been using a transducer that is a differential transformer. The transducer used in our laboratory for recording the carotid artery pulse, jugular venous pulse, and apexcardiogram is the Hewlett–Packard APT-16 differential transformer. This unit has the advantage of eliminating air leaks, and it has a long time constant (Fig. 2.4).

When microphones are positioned properly on the chest wall, the signal is amplified on the phonocardiographic amplifier, a matching unit that converts volts to watts (electromotive force to power). The tracing is displayed on an oscilloscope and a photographic paper recording, direct write-out or storage on magnetic tape can then be accomplished. Most units employ a cathode ray tube for photographic recording or a galvanometer. A galvanometer is a moving coil that oscillates in response to electrical impulses. One disadvantage of the galvanometer is that it has significant inertia, which limits the recordings of high and low frequency vibrations. However, recent direct writer–recorders are adequate for clinical phonocardiography because electronic improvements have resulted in better frequency response. Direct writer–recorders must have a flat frequency response at a minimum of 10–20 to 200–500 Hz without causing significant loss in amplitude of the vibratory waves, or elimination of vibrations above that range. Some galvanometers can be equipped with a mirror connected to a photographic unit so that high frequency vibrations are properly recorded.

Recording devices that use a cathode ray tube are the most popular and probably represent the best unit available for recording phonocardiograms and pulse waves. They amplify the heart sounds and murmurs, causing deflection of the electronic beam on the oscilloscope. This deflection is proportional to the strength of the wave. On these units, frequency response is quite high. Attachments for rapid processing are available for immediate analysis of the records. Tracings illustrated in this book were recorded on an Electronics for Medicine DR-8 oscilloscopic photographic recorder or the Irex phonocardiographic unit.

LABORATORY REQUIREMENTS

Noninvasive evaluation of a patient with cardiovascular disease should include phonocardiograms at multiple precordial areas recorded simultaneously with a carotid pulse tracing, jugular venous tracing, or apexcardiogram (Fig. 2.4).

TECHNIQUE FOR RECORDING CAROTID PULSE TRACINGS

The transducer can be placed over the right or left common carotid artery. We normally place it over the right carotid artery, one to two inches below the jaw. For a short recording, the transducer can be held by hand, applying slight pressure. The best recordings are obtained when the patient's head is turned slightly to the left and the neck is slightly hyperextended (Fig. 2.4). For recordings of the left carotid artery pulse tracing, the patient's head should be turned slightly to the right. This method brings the carotid artery closer to the skin and moves the sternocleidomastoid muscle away from the carotid artery. The patient's head should be elevated at a 30–50° angle. Encourage the patient to relax, assuring him that the test is not painful. The patient should hold his breath during the phase of the respiratory cycle you wish to record, i.e., held expiration. It is useful to have the patient practice holding his breath prior to recording.

Another technique for recording the carotid pulse tracing is attaching the transducer to a cuff placed around the neck. There is no particular advantage to this technique for short recordings, but it is advantageous if records are to be obtained continuously or intermittently for prolonged periods of time. Be sure not to apply too much pressure over the carotid artery. Many patients, particularly those past age 60, have a sensitive carotid sinus and the pressure can cause marked slowing of the heart rate and/or cardiac arrest.

JUGULAR VENOUS PULSE TRACINGS

Good recordings of the jugular venous pulse require practice, patience, and experience. The best anatomical area in which to record this pulse wave is over the supraclavicular area near the sternum (manubrium) or the area 2–3 cm below the jaw (Fig. 2.4). The transducer should be held by hand with very slight pressure applied. The patient's head should be turned to the left with slight hyperextension of the neck. The head should be elevated slightly with a pillow placed under the neck and the head making an angle of about 30–50° in relation to the chest. This moves the sternocleidomastoid muscle away from the junction of the jugular and subclavian veins. When a good pattern is recognized on the oscilloscope, ask the patient to relax the neck muscles and hold his breath. The tracing should be monitored on the oscilloscope for recognition of the two most important waves on this tracing, the A and V waves. A technically satisfactory jugular venous pulse tracing can be obtained in most patients with cardiovascular diseases and a large number of normal subjects. However, good jugular venous recordings cannot be obtained in approximately 10–20% of subjects. Applying too much pressure on the transducer can cause an artifactual reading, which will be "contaminated" with a carotid pulse wave as shown in Figure 2.5.

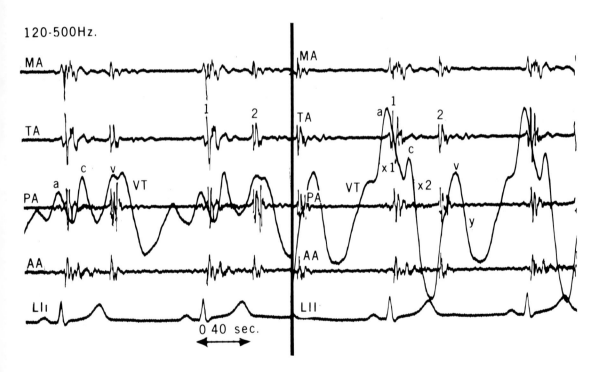

Figure 2.5. *Left:* Simultaneously recorded phonocardiogram at the mitral (MA), tricuspid (TA), pulmonic (PA), and aortic areas (AA), lead II (LII) of the electrocardiogram and an artifactual venous pulse tracing (VT). Note that the C wave is quite prominent and is probably due to too much pressure applied to the transducer over the jugular pulse. *Right:* Simultaneously recorded phonocardiogram at the mitral (MA), tricuspid (TA), pulmonic (PA), and aortic areas (AA), lead II (LII) of the electrocardiogram and a normal, properly recorded venous pulse tracing (VT). Note that the A wave exceeds the C point, which indicates a normal venous pulse.

APEXCARDIOGRAM RECORDINGS

Recording the precordial pulsations has gained increasing popularity because of their value in timing various events of the cardiac cycle such as clicks and opening snaps, for the diagnosis of various disease states. In order to obtain a technically satisfactory apexcardiogram, good recording technique is essential. The transducer should fulfill the electronic characteristics described earlier in this chapter. Techniques for recording precordial pulsations have been developed by several investigators. The apexcardiogram is the recording that has gained the greatest acceptance for clinical use. It is also called a mechanocardiogram. A good recording of the apexcardiogram can be obtained with the patient in a left lateral decubitus position with the left arm placed behind the head. It is important for the patient to be relaxed, and it is quite helpful to place a pillow behind the patient's back and head. The tracing should be displayed continuously on the oscilloscope in order to recognize artifacts and for reproducibility of the various components of the apexcardiogram. Initially, the point of maximal cardiac impulse must be carefully palpated by hand. Subsequently, one should identify the center of that maximal cardiac impulse, which is represented by the most forceful contraction of the heart against the chest wall. The transducer is then placed at the center of the maximal impulse and held by hand except for prolonged recordings (Fig. 2.4). The position of the transducer is very critical. Different wave form configurations can be recorded in one subject simply by changing the position of the transducer as shown in Figure 2.6. The patient is instructed to take a short inspiration followed by a short, held expiration. Adequate, reliable, and reproducible tracings can be obtained in approximately 80–90% of patients with cardiovascular disease and in most normal subjects. In many instances, it is difficult to decide which is the best recording. Our earlier work in this field was done utilizing a barium titanate piezoelectric transducer bell connected by rubber tubing to the side of the bell because a phonocardiogram could be recorded simultaneously with the apexcardiogram from the same area. We have abandoned this technique because of problems with poor frequency response, short time constant, and air leaks. It is very desirable to obtain a phonocardiogram at the precordial area where the heart mumur is present along with the apexcardiogram. Therefore, the technician must know the diagnosis of the patient in order to obtain an apexcardiogram and phonocardiogram with the heart murmurs or sounds clearly defined.

Recordings of precordial motion such as in patients with right ventricular hypertrophy can be obtained by placing the transducer along the left sternal border at the third or fourth intercostal space or over the subxyphoid area, with the patient lying flat on his back. Other anatomical locations for recording the apexcardiogram in patients with coronary artery disease, left ventricular aneurysm, and other conditions will be discussed in subsequent chapters.

A highly skilled technician, well versed in the characteristics of heart sounds, murmurs, pulse wave forms, and the techniques for recording them is necessary to obtain good tracings. This requires a basic knowledge of cardiac anatomy and the basic characteristics of various cardiac diseases. A physician must be present during maneuvers or administration of pharmacologic agents used to induce changes in cardiac function that may be important in differential diagnosis. The technician should not assume the responsibility for administration of pharmacologic agents, which can be dangerous in patients with some disease states.

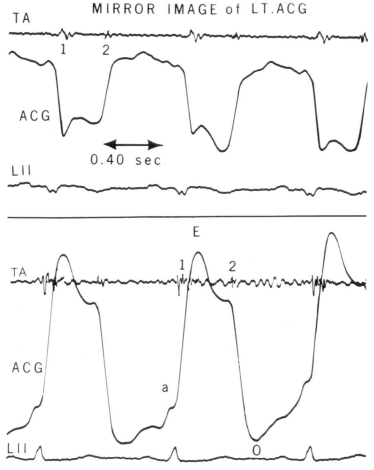

120-500Hz.

MIRROR IMAGE of LT.ACG

TA

1   2

ACG

0.40 sec.

LII

E

TA

1   2

ACG

a

LII   O

Figure 2.6. *Top:* Phonocardiogram and mirror image of a normal apexcardiogram (ACG) obtained purposely. This is an artifactual apexcardiogram obtained when the transducer is located outside of the apex beat rather than at the center of it, causing paradoxical motion. The first (1) and the second (2) heart sounds are normal at the tricuspid area (TA). *Bottom:* Phonocardiogram and apexcardiogram of the same patient demonstrating a normal apexcardiogram. Note that the E point follows the first heart sound and then the tracing reaches the baseline at the point called the O point. There is also a small A wave.

CLASSIFICATION OF MURMURS

Heart Murmurs

All heart murmurs are the result of turbulent blood flow across either the cardiac valves or the blood vessels as described earlier in this chapter.

Systolic Murmurs

There are two types of systolic murmurs, ejection and regurgitant. Ejection murmurs are due to ejection of blood through the aorta and pulmonary arteries.

An ejection murmur usually has a diamond configuration with a maximal peak in systole, terminating with the aortic component of the second heart sound if it originates in the aortic valve, or with the pulmonic component of the second heart sound if it originates from the pulmonic valve in patients with severe narrowing of that valve (Fig. 2.7). This type of murmur also has a characteristic that is quite peculiar. It usually has a silent interval between the first heart sound and the beginning of the murmur. Systolic regurgitant murmurs are due to insufficiency of either the mitral or tricuspid atrioventricular valves, and have high frequency characteristics. A systolic regurgitant murmur starts with the first heart sound, reaching an early systolic peak, followed by a systolic plateau and terminating with the second heart sound.

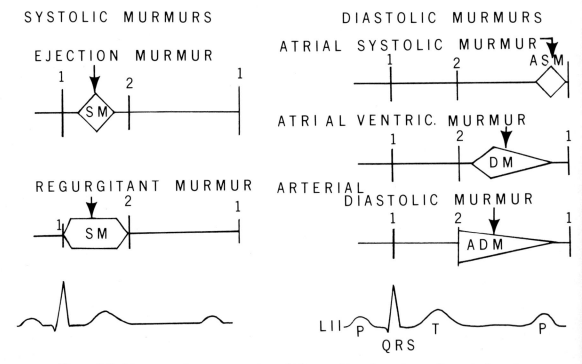

Figure 2.7. Diagrammatic representation of the configuration of systolic and diastolic murmurs. *Left:* Systolic ejection and regurgitant murmurs. Note that the ejection murmur has a silent interval between the first heart sound and the beginning of the murmur, and the murmur has a diamond shaped characteristic. It reaches a peak in systole and terminates prior to the second heart sound. The regurgitant systolic murmur starts with the first heart sound, reaching a maximal peak in early systole. This is followed by a plateau and the murmur terminates with the second heart sound. *Right:* Atrial systolic murmurs are due to active atrial contraction. They usually start after the P wave of the electrocardiogram and terminate before the QRS complex. These murmurs are seen in patients with mitral and tricuspid stenosis. Atrioventricular diastolic murmurs begin shortly after the second heart sound, reaching a maximal peak in early or mid-diastole and terminating prior to the P wave of the electrocardiogram. These murmurs are due to tricuspid or mitral stenosis or increased flow across the mitral or tricuspid valves in patients with congenital heart disease. The arterial diastolic murmur begins with the second heart sound and terminates with the P wave of the electrocardiogram. This murmur is due to aortic or pulmonic insufficiency.

Diastolic Murmurs

The diastolic murmurs are of three types—arterial, atrioventricular and atriosystolic. The high frequency arterial diastolic murmur is easily recognizable by the fact that it starts with the aortic or pulmonic component of the second heart sound. These murmurs are seen in patients with aortic and pulmonic insufficiency. The low frequency atrioventricular murmur starts a little late in diastole, approximately 0.14 to 0.16 sec after the second heart sound, and terminates prior to atrial contraction. These murmurs are usually seen in patients with mitral or tricuspid stenosis. The high frequency atriosystolic murmur, seen only in patients with sinus rhythm, is due to active atrial contraction. They are present in patients with mitral and/or tricuspid stenosis (Fig. 2.7).

SUMMARY AND PRACTICAL INFORMATION—ARTIFACTS

1. Be aware of sixty cycle interference, and learn to identify it (Fig. 2.2).
2. Somatic tremor can be avoided in most patients except those with a disease associated with muscle tremor, in which case the phonocardiogram is of no help (Fig. 2.2).
3. Loose microphone attachments: Be sure to use water soluble gel for good contact with the skin. Also, be sure to clean the edges of the microphone after the tracings are recorded.
4. Conversation during recording: There should not be conversation during the recording. If a telephone is installed in the phono room, either make sure that the bell sound is very low or take the telephone off the hook.
5. Routine for recording phonocardiogram and pulse waves: Establish a good routine. Have a work sheet and mark events carefully so that when the paper is processed you can readily identify what you recorded.
6. Be alert for unexpected findings. A good technician should record unexpected findings such as cardiac arrhythmias. Do not discard these tracings. They are very valuable to the physician. Important information can be obtained by analyzing the heart sounds and murmurs during and after cardiac arrhythmias. In many cases the diagnosis of prosthetic valve malfunction has been diagnosed in our own laboratory because of unusual murmurs and clicks that occurred during cardiac arrhythmias.
7. Request a doctor's presence if pharmacologic agents are used.
8. Shave patient's hair in the anatomical area at which you are going to record the tracing.

BIBLIOGRAPHY

Aronow, W.S.:   Effect of position on the resting and postexercise phonocardiogram. Chest, *61*:439, 1972.

Benchimol, A.:   Non-invasive diagnostic techniques in cardiology. Baltimore: Williams & Wilkins, 1977.

Benchimol, A., and Desser, K.B.:   Diagnostic value of arterial and venous wave forms. Cardiovasc. Clin., 6:73–92, 1975.

Benchimol, A., and Dimond, E.G.:   The apexcardiogram in normal older subjects and in patients with arteriosclerotic heart disease. Effect of exercise on the "a" wave. Am. Heart J., 65:789, 1963.

Benchimol, A., and Dimond, E.G.:   The normal and abnormal apexcardiogram. Its physiologic variation and its relationship to intracardiac events. Am. J. Cardiol., 12:368, 1963.

Benchimol, A., Dimond, E.G., and Carson, J.C.:   The value of the apexcardiogram as a reference tracing in phonocardiography. Am. Heart J., 61:485–493, 1961.

Benchimol, A., Fishenfeld, J., and Desser, K.B.:   The influence of atrial contraction on the apexcardiogram during atrioventricular dissociation: Apical "Cannon Waves." Chest, 64:647–648, 1973.

Benchimol, A., Fishenfeld, J., and Desser, K.B.:   Influence of atrial systole on first derivative of the apexcardiogram. Chest, 65:446–447, 1974.

Benchimol, A., and Maroko, P.:   The apex cardiogram. Dis. Chest, 54:378–380, 1968.

Bertrand, C.A., Miline, I.G., and Hornick, R.:   A study of heart sounds and murmurs by direct heart recordings. Circulation, 13:49, 1956.

Bramwell, C.:   Use of the phonocardiograph in clinical cardiology. Br. Heart J., 10:98, 1948.

Braunwald, W., Fishman, A.P., and Cournand, A.:   Time relationship of dynamic events in the cardiac chambers, pulmonary artery and aorta in man. Circ. Res., 4:100, 1956.

Cowan, E.D.H., and Parnum, D.H.:   The phonocardiography of heart murmurs; I. Apparatus and technique. Br. Heart J., 11:356, 1949.

Desser, K.B., and Benchimol, A.:   The apexcardiogram in patients with the syndrome of midsystolic click and late systolic murmur. Chest, 62:739–740, 1972.

Desser, K.B., Benchimol, A., and Schumacher, J.A.:   The postextrasystolic apexcardiogram. Chest, 64:747–748, 1973.

Dimond, E.G., and Benchimol, A.:   Phonocardiography. Calif. Med., 94:139, 1961.

Dimond, E.G., Duenas, A., and Benchimol, A.:   Apex cardiography: A review. Am. Heart J., 72:124–130, 1966.

Grant, R.P.:   Architectonics of the heart. Am. Heart J., 52:944, 1956.

Groom, D., and Boone, J.A.:   The recording of heart sounds and vibrations; II. The application of an electronic pickup in the graphic recording of subaudible and audible frequencies. Exp. Med. Surg., 14:255, 1956.

Hartman, H.:   Differentiation between the influence of the right and left ventricle in the phonocardiogram, with the aid of pulsation curves (Abstracts of papers, p. 127). Second European Congress of Cardiology, 1956.

Hillard, J.K., and Fiala, W.T.:   Condenser microphones for measurement of high sound pressures (mimeograph). Altec Lansing Corporation, 9356 Santa Monica Blvd., Beverly Hills, California.

Holldack, K., Luisada, A.A., and Ueda, H.:   Standardization of phonocardiography. Am. J. Cardiol., 15:419, 1965.

Kelly, J.J. Jr.:   Symposium on cardiovascular sound. Circulation, 16:270, 1957.

Kotis, J.B.:   The value of the ultrasonic Doppler method and apexcardiography as reference tracing in phonocardiography. Am. Heart J., 84:634, 1972.

Leatham, A.:   Phonocardiology. Br. Med. Bull., 8:333, 1952.

Luisada, A.A., and Gamna, G.:   Clinical calibration in phonocardiography. Am. Heart J., 48:826, 1954.

Luisada, A.A., Richmond, L., and Aravanis, C.: Selective phonocardiography. Am. Heart J., *51*:221, 1956.

McKusick, V.A., Jenkins, J.T., and Webb, G.N.: Acoustic basis of the chest examination. Am. Rev. Tuberc., *72*:12, 1955.

Miller, A., and White, P.D.: Crystal microphone for pulse wave recording. Am. Heart J., *21*:504, 1941.

Mounsey, J.P.D.: The impulse cardiogram and the phonocardiogram. Cardiologia, *48*:203, 1966.

Rappaport, M.B., and Sprague, H.B.: Physiologic and physical laws which govern auscultation and their clinical application: the acoustic stethoscope and the electrical amplifying stethoscope and stethograph. Am. Heart J., *21*:257, 1941.

Tavel, M.E.: Clinical phonocardiography and external pulse recording. 2nd ed. Chicago: Year Book Medical Publishers, 1972.

Weissler, A.M. (Ed.): Non-invasive cardiology. New York: Grune & Stratton, 1974.

Zoneraich, S. (Ed.): Non-invasive methods in cardiology. Springfield, Ill.: Charles C. Thomas, 1974.

3
Vectorcardiography

The vectorcardiogram records the electrical forces of the heart. It is essential to understand the anatomy of the conduction system of the heart to record properly the vectorcardiogram (Figs. 3.1, 3.2). The definition of a vector in terms of physics is a force that has three fundamental characteristics: (1) magnitude (size); (2) rotation of the loop, which will be clockwise, counterclockwise, or figure-of-eight; (3) direction, expressed in degrees. The vectorcardiogram records a three-dimensional display of the electrical activity of the heart, whereas the electrocardiogram records electrical forces in a single plane. A plane uses the combination of two axes, which are displayed in the horizontal or transverse, frontal and sagittal projections (Figs. 3.3, 3.4). Despite the fact that there are a number of systems for electrode placement, they all use the X, Y, and Z axes. The X (horizontal) is the right-left axis. The Y (longitudinal) is the head-foot axis. The Z is the anterior-posterior or front-back axis. The combination of these axes forms a plane. There are three planes in vectorcardiography:

1. The frontal plane combines the Y (head–foot) and the X (right–left) axes.
2. The sagittal plane is a combination of the Y (head–foot) and Z (front–back) axes.
3. The horizontal plane is a combination of the X (right–left) and Z (front–back) axes.

There are a number of lead systems for recording the electrical forces of the heart. However, you must satisfy certain characteristics in order to obtain a high degree of fidelity. These are:

1. The lead system utilized must be parallel to the coordinate axis of the body.
2. The magnitude of these leads should be equal as far as the vectorial expressions are concerned.
3. The vectors that result from the combination of these leads should have equal magnitude and also be perpendicular to a single point within the heart.

In addition, they must retain identical magnitudes and directions for many infinite points where the electromotive forces are generated.

If the lead systems used satisfy requirements 1 and 2, they are called orthogonal leads. The ones that satisfy all the above requirements are known as corrected orthogonal lead systems. Those that do not satisfy the requirements of 1, 2, and 3 are called uncorrected systems.

26

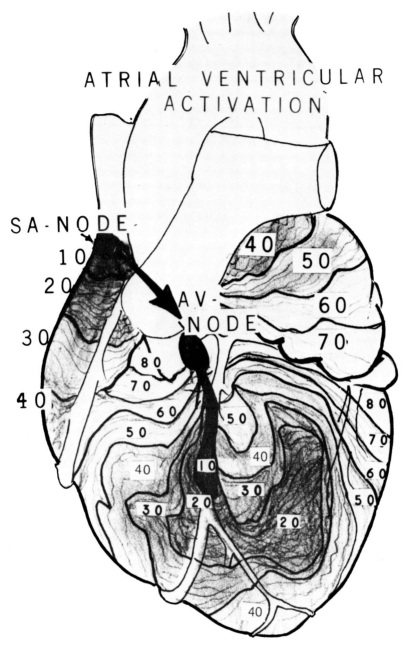

Figure 3.1. A schematic representation of the conduction system of the heart and the sequence of activation. Activation starts in the sinus node, which is located at the junction of the superior vena cava and the right atrium. From there it spreads through the walls of the right atrium and finally reaches the left atrium at 40, 50, 60, and 70 msec time intervals. Then there is a delay at the level of the AV node, followed by depolarization of the bundle of His. Notice that both the right and left ventricles depolarize at the same time through the various branches of the left and right bundles. Although the activation of both ventricles occurs at the same time, most of the electrical forces of the heart are seen as the QRS complex on the electrocardiogram and as the QRS loop on the vectorcardiogram. They represent electrical forces of the left ventricle because the left ventricle has a much greater muscle mass compared with the right ventricle.

27

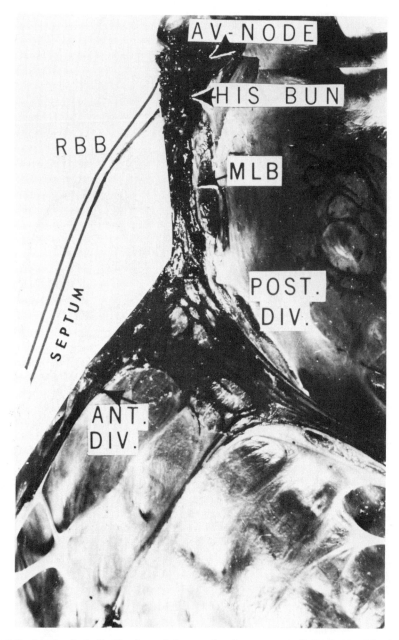

Figure 3.2. Anatomical distribution of the conduction system of the heart. The left conduction system has been injected with India ink and the endocardial surface of the left ventricle has been removed. One can clearly see the main left bundle and its anterior and posterior divisions. Note that the anterior division of the left bundle is long and thin, and the posterior division is quite broad. The left side of the picture is a diagrammatic representation of the position of the right bundle and the AV node. (From A. Benchimol: Vectorcardiography. Copyright 1973 by The Williams & Wilkins Company, Baltimore. Used by permission.)

28

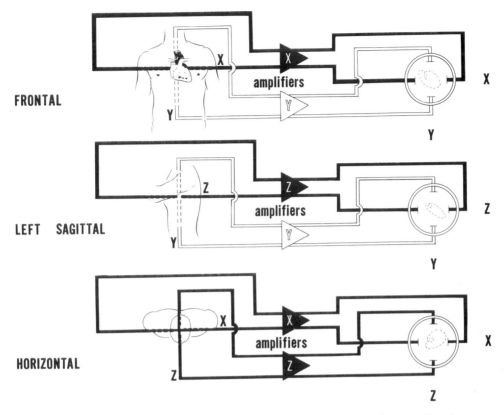

Figure 3.3. Diagrammatic representation of the principles involved in recording the vectorcardiogram in three planes with the corresponding QRS loop. (From A. Benchimol: Vectorcardiography. Copyright 1973 by The Williams & Wilkins Company, Baltimore. Used with permission.)

The most popular and simplified corrected system is the Frank system, which uses seven electrodes plus one ground electrode. The position of the electrodes is shown in Figure 3.5. Four electrodes are placed on the chest at the fourth intercostal space, the fifth in the middle of the back at the level of the fourth intercostal space, the sixth on the back of the neck or forehead, and the seventh on the left leg. An eighth electrode is placed on the right leg as a ground. The use of the fourth or fifth intercostal space is based on preference and we prefer the fourth intercostal space.

We find the Frank system most advantageous because: (1) it is simple and provides the orthogonality that is necessary; (2) electrode placement is fast and simple and the number of electrodes is small as compared with the other orthogonal systems: (3) position of the chest electrodes is not as critical as it is with other corrected systems. We do not measure the angle between the C and X electrodes. We roughly calculate and have found that it works out quite well.

The other corrected systems are the McFee and Parungao, and the Schmitt and Simonson Stereovectorelectrocardiography Lead 3 System (SVEC-III). There are other systems that are rarely used in clinical practice.

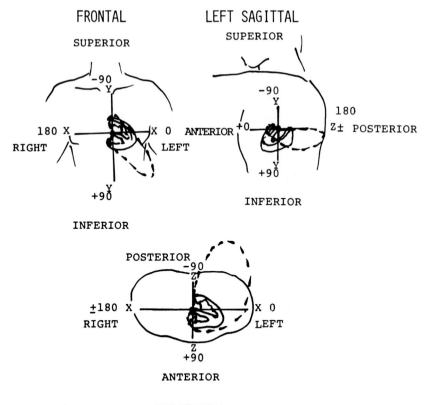

Figure 3.4. Diagrammatic representation of the QRS loop and polarity of the lead axis with the Y lead in the frontal, left sagittal, and horizontal planes. Arrows indicate the direction of rotation of the QRS loop. (From A. Benchimol: Vectorcardiography. Copyright 1973 by The Williams & Wilkins Company, Baltimore. Used by permission.)

The most popular uncorrected system is the Cube system developed by Grishman (Fig. 3.6). It is a simple system but it does not provide orthogonality. It has proved to be a very good system for detecting early signs of right ventricular hypertrophy.

PRINCIPLES

In all systems used for recording vectorcardiograms, regardless of electrode placement, the electrical vectorial forces generated by the heart are displayed on a cathode ray tube for photographic or direct writer recording. The cathode ray tube consists of two sets of plates that control horizontal and vertical deflections of the electronic beam. The electronic circuits of the oscilloscope are shown in Figure 3.3. For the frontal and horizontal planes they all have essentially the same set connections and display. However, sagittal plane can be seen on the oscilloscope and recorded on paper from either the left or right side. There is no particular

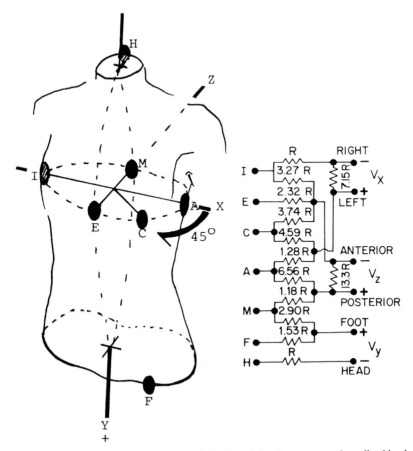

Figure 3.5. Diagrammatic representation of the Frank lead system as described in the text. Electrode H is placed at the back of the neck or on the forehead. Electrode F is placed on the left leg. Five electrodes are placed on the trunk at the level of the fourth intercostal space. Electrode I is placed at the right midaxillary line, Electrode A at the left anterior midaxillary line, Electrode M is placed on the back overlying the thoracic spine, and Electrode E in front of the sternum. Electrode C is placed at the fourth intercostal space 45° between Electrodes E and A. In addition, we place an electrode on the right leg as a ground. Schematics of the electronic circuits are shown on the right side of the illustration. (From A. Benchimol: Vectorcardiography. Copyright 1973 by The Williams & Wilkins Company, Baltimore. Used by permission.)

advantage to the right sagittal plane. We use the left sagittal projection as recommended by the American Heart Association. A diagrammatic representation of each plane and polarity (+ −) of the leads is shown in Figure 3.3.

TECHNIQUE AND INSTRUMENTATION

Among the vectorcardiographic units available for practical use, the majority of them provide oscillographic display of the loop. Some have a Polaroid camera attached in front of the oscilloscope. However, we have found that the small

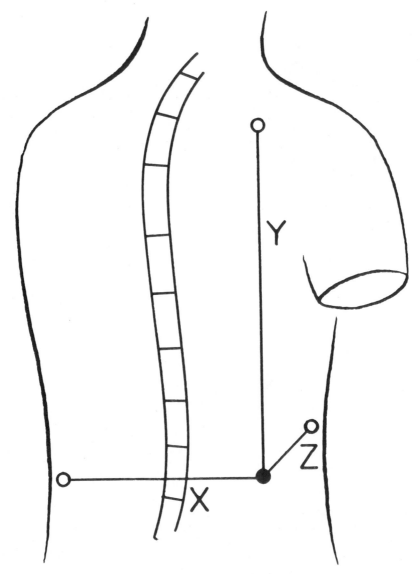

Figure 3.6. Diagrammatic representation of electrode placement for the cube system developed by Grishman. (From A. Benchimol: Vectorcardiography. Copyright 1973 by The Williams & Wilkins Company, Baltimore. Used by permission.)

screen on these units does not allow for enlargement of the initial and terminal components of the QRS or P loop, which is a major limitation to the use of the Polaroid camera for permanent recordings. Requirements for vectorcardiographic units in order to obtain the maximal diagnostic value include:

1. The vectorcardiographic unit should have a high frequency response from 0.1 to over 500 Hz.

2. It should display the vectorcardiogram on a time scale with varying speed for study of cardiac arrhythmias and determination of heart rate.

3. Interruption of the loop at about 2 or 2.5 msec and/or 4 msec is desirable to study initial and terminal forces of the QRS, P and T loops, and ST vectors.

4. It should have a gate system that selectively eliminates some segments of the cardiac cycle and records only the initial and terminal portions of the QRS loop.

Most of the vectorcardiograms shown in this book were recorded with an Electronics for Medicine DR-8 oscilloscopic photographic recorder using the Frank system. The amplifier we use has a frequency response of 0.1 to 500 Hz and we have the ability to filter at 25, 50, 500, and 2500 Hz. The QRS loops are interrupted at each dot or comet, which measures 2 msec. The thin part of the "comet" indicates the direction of the loop on both the Instruments for Cardiac Research (ICR) direct writing unit, and the Electronics for Medicine (EFM) unit. Our standard technique for recording a vectorcardiogram is as follows:

1. Obtain the QRS loop in a single plane or in two planes simultaneously with 1 millivolt (mv) calibration, which corresponds to 5 or 6 cm of deflection.

2. Amplify initial and terminal segments of the QRS forces and the P and T loops so that 0.50 mv corresponds to 5 cm of deflection. This allows for a very good analysis of the initial forces of the vectorcardiogram, which is extremely useful in patients with myocardial infarction and/or ventricular hypertrophy. If the unit does not provide this degree of magnification, the vectorcardiogram is not of much use. One should be able to isolate clearly the very first few milliseconds of electrical activity of the heart (depolarization). This can only be obtained if a major degree of magnification is obtained.

3. A third degree of magnification is routinely used for analyzing the P or T loops. The gate begins with the P loop and terminates with the QRS loop. When analyzing the ST segments and T loops, the gate should begin after the QRS loop and end after inscription of the T loop.

4. Timed vectorcardiography is gaining importance. This technique is also called "running loops." We record running loops in two planes simultaneously, frontal and horizontal, at a paper speed of 75 to 100 mm per sec. This technique provides a very clear definition of cardiac arrhythmias.

5. X, Y, and Z leads are recorded simultaneously at a paper speed of 100 mm per sec. The time required to obtain a complete vectorcardiographic study is approximately 20 minutes.

POINTS OF CAUTION AND IMPORTANCE

1. If you have the problem of 60 cycle interference, be sure to record a tracing that is unfiltered even though the QRS loops are not quite satisfactory. Filtering will certainly eliminate some important features of the vectorcardiogram as shown in Figures 3.7, 3.8, and 3.9.

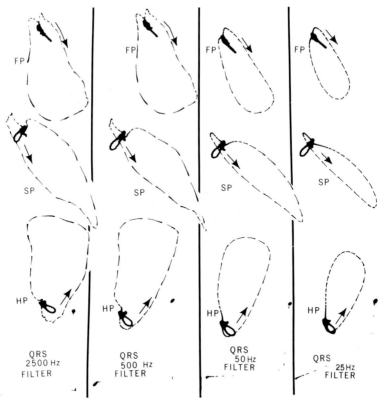

Figure 3.7. Normal vectorcardiogram in the frontal, horizontal, and sagittal planes, showing the effect of filtering on the QRS loop. In the tracings recorded at a wide bandpass filter setting of 2500 Hz the loops have notching and some irregularities. This is the way tracings should be obtained. As the setting is increased to 500, 50, and 25 Hz, there are major changes in the configuration and magnitude of these vectors completely distorting the important features of the vectorcardiogram. Compare with Figure 3.8.

2. Try to record the tracing when the patient is quite relaxed and during quiet breathing. Do not ask the patient to take deep inspiration or expiration because it may modify the configuration of the QRS loop as shown in Figure 3.18.

3. If a filter system is used, try to obtain a minimal degree of filtering. Increased filtering results in greater distortion of the loop as shown in Figure 3.8.

4. If the patient has a disease that is associated with muscular tremor such as Parkinson's disease or other conditions that affect the peripheral muscles, try to obtain one tracing without filtering and a second tracing with filtering. Also obtain an enlargement of the initial QRS forces so that you have a clear definition of the direction and magnitude of the initial forces.

5. Be sure that electrodes are placed in the right anatomical position. Figure 3.10 shows a tracing in which the leads were reversed. You will have the same problem as in electrocardiography. This tracing simulates dextrocardia (heart on right side of chest).

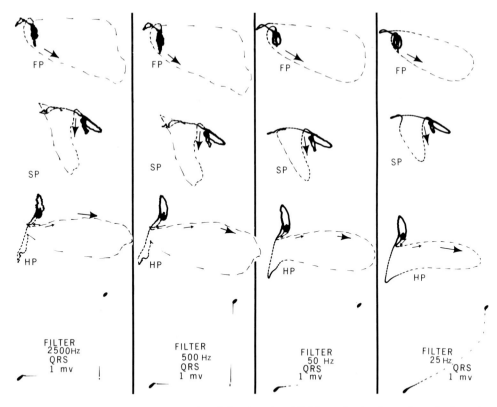

Figure 3.8. This is another example of filtering the QRS loop in the frontal, sagittal, and horizontal planes in a patient with heart disease and right bundle branch block. In the unfiltered loop recorded at 2500 Hz, you can see irregularities in the inscription of the various comets. This is particularly well seen in the frontal and horizontal planes. Pay particular attention to the terminal portion of the QRS loop and its relationship to the O point. This is a typical delay for right bundle branch block where the comets are inscribed closer to one another. With progressive increase in filtering at 500 Hz, there are less comets in that area. At 50 Hz, not only do the comets become less visible, but they also move to the front. At filtering of 25 Hz, the loop becomes completely open in the horizontal plane. Compare with Figure 3.7.

6. Be sure the vertical and horizontal deflections have identical magnitudes. If they do not, the recorded vectorcardiogram will be distorted (Fig. 3.12).

ATRIAL AND VENTRICULAR ACTIVATION

In order to understand vectorcardiograms properly and perform pattern analysis, knowledge of the depolarization (electrical disbursement) and repolarization (regaining the electrical activity) processes of the heart is very important.

The site of impulse formation is in the sinoatrial node (node of Keith and Flack) as described in Chapter 1. After that it spreads through the atrial walls as shown in Figures 3.1 and 3.2 and depolarizes first in the right atrium and then in the left

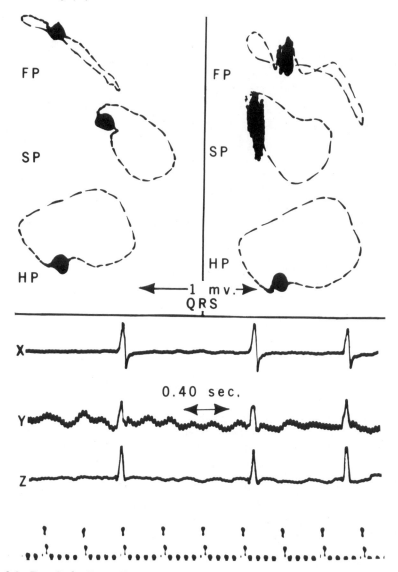

Figure 3.9. *Top Left:* Recording of the vectorcardiogram in the frontal, sagittal, and horizontal planes showing the effect of the filtering on the QRS loops. The rotation becomes definitely abnormal when the tracing is filtered. *Top Right:* In the tracing with AC (alternating current) interference, the initial and terminal forces are obscured by the multiple 60 cycle current (upper right panel). *Bottom:* The X, Y and Z leads are shown. Most of the 60 cycle interference is in lead Y.

atrium. It is important to remember that the right atrium is the chamber that is located in the front (anteriorly) and to the right and the left atrium is the chamber located in the back (posteriorly) and to the left. Therefore, vectors originating in the right atrium are oriented in the direction of that chamber, i.e., the vectors from the right P loop are located anteriorly and either to the right or left. The vectors from the left atrium are located posteriorly and to the left. After that, the electrical

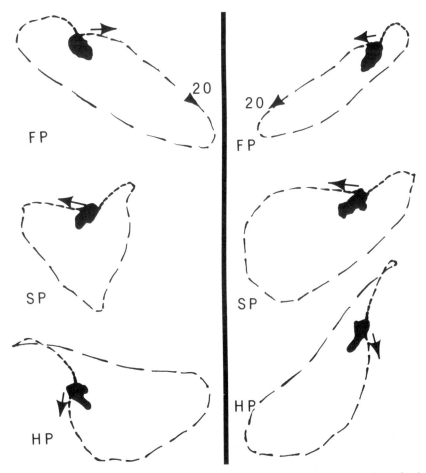

Figure 3.10. *Left:* Normal recording of the vectorcardiogram in the frontal, sagittal, and horizontal planes. *Right:* Recording of the vectorcardiogram in the three planes with the leads reversed. The tracing is almost a mirror image of normal simulating dextrocardia (heart located on the right side of chest).

impulse reaches the atrioventricular node or junction (called the node of Aschoff and Tawara). The beginning of atrial depolarization is conventionally called the E point. It is followed by the first deflection that corresponds to activation of the right atrium. These comets or electrical vectors are located anterior to the O point and to the right or left. After the electrical impulse reaches the AV node, the right and left ventricles are depolarized. Remember that the right ventricle is located anteriorly and to the left side with a small segment on the right side; therefore, electrical forces in this chamber are anterior and to the right or left. There are a few exceptions that will be mentioned in subsequent chapters. The left ventricle is the chamber located posteriorly and to the left. The activation process proceeds from the AV node through the septum.

In normal subjects, the left atrium and left ventricle dominate the electrical field simply because they have increased muscle mass, although both the right and left atrium depolarize almost at the same time. Most of the vectorial forces seen in normal subjects represent left atrial and left ventricular forces. From the AV junction, the electrical impulses pass through the specialized conduction system called the bundle of His and its branches and finally through the Purkinje fibers, which penetrate into the ventricular muscle fibers to depolarize the ventricles, creating the QRS loop through a complex biochemical process. The repolarization process is responsible for the T loop and ST vectors.

ATRIAL ACTIVATION

P Loop

A normal P loop is shown in Figure 3.11. The right atrial forces are best seen in the horizontal projection. They are located anteriorly and to the left of the O point. Most of the posterior forces are due to the left atrial depolarization.

VENTRICULAR ACTIVATION

QRS Loop

Ventricular activation is responsible for the QRS loop. As the activation process reaches the AV node and the bundle of His, the ventricle begins to depolarize. As indicated in the section on atrial activation, although the right ventricle is depolarized at about the same time as the left ventricle, most of the vectorial forces that originate in the right ventricle in the normal subjects are not seen on the vectorcardiogram. These vectors are represented by left ventricular forces because they dominate the electrical field of the heart.

The first portions of the ventricular muscle to be activated are the middle and lower segments of the interventricular septum near the left ventricle. These forces, best appreciated in the horizontal plane, are located anteriorly, to the right and superiorly or inferiorly. Septal activation lasts approximately 10 to 20 msec and is followed by activation of the free anterior wall of the left ventricle which lasts from the 20 to 30 msec QRS vectors (Figs. 3.13, 3.14, 3.15). These vectors are located to the front toward the head and foot. The QRS loop will have a counterclockwise rotation in the horizontal and left sagittal planes and a variable rotation in the frontal plane. Subsequently, the activation moves quite rapidly toward the apex spreading to both right and left ventricular surfaces. The posterior wall of the left ventricle is depolarized at about 40 to 50 msec and this is quite important in diagnosing coronary artery disease involving the posterior wall of the left ventricle.

Figure 3.1 shows the normal sequence of ventricular depolarization. The total time for activation of the right and left ventricles is between 80 and 100 msec. The time needed for completion of activation of the left and right ventricle is not the same for every patient. In some cases, there is late activation of the outflow tract of the right ventricle and the upper third of the interventricular septum. In this case, one might record a QRS loop that simulates an RSR' pattern on the electrocardiogram, which is usually interpreted as incomplete right bundle branch block.

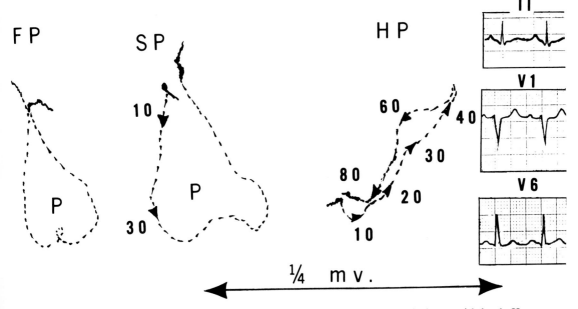

Figure 3.11. Magnified P loop in the frontal, sagittal, and horizontal planes with leads II, V1, and V6 of the electrocardiogram. Most of the P loop is directed inferiorly, posteriorly and to the left, representing forces originating in the left atrium.

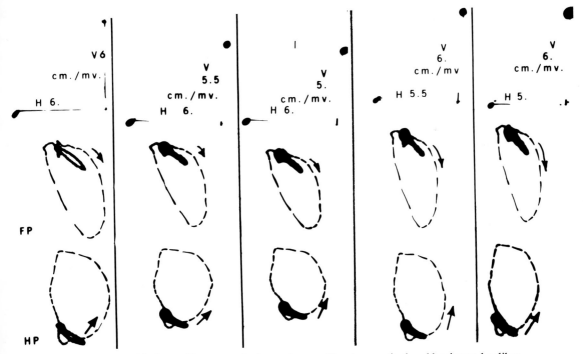

Figure 3.12. This figure illustrates the importance of having vertical and horizontal calibration of exactly the same length. In the first QRS loop recorded in the frontal and horizontal planes (*left*) with horizontal and vertical calibrations of 6 cm/mv, the loops have an essentially normal configuration. In the subsequent panels changes of the horizontal or vertical calibrations cause marked distortion of the QRS loop.

39

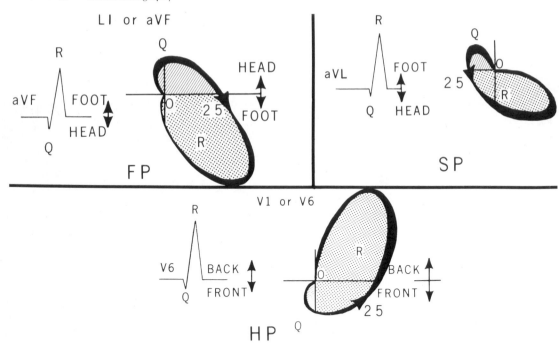

Figure 3.13. Diagrammatic comparison of the vectorcardiogram with the electrocardio-gram. *Top Left:* The frontal plane is compared with leads I and aVF. The patient has a QR pattern on the electrocardiogram. The Q wave represents forces directed toward the head on the electrocardiogram and corresponds with the forces going above the O point until they cross the horizontal line on the vectorcardiogram. The R wave of the electrocardio-gram, which is positive, is the force going toward the foot. On the vectorcardiogram this is the R loop, which is located to the left and inferiorly as shown in the dotted area. *Top Right:* The sagittal plane is very difficult to compare with the electrocardiogram. The one lead that comes close is aVL where the Q wave represents forces going to the head and the R wave represents forces going to the foot. On the vectorcardiogram, the Q wave is represented by the diagonal lined area above the O point. The dotted area represents the R loop forces directed inferiorly and posteriorly. *Bottom:* The horizontal plane is compared with leads V1 or V6. In lead V6, the Q wave represents forces coming to the front of the heart and the R wave is the forces going to the back of the heart. On the vectorcardiogram, the Q waves are represented by the diagonal lined area and the forces are directed anterior to the O point. The forces going to the back represent R deflection on the electrocardiogram and on the vectorcardiogram they are located posterior to the O point.

This may not represent an actual anatomical block but could simply be a disparity in the activation of the two ventricles.

In most cases, one can analyze the three major components of the QRS loop. The first, called vector 1, represents depolarization of the middle segment of the interventricular septum and usually lasts from the 1 to 20 msec QRS vectors. It is best appreciated in the horizontal plane. These forces are located in front of and to the right of the O point, corresponding to the R wave in V1 and Q wave in V6 on the electrocardiogram. Vector 2 represents simultaneous activation of the free wall of the right and left ventricles causing a large deflection of the QRS loop. As

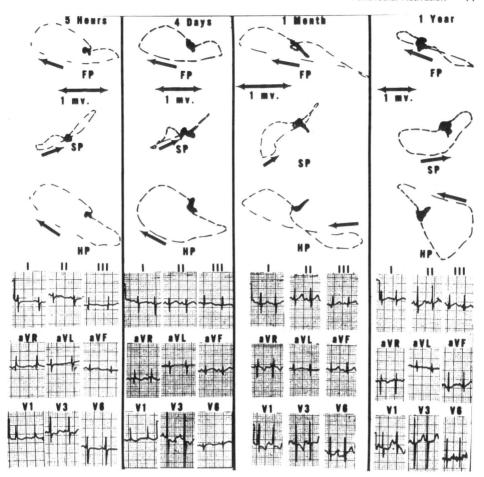

Figure 3.14. Evolutionary changes on the vectorcardiogram of a normal infant recorded at 5 hours, 4 days, 1 month, and 1 year of life. In the tracings recorded 5 hours and 4 days after birth, the horizontal plane QRS loop rotates clockwise because at that time the right ventricle dominates the electrical field. At 1 month of life, the loop rotates in a "figure-of-eight." It rotates counterclockwise in the horizontal plane at one year of age. Somewhat similar changes can be seen on the electrocardiogram in the precordial leads. (From A. Benchimol: Vectorcardiography. Copyright 1973 by The Williams & Wilkins Company, Baltimore. Used by permission.)

indicated, the left ventricle dominates the electrical field of the heart. Most of the forces seen in normal subjects are located at the left ventricle, i.e., posteriorly and to the left. These forces are oriented to the back toward the foot and to the left side as shown in Figures 3.13, 3.14, and 3.15. Vector 3 represents the terminal QRS vectors, which are usually the result of depolarization of the upper portion of the interventricular septum and the outflow tract of the right and left ventricles. These vectors are located to the back, upward and to the right. The normal direction and magnitude of the QRS vector is shown in Table 3.1.

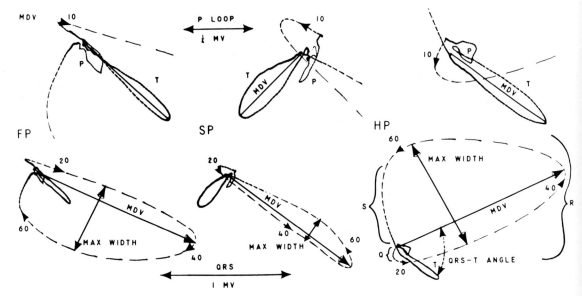

Figure 3.15. Vectorcardiogram in a normal subject showing how measurements of the QRS and T loops can be made at the time of inscription of the QRS vectors. Place a line from the O point to the maximal distance of the QRS loop. Then draw a second line from the O point to the maximal distance of the T loop. The difference in angle between these two lines is the QRS-T angle. The maximum width vector does not have much clinical significance. (From A. Benchimol: Vectorcardiography. Copyright 1973 by The Williams & Wilkins Company, Baltimore. Used by permission.)

Table 3.1. Direction and Magnitude (in Millivolts) of the Various QRS Vectors in the Frontal (FP), Left Sagittal (SP), and Horizontal (HP) Planes in a Group of 50 Normal Adult Subjects With Ages Ranging From 30 to 50 Years. (From A. Benchimol: Vectorcardiography. Copyright 1973 by The Williams & Wilkins Company, Baltimore. Used by permission.)

Plane		10	20	30	40	50	60	70	80	Max.
FP	Dir.	−79°	+12°	+32°	+42°	+50°	+46°	+73°	+16°	+38°
	Mag.	.08	.22	.70	.87	.51	.19	.09	.07	1.1
SP	Dir.	−19°	+19°	+96°	+133°	+153°	+162°	+164°	+41°	+134°
	Mag.	.11	.21	.43	.75	.67	.35	.14	.07	.86
HP	Dir.	+106°	+61°	+1°	−31°	−65°	−93°	−94°	−19°	−29°
	Mag.	.10	.23	.56	.88	.66	.35	.15	.07	.96

T Loop

Repolarization or the reactivation process of the heart is represented by the ST vectors and T loops. The origin of the T loop is not well understood, but it should follow the direction of the QRS loop. Measurement of the angle formed between the T and QRS loops, as shown in Figure 3.16, is important in the diagnosis of myocardial ischemia, ventricular hypertrophy and strain, metabolic disturbances, and other conditions.

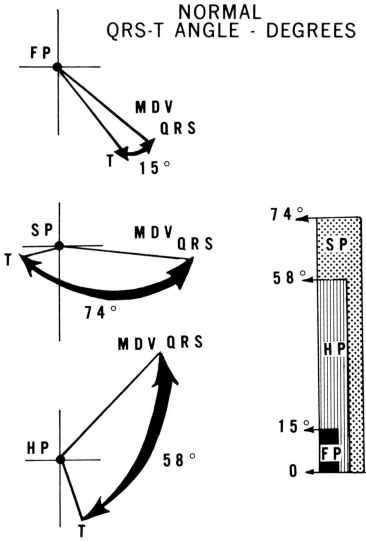

Figure 3.16. Diagrammatic representation of the QRS-T angles measured in the frontal, sagittal, and horizontal planes. The diagram on the right side shows the maximal average for a number of subjects that we studied. The frontal plane has the narrowest QRS angle, the sagittal plane is the widest and the horizontal plane is halfway between.

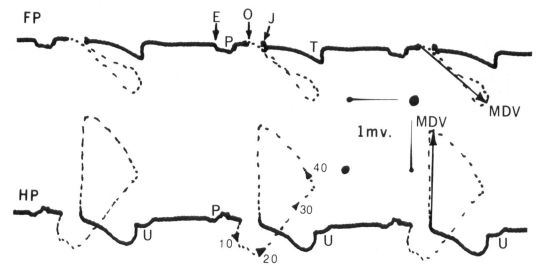

Figure 3.17. Simultaneously recorded timed vectorcardiogram in the frontal and horizontal planes in a 38-year-old subject with a normal heart. The E point is followed by the P loop. The E–O interval corresponds to the P–R interval on the electrocardiogram. The O point represents the beginning of the QRS loop. The J point represents the end of the QRS loop. This is followed by the ST vector and T loop. The U loop follows the T loop. The 10, 20, 30, and 40 msec QRS vectors are indicated in the horizontal plane.

U Loop

Analysis of the U loop (Fig. 3.17) on the vectorcardiogram has been reported but it is difficult. It is supposed to represent electrical forces after the entire heart has been depolarized and repolarized. Occasionally we find large U loops, especially in athletic hearts and in some patients with kidney disease or myocardial ischemia due to blockages in the blood vessels of the heart.

QRS-T Angle

The QRS-T angle is measured from the maximal deflection vector of the QRS loop. Place a line from the O point to the maximal distance of the QRS loop as shown in Figure 3.16. Then draw a second line from the O point to the maximal distance of the T loop. The difference in angle between these two lines is the QRS-T angle. The QRS-T angle is quite important in diagnosing myocardial ischemia of the various walls of the left ventricle. The angle is usually quite narrow in the frontal plane, very wide in the sagittal plane, and in the horizontal plane the angle is halfway between the frontal and sagittal plane angles. The normal values for the QRS-T angle are shown in Figure 3.16.

EVOLUTION OF THE VECTORCARDIOGRAM

Figure 3.14 demonstrates how the vectorcardiogram evolves from birth through the first few years of life. At birth, the right ventricle carries most of the overload;

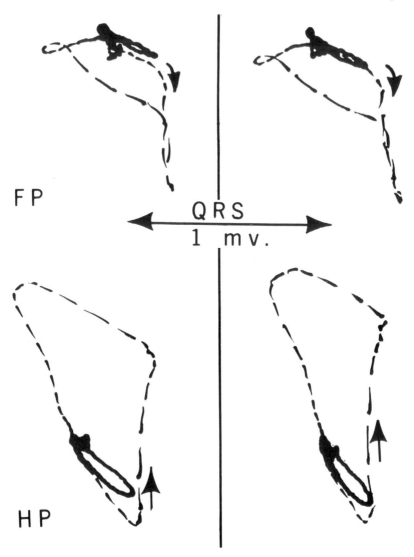

Figure 3.18. Vectorcardiogram in the frontal and horizontal planes recorded during quiet respiration (*left*) and during deep inspiration (*right*). Note changes in the configuration of the QRS loop particularly well seen in the horizontal plane, where most of the comets are located posterior and to the left.

therefore, the right ventricle dominates the electrical field and the forces are oriented toward this chamber, i.e., anteriorly and to the right or left. With subsequent age progression, the loops become oriented toward the back and to the left because the right ventricle becomes smaller and has less pressure and the left ventricle dominates the electrical field. Therefore, the QRS forces are oriented toward the left ventricle or posteriorly and to the left.

The P loop is usually located anterior and to the right or left because of increased right atrial pressure at birth, but within three to four years, the loop reaches the normal pattern and is located posteriorly and to the left where the left atrium is anatomically located. A typical example of a normal vectorcardiogram in adult life is shown in Figure 3.15. In Table 3.1, the direction and magnitude of the various QRS vectors are indicated.

PHYSIOLOGICAL VARIABLES

Physiological variables are seen with heavy body build in which one might record QRS loops that sometimes simulate right ventricular hypertrophy as shown in subsequent chapters. This is usually best appreciated in the frontal and horizontal planes.

The influence of respiration is shown in Figure 3.18. Be sure to record the tracing during quiet respiration and instruct the patient to relax as much as possible.

BIBLIOGRAPHY

Ainger, L.E., and Skinner, W.R.:   Normal maturation of spatial QRS curve characteristics in early infancy. Am. Heart J. *77*:5, 1969.

Benchimol, A.:   Vectorcardiogram. ACCESS Tape; Supplement Tape No. 1, March, 1970. American College of Cardiology, Bethesda, Md.

Brody, D.A., Cox, J.W., McEachran, A.B., Giles, H.H., and Ruesta, V.J.:   Spatial parameters and shape factors of the normal atrial vectorcardiogram and its scalar components. Circulation *39*:229, 1969.

Castellanos, A., Jr., Salhanick, L., Lemberg, L., and Cohen, R.:   The T loop in normal children. Am. J. Cardiol. *16*:336, 1965.

Chou, T., and Helm, R.A.:   Clinical Vectorcardiography. 2nd ed. New York: Grune & Stratton, 1974.

Chou, T., Helm, R.A., and Lach, R.:   The significance of a wide TsE loop. Circulation *30*:400, 1964.

Draper, H.W., Peffer, C.J., Stallmann, F.W., Lettmann, D., and Pipberger, H.V.:   The corrected orthogonal electrocardiogram and vectorcardiogram in 510 normal men (Frank lead system). Circulation *30*:853, 1964.

Durrer, D.:   Electrical aspects of human cardiac activity; a clinical–physiological approach to excitation and stimulation. Cardiovasc. Res. *2*:1, 1968.

Durrer, D., Van Dam, R.T., Freud, G.E., Janse, M.J., Meijler, F.L., and Arzbaecher, R.C.:   Total excitation of the isolated human heart. Circulation *41*:899, 1970.

Forkner, C.E., Jr., Hugenholtz, P.G., and Levine, H.D.:   The vectorcardiogram in normal young adults; Frank lead system. Am. Heart J. *62*:237, 1961.

Frank, E.:   An accurate, clinically practical system for spatial vectorcardiography. Circulation *13*:737, 1956.

Grishman, A., Borun, E.R., and Jaffe, H.L.:   Spatial vectorcardiography; technique for the simultaneous recording of the frontal, sagittal and horizontal projections. Am. Heart J. *41*:483, 1951.

Gunther, L., and Graf, W.S.:   The normal adult spatial vectorcardiogram; the timed sequence of inscription of the QRSsE of the cube and Frank systems. Am. J. Cardiol. *15*:656, 1965.

Johnston, F.D.:   The clinical value of vectorcardiography. Circulation *23*:297, 1961.

Kennedy, R.J., Varriale, P., and Alfenito, J.C.:   Textbook of vectorcardiography. New York: Harper & Row, 1970.

Khoury, G.H., and Fowler, R.S.:   Normal Frank vectorcardiogram in infancy and childhood. Br. Heart J. *29*:563, 1967.

Lal, S., Fletcher, E., and Binnion, P.:   Frank vectorcardiogram correlated with hemodynamic measurements. Br. Heart J. *31*:15, 1969.

Lamb, L.E.:   Electrocardiography and vectorcardiography. Philadelphia: W.B. Saunders, 1966.

Lyon, A.F., and Belletti, D.A.:   The Frank vectorcardiogram in normal men, norms derived from visual and manual measurement of 300 records. Br. Heart J. *30*:172, 1968.

McCall, B.W., Wallace, A.G., and Estes, E.H.:   Characteristics of the normal vectorcardiogram recorded with the Frank lead system. Am. J. Cardiol. *10*:514, 1962.

Mori, H., Nakagawa, K., Dahl, J.C., Schmitt, O.H., and Simonson, E.:   A quantitative study of initial and terminal QRS vectors in a group of normal older men. Am. Heart J. *59*:374, 1960.

Namin, E.P., Arcilla, R.A., Cruz, I.A., and Gasul, B.M.:   Evolution of the Frank vectorcardiogram in normal infants. Am. J. Cardiol. *13*:757, 1964.

Report of Committee on Electrocardiography, American Heart Association: Recommendations for standardization of leads and of specifications for instruments in electrocardiography and vectorcardiography. Circulation *35*:583, 1967.

Selvester, R.H., Collier, C.R., and Pearson, R.B.:   Analog computer model of the vectorcardiogram. Circulation *31*:45, 1965.

Sodi-Pallares, D., Medrano, G.A., Bisteni, A., and Jurado, J.P.L.:   Deductive and polyparametric electrocardiography. Instituto Nacional de Cardiologia de Mexico, Mexico D.F., Mexico, 1970.

Witham, A.C., and Lahman, J.E.:   Vectorcardiogram past forty. Am. Heart J. *79*:149, 1970.

4
Echocardiography and the Doppler Flowmeter

Sound with a frequency greater than 20,000 cycles per second, which is beyond the capability of human hearing, is defined as ultrasound. For echocardiography we utilize frequency ranges of millions of cycles per second (mega Hertz). Ultrasound travels in straight lines unless it is reflected or refracted by an interface or junction. An interface is defined as tissue refracting sound at different variations. The ultrasound beam must be perpendicular to the cardiac structure being analyzed. This is a very valuable concept in echocardiography that is necessary to obtain good, accurate recordings of the valvular structures, septal and posterior wall motion.

Certain tissues transmit or conduct ultrasound better than others. Muscle, blood and fat conduct very well, while bone and air conduct very poorly. Therefore, if the ultrasonic beam passes through the sternum, ribs, or lungs, it will be difficult or almost impossible to obtain a good echocardiographic recording of the cardiac structures.

If the technician avoids the bone and lungs through proper transducer placement, it is possible to differentiate the various cardiac structures because they have different densities. Any difference in density is seen as a junction or interface, and it will reflect an echo. An echo is defined as the repetition of a sound caused by reflection of sound waves. The clarity or resolution needed to define structures precisely will depend upon the ability to detect very small interfaces. The higher frequency transducers produce better resolution to define clearly these small interfaces, but have less penetration power. Lower frequency transducers penetrate more deeply but have less resolution for defining small interfaces. Echocardiographic recordings in infants and children do not require as much penetration power and a high frequency transducer, i.e., 5 mHz or 7.5 mHz, which has a small wave length, is used. For most adults deeper penetration is achieved by using a lower frequency transducer (2.25 mHz).

Echocardiographic (Fig. 4.1) and Doppler flowmeter transducers have a piezoelectric crystal that changes shape with variations in electrical fields. The transducer is an instrument that changes one form of energy into another. In echocardiography reflected sound energy is transformed into electrical energy, which can be expressed as changes in voltage. Rapid alternation of the electrical

48

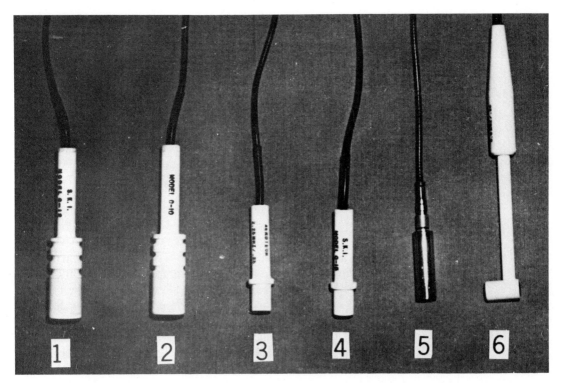

Figure 4.1. Various types of transducers that can be used for echocardiographic examination. Numbers 1 and 2 are most commonly used in adults, numbers 3, 4, and 5 are primarily for pediatric echocardiography, and number 6 is used for the suprasternal approach. (From A. Benchimol: Non-Invasive Diagnostic Techniques in Cardiology. Copyright 1977 by The Williams & Wilkins Company, Baltimore. Used by permission.)

field around the crystal causes it to vibrate and produce the ultrasonic beam. The echocardiographic units available today emit ultrasonic beams in very short bursts to reduce the total exposure to the ultrasound. Transducers used in these units act as a receiver 99.9% of the time and as an emitter only 0.1% of the time. Pulsed ultrasound has proven to be practically free of power damaging to the body tissues.

When the ultrasonic beam leaves the transducer, it remains parallel for a given distance before it begins to diverge. Objects recorded in a widely divergent beam will be fainter and may appear to lie on top of each other when they are actually side by side. It is advantageous to use a transducer with a concave focusing lens to minimize this effect. As the transducer senses the returning echoes, it generates electrical impulses that correspond in timing to a particular depth from the chest wall. These signals are then amplified and displayed as spikes on the oscilloscope of the echocardiograph. This display is called the "A-mode," and it does not indicate the motion of the object. The "M-mode," or "motion-mode," displays the object moving toward and away from the transducer. The "M-mode" is the most valuable in single plane echocardiography because the various cardiac structures can be identified by their characteristic motions.

Several types of recording units are available for permanent recordings. The echocardiogram can be obtained with polaroid cameras, strip chart recorders, or various hard copiers. The use of Polaroid cameras to record the echoes is limited because only a few beats may be seen at one time and a good scan cannot be easily obtained. Strip chart recorders allow a larger number of uninterrupted beats to be recorded enabling us to establish the interrelationships of the intracardiac structures when scanning from one area of the heart to another. A further advantage of strip chart recorders is that they may be equipped with additional amplifiers that allow for simultaneous recording of the echocardiogram with an electrocardiogram, carotid or jugular venous pulse tracing, phonocardiogram or apexcardiogram. This type of unit is very well suited for noninvasive diagnosis and evaluation of patients with cardiovascular disease.

The echocardiograph controls are nearly identical in most commercially available instruments. At our institution, we use a Smith-Kline Ekoline 20 unit (Fig. 4.2) interfaced with an Electronics for Medicine DR-8 recorder, an Irex echocardiograph and a Smith-Kline Ekoline 20 interfaced with a Honeywell 1856 strip chart recorder. The coarse gain switch controls the overall amplitude of all echoes (Fig. 4.3). Increasing or decreasing this setting will effect all echoes to the same degree. The near gain control sets the gain or brightness of the echoes seen in the near field only (Fig. 4.4).

Also in the control panel of the echocardiographic units are switches that can modify the depth, delay, ramp rate and depth compensation. The depth control

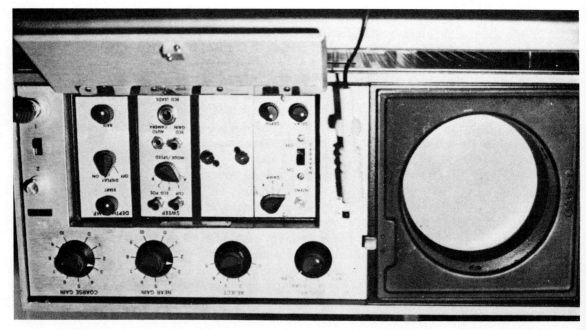

Figure 4.2. Smith-Kline Ekoline control panel, one of several commercially available echocardiographic units. See text for description of the various controls. (From A. Benchimol: Non-Invasive Diagnostic Techniques in Cardiology. Copyright 1977 by The Williams & Wilkins Company, Baltimore. Used by permission.)

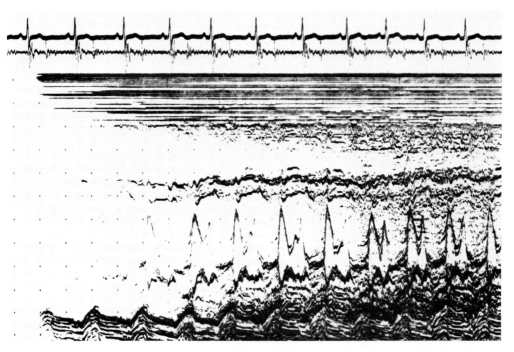

Figure 4.3. Echocardiogram of the mitral valve showing the changes in the recording when the coarse gain is increased from 0 to 10. The best recording is located in the center of the illustration where the mitral valve and interventricular septum are well seen.

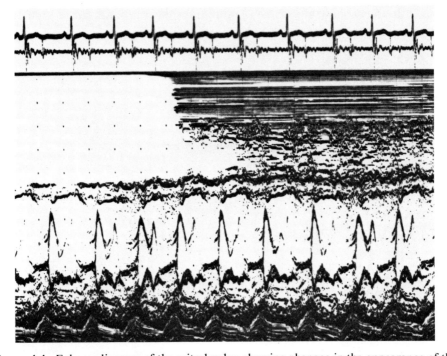

Figure 4.4. Echocardiogram of the mitral valve showing changes in the appearance of the intracardiac structures when the near gain control is increased from 0 to 5. The best recording of the mitral valve and interventricular septum is near the center of the illustration.

51

expands or contracts the field of echoes making the record easier to visualize (Fig. 4.5). The depth compensation (also called time gain or electronic distance compensation) is an electronic circuit for suppressing near field echoes and enhancing the weaker far field echoes. This device is represented on the "A-mode" as a ramp on the depth scale with a variable slope. All echoes to the left of the ramp are suppressed in relation to echoes on the right. The ramp itself represents increasing depth compensation. All echoes to the left of the top of the ramp fall within the control of the near gain, whereas all those to the right are outside the control of the near gain switch.

The damping control acts much like the coarse gain (Fig. 4.6). By increasing the damping, most echoes are suppressed and only the most dominant ones remain.

The reject control switch selectively eliminates low amplitude echoes (Fig. 4.7). Unlike the coarse gain or damping control, it does not diminish the stronger signals. The net effect is to make dominant structures appear as sharper lines by eliminating the smaller echoes.

The depth control regulates the depth of the echocardiographic field, as shown in Figure 4.5. For most adult echocardiograms, it is set at approximately 15 cm or less. Obviously, by setting the depth too shallow, only the anterior cardiac structures will be recognized. On the other hand, if the setting is too deep, the tracing will be abnormally crowded and the structures will not be easily recognizable or measurable.

The delay control is not important unless it is set incorrectly. In that event, the anterior structures will be completely cut off (Fig. 4.8). While using the "A-mode," the delay should be set so that the transducer artifact can be seen and all echoes will be present on the screen.

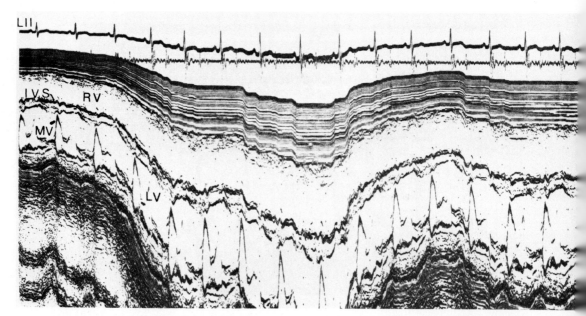

Figure 4.5. Echocardiogram of the mitral valve showing variations in the configuration of the valve and intracardiac structures when the depth control is changed. The best recording is toward the right side.

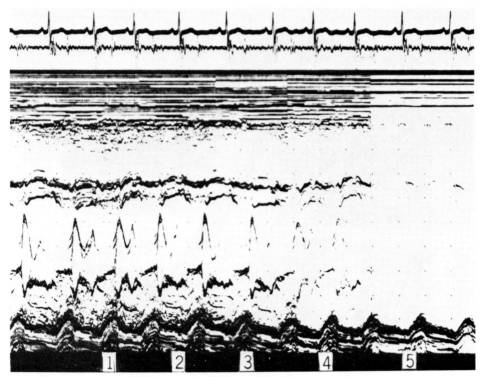

Figure 4.6. Echocardiogram of the mitral valve showing changes in the cardiac structures when the damp control is increased from 1 to 5.

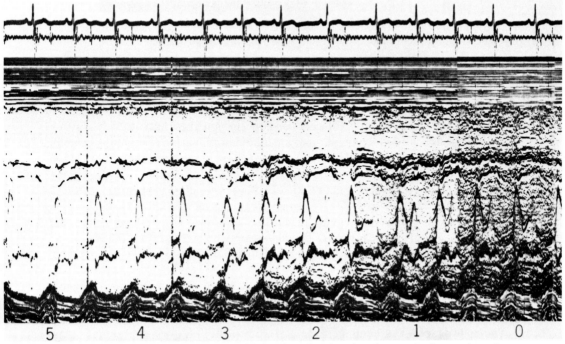

Figure 4.7. Echocardiogram of the mitral valve showing the changes in the tracing when the reject control is moved from position 5 to 0. The best recording is around position 2.

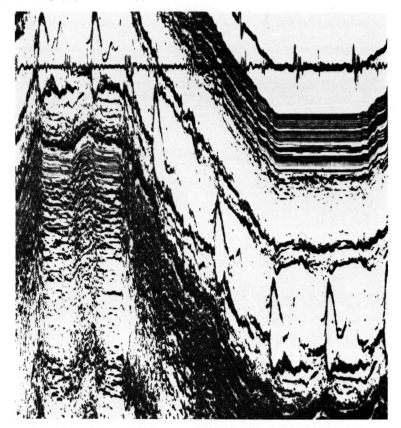

Figure 4.8. Echocardiogram of the mitral valve showing the effect of changes in the delay control. The best recording is toward the right side of the illustration.

It is very important for echocardiographic technicians to have a good under-standing of cardiac anatomy and normal and abnormal cardiac function such as valve abnormalities, congenital heart defects, etc. In most centers, the physicians are not trained to record a good echocardiogram and they have to rely on the tracing recorded by the technician. Among all the noninvasive techniques used in diagnosing cardiovascular diseases, the one requiring the technician with the most knowledge of cardiac structure and function is echocardiography. Artifacts can result from poor technique. Failure to record good quality echocardiograms is quite common and is often due to inexperience, poor technique used by the technician, or a lack of knowledge of cardiac anatomy. In our laboratory, the recordings are done by technicians. The physician who will interpret the echoes is expected to be familiar with the instrumentation and be able to recognize good and bad recordings.

The first step in learning to perform a good study is recognizing a normal echocardiogram. This requires a basic understanding of cardiac anatomy and pathophysiology (Fig. 4.9).

The right side of the heart lies anterior and to the left. In a horizontal cross section of the heart, the pulmonic valve lies anterior and to the left of the aortic valve, and the mitral valve to the left of the tricuspid valve (Figs. 4.9, 4.10). The

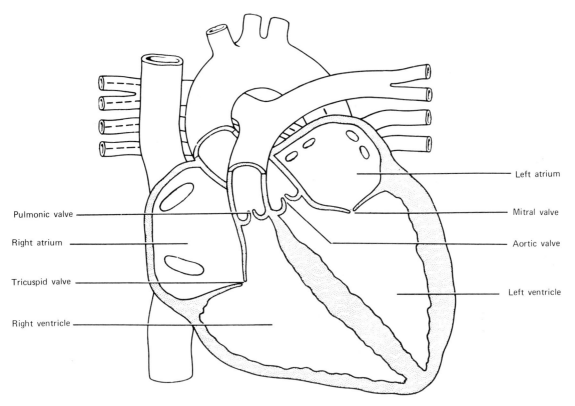

Pulmonic valve

Right atrium

Tricuspid valve

Right ventricle

Left atrium

Mitral valve

Aortic valve

Left ventricle

Figure 4.9. Frontal view of the heart showing the various intracardiac chambers. LA = left atrium, LV = left ventricle, AV = aortic valve, PV = pulmonic valve, MV = mitral valve, TV = tricuspid valve, RA = right atrium, RV = right ventricle.

interventricular septum is continuous with the anterior aortic wall. Figure 4.10 is a normal echocardiographic scan showing cross-sectional representations of the heart as seen with the echocardiographic transducer placed at the fourth intercostal space and to the left of the sternum. The right part of this diagram is the left sagittal cross section of the chest. Figure 4.11 shows the position of the transducer and the corresponding echo for the suprasternal and subxyphoid approaches.

There are four traditional positions for transducer placement on the chest wall (Fig. 4.10). In position 1, the ultrasonic beam passes through the chest wall, anterior right ventricular apex, and posterior papillary muscle. In position 2, it passes through the anterior right ventricle, right ventricular cavity, interventricular septum, left ventricle, chordae tendineae, and posterior left ventricular wall. In position 3, the structures seen are the anterior chest wall, right ventricle, interventricular septum, the M-shaped anterior mitral leaflet, the posterior mitral leaflet, posterior left ventricular wall, pericardium, and finally the lung and posterior mediastinal structures behind the heart. In position 4, the beam passes through the right ventricular outflow tract, the anterior wall of the aorta, aortic cusps, posterior aortic wall, and the left atrium.

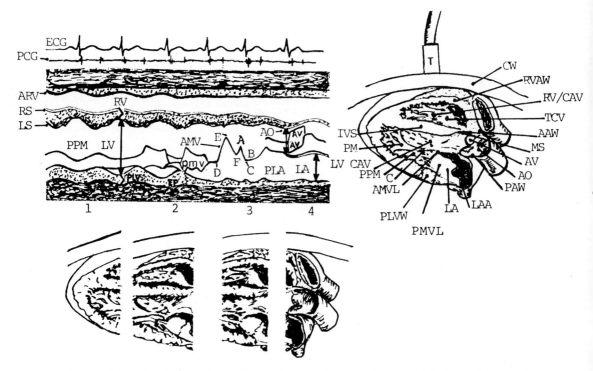

Figure 4.10. *Top Left:* Echocardiographic scan from the left ventricle toward the aorta showing the various intracardiac structures. *Bottom Left:* Corresponding anatomic site of the heart through which the ultrasonic beam crosses to obtain the recording. *Right:* Sagittal view of the heart showing the position of the transducer to the various intracardiac structures. ECG = electrocardiogram; ARV, RVAW = anterior right ventricular wall; RV, CAV, RV = right ventricle cavity; TCV = tricuspid valve; RS = right septal surface; IVS = interventricular septum; LS = left septal surface; LV, LV CAV = left ventricular cavity; PM = anterior papillary muscle; PPM = posterior papillary muscle; C = chordae; AMV, AMVL – anterior mitral leaflet; PMV = posterior mitral valve leaflet; PLVW, PLV = posterior left ventricular wall; EN = endocardium; EP = epicardium; PER = pericardium; A, B, C, D, E, F = points and slopes of anterior mitral valve leaflet motion; PLA = posterior left atrial wall; LA = left atrium; LAA = left atrial appendage; MS = membranous septum; AAW = anterior aortic wall; AV = aortic valve; AO = aorta; PAW = posterior aortic wall; CW = chest wall. (From S.J. Goldberg, H.D. Allen and D.J. Sahn: Pediatric & Adolescent Echocardiography: A Handbook. Copyright 1975 by Year Book Medical Publishers, Inc., Chicago. Used by permission.)

Examination of mitral valve motion shows that with rapid ventricular filling, the mitral leaflets open maximally and in opposite directions. The time of mitral valve opening is called the E point (Fig. 4.12). The leaflets then drift together into a semiclosed position, called the F point. There is frequently a second, low frequency vibration just after the F point that is seen in longer diastolic intervals. Subsequently, with atrial contraction, the valve reopens and this is called the A point or A wave. With the onset of ventricular systole, the mitral valve closes at point C. The closed valve echoes should form an anteriorly directed line during ventricular systole.

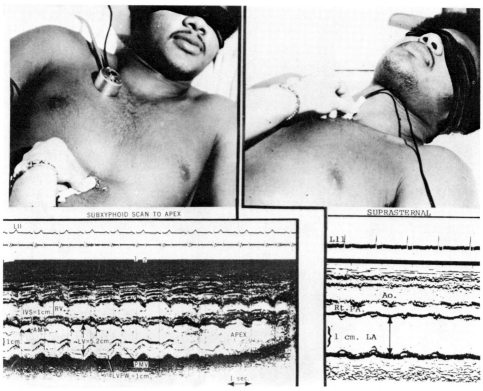

Figure 4.11. *Top Left:* Position of the transducer for the subxyphoid approach, with a microphone placed at the aortic area. *Bottom Left:* Corresponding scan from the mitral valve toward the apex of the heart. *Top Right:* Position of the transducer for the suprasternal approach. *Bottom Right:* Echocardiogram using the suprasternal approach showing a good recording of the aorta, right pulmonary artery, and left atrium.

Figure 4.10 is a scan from the aorta to the left ventricular apex in a normal subject showing normal motion of the various cardiac structures. During ventricular systole, the septum moves posteriorly as the left ventricular posterior wall moves anteriorly (Figs. 4.13, 4.14). This simply means that the walls of the left ventricle contract toward each other with each heart beat. Normal interventricular septal thickness should not exceed 1.1 cm and it normally moves less than the posterior left ventricular wall. The normal range of septal motion measured from the standard position is 0.3 to 0.8 cm. The amplitude of motion of the left ventricular posterior wall through this same area should be 0.9 to 1.4 cm. It is important to measure these structures from a standard location, just below the mitral valve level where the chordae echoes are seen, because interventricular septal motion is usually paradoxical as one angles the transducer too far superiorly. This is because the septum follows the normal motion of the aortic root.

The best recording of the aortic valve is obtained from position 4 (Fig. 4.10). This can be accomplished by angling the transducer medially and toward the right shoulder. In this position, the ultrasonic beam passes first through the right

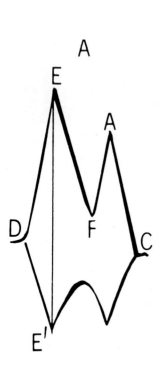

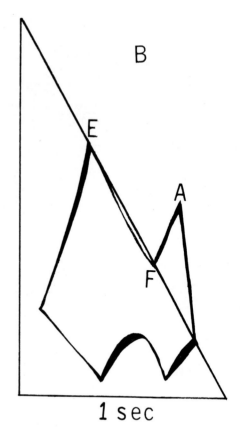

1 sec

Figure 4.12. *A:* Diagrammatic representation of the echocardiogram at the mitral valve showing the various labelings for the waveforms of the valve during diastole. *B:* Diagrammatic representation of the mitral valve showing how to measure the E-to-F slope.

ventricular outflow tract, the anterior wall of the aorta, and the aortic cusps. These cusps form a box-shaped structure during systole and a single line during diastole (Fig. 4.15). Behind the aortic valve is the posterior wall of the aorta. Note that the normal aortic echoes are thin and occupy the major portion of the aortic root during systole.

The standard left atrial measurement should be made at the end of systole, at the time of aortic valve closure from the posterior aortic wall and left atrial wall (Fig. 4.15). Simultaneous recording of the phonocardiogram with the echocardiogram helps to identify the second heart sound and this measurement should be made at the time of inscription of the first high frequency vibration of the second heart sound. In general, the aortic root and the left atrial dimension should be somewhat the same.

A recording of the pulmonic valve echoes is shown in Figure 4.16. Like the aortic valve, the pulmonic valve opens during systole and closes during diastole. Usually, only the posterior leaflet of the pulmonic valve is recordable. The complete box-shaped valve with motion similar to the aortic valve is rarely recorded in normal subjects. The downward deflection of the pulmonic valve,

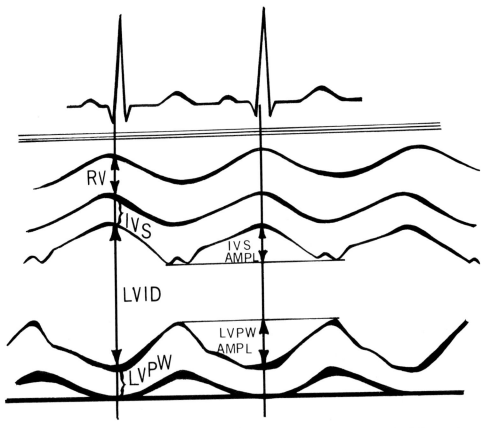

Figure 4.13. Diagrammatic representation of the ultrasonic beam crossing the left ventricle. This illustrates how to measure the right ventricular dimension, interventricular septal thickness and amplitude of motion, left ventricular internal dimension, posterior wall thickness, and left ventricular posterior wall amplitude of motion.

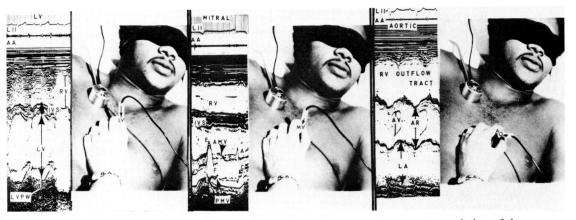

Figure 4.14. *Left:* Echocardiogram of the left ventricle showing correct angulation of the transducer for proper recording, with a microphone placed at the aortic area. *Middle:* Echocardiogram of the mitral valve showing angulation of the transducer with a microphone placed at the aortic area. *Right:* Echocardiogram of the aortic valve showing angulation of the transducer for a good recording of the aortic valve, aortic root, and right ventricular outflow tract. A microphone is placed at the aortic area.

59

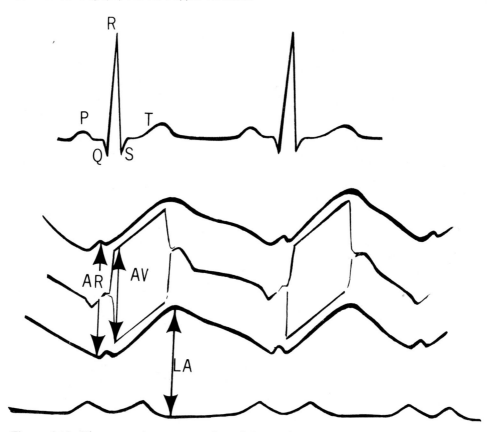

Figure 4.15. Diagrammatic representation of the aortic root, aortic valve, and left atrium indicating how measurements of these structures should be made. A diagrammatic representation of the electrocardiogram is shown at the top of the illustration.

caused by right atrial contraction, is called the A wave or A dip. As the pulmonic valve opens, it forms the box-shaped structure.

A recording of the tricuspid valve is shown in Figure 4.16. This valve motion is similar to mitral valve motion. Artifacts can be created by using improper techniques as shown in Figures 4.17, 4.18, and 4.19.

After emphasizing the technical aspects and normal motion of the cardiac structures as seen with sonic echocardiography, it is important to mention briefly other methods currently under evaluation by many investigators. These modalities include the two-dimensional sector scan concept and the linear array multielement transducer technique. Both methods produce two-dimensional images of the heart in real time. Current investigational studies indicate that these methods may have certain advantages over the single element unidimensional technique. These studies have suggested an improvement in visualizing structural cardiac abnormalities in patients with congenital heart disease, a more qualitative analysis of valve motion in patients with valvular heart disease, and the ability to recognize left ventricular wall motion more accurately, as well as better accuracy in determining the mitral valve orifice.

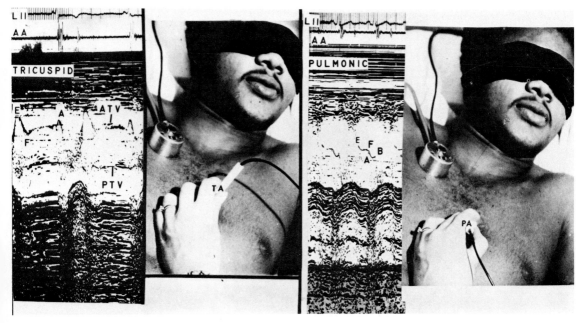

Figure 4.16. *Left:* Echocardiogram of the tricuspid valve showing the position of the transducer for proper recording. A microphone is placed at the aortic area. *Right:* Echocardiographic image of the pulmonic valve showing the position of the transducer with proper angulation for a good recording of the valve. A microphone is placed at the aortic area.

HOW TO MAKE ECHOCARDIOGRAPHIC MEASUREMENTS

Aortic Root

Measure the root size where the aortic valve cusps are well seen. With the peak of the R wave of the electrocardiogram, measure the vertical distance between the anterior and posterior aortic walls. Using the echoes observed from the inside dimension will avoid errors due to transducer angulation (Fig. 4.15). Normal adult range is 2.0 to 3.7 cm with a mean of 2.7 cm.

Aortic Leaflet Opening

Measure the maximal opening of the valve cusps in initial systole, using the internal borders of the cusp echoes (Fig. 4.15). Normal adult range is 1.6 to 2.6 cm with a mean of 1.9 cm.

Left Atrial Dimension

Measure the vertical distance between the posterior aortic wall and the posterior wall of the left atrium at its widest excursion point. This usually occurs at the time of the downslope of the T wave on the electrocardiogram. The left atrium should be measured where the aortic valve cusps are seen in the aortic root and proper damping should be utilized to clear echoes at the level of the posterior aortic and

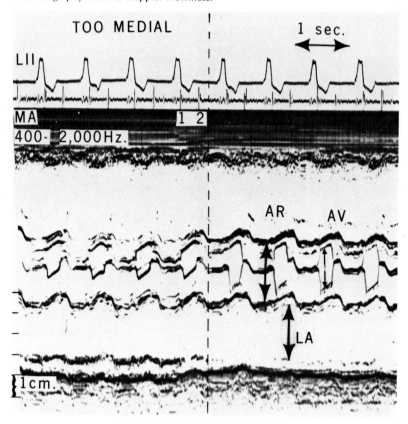

Figure 4.17. *Left:* Echocardiogram showing an artifactual recording of the aortic valve when the transducer is angulated too medially. *Right:* When the transducer is angulated properly, the valve has a perfectly normal configuration.

left atrial walls (Fig. 4.15). Normal adult range is 1.9 to 4.0 cm with a mean of 2.9 cm.

Left Ventricular Internal Dimension

The left ventricular internal dimension should be measured just below the mitral valve level, where only portions of the mitral valve apparatus and the chordae echoes are seen. A clear left septal echo and endocardial echo of the posterior wall should be seen consistently in systole and diastole. Measure the vertical distance from the left side of the septum to the endocardial surface of the left ventricular posterior wall with the peak of the R wave of the electrocardiogram (Fig. 4.13). Normal adult range is 3.5 to 5.6 cm with a mean of 4.7 cm.

Left Ventricular Posterior Wall Thickness

At end-diastole or with the peak of the R wave of the electrocardiogram, measure the vertical distance from the epicardium of the left ventricular posterior wall to the endocardium at the same area where the left ventricular internal dimension is measured (Fig. 4.13). Normal adult range is 0.6 to 1.1 cm with a mean of 0.9 cm.

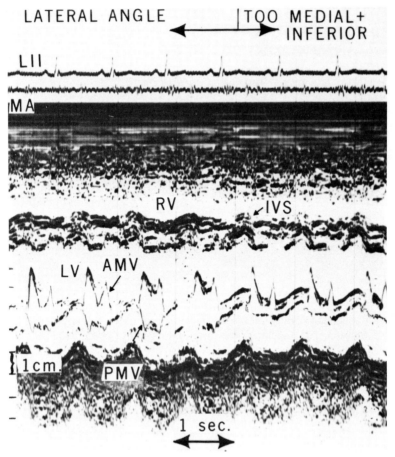

Figure 4.18. Echocardiogram of the mitral valve. The transducer is angulated too far medial and inferior on the right side of the picture and the valve becomes distorted. The proper recording of the valve is on the left.

Left Ventricular Posterior Wall Amplitude of Excursion

Where the left ventricular posterior wall thickness is determined, draw a horizontal line on the most anterior excursion of the left ventricular posterior wall in systole and measure the vertical distance from this line to the endocardium of the left ventricular posterior wall at the point corresponding to the peak of the R wave of the electrocardiogram (Fig. 4.13). Normal excursion is 0.9 to 1.4 cm with a mean of 1.2 cm. Normal motion is anterior in systole and posterior in diastole.

Interventricular Septal Thickness

Measure at the same point where the left ventricular posterior wall thickness was determined. The left and right sides of the septum should be seen clearly in systole and diastole. Measure the vertical distance from the right side of the interventricular septum to the left side at end-diastole or with the peak of the R wave of the electrocardiogram (Fig. 4.13). Normal adult range is 0.6 to 1.1 cm with a mean of 0.9 cm.

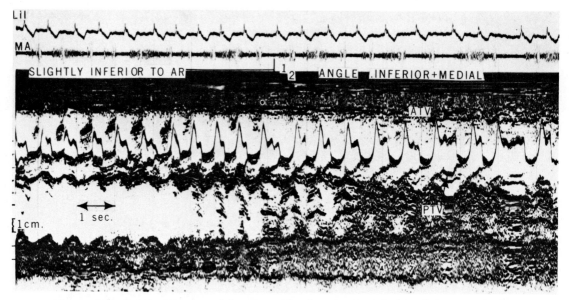

Figure 4.19. Echocardiogram of the tricuspid valve. On the left side of the recording the transducer is angulated slightly inferior to the aortic root (AR). Toward the right side of the picture the transducer is angulated inferiorly and medially, and a good recording of the tricuspid valve is obtained.

Interventricular Septum Amplitude of Excursion

At the point where the septal measurements are made, draw a horizontal line on the most posterior point of the left septum during systole and then measure the vertical distance from the line to the left septal surface at a point corresponding to the peak of the R wave of the electrocardiogram (Fig. 4.13). Normal excursion is 0.3 to 0.8 cm with a mean of 0.5 cm. Normal motion means the septum moves posteriorly in systole and anteriorly in diastole.

Right Ventricular Dimension

Measure the vertical distance from the right side of the interventricular septum to the anterior right ventricular wall at the same area where the left ventricular internal dimension was measured. Measure with the R wave of the electrocardiogram. Measurements should be made on the tracing if the patient was in a supine position during the recording. Left lateral measurements may be distorted due to rotation of the heart (Fig. 4.13). Normal adult range is 0.7 to 2.3 cm with a mean of 1.5 cm in the supine position.

Mitral Valve

Make all measurements of the anterior mitral leaflet that show maximal amplitude of motion, which is well recorded with the transducer placed perpendicular to the chest wall.

Mitral Valve Opening Amplitude

This is determined by drawing a verticle line from the E point of the mitral valve anterior leaflet to the E point of the posterior mitral valve leaflet (Fig. 4.12). The normal range is 2.6 to 3.7 cm.

E to F Slope Velocity

Draw a diagonal line from the peak of the E point to the F point. Draw a horizontal line near the bottom of the tracing where it intersects the diagonal line drawn from the E and F points. From the point where the horizontal line intersects the diagonal, measure horizontally for one second. At that point, measure the vertical distance to the diagonal line (Fig. 4.12). The velocity is equal to the distance in mm/sec. Normal range is greater than 35 mm/sec.

P–R Minus A–C Interval

For this to be calculated, the anterior and posterior mitral valve leaflets must have been recorded with a clear closing point called the C point. Measure the horizontal distance from the A point to the C point of the echocardiogram and subtract this from the P–R interval of the electrocardiogram. Normally, the P–R interval is 0.06 second greater than the A–C interval. If it is less than 0.06 second, it is an abnormal measurement (Fig. 4.20).

Tricuspid Valve

Measurements of the tricuspid valve are the same as those described for the mitral valve.

Pulmonic Valve

The whole diastolic portion of the pulmonic valve must be seen to calculate pulmonic valve motion.

"a" Wave Depth or "a" Dip

This is determined by drawing a horizontal line at the "f" point and another at the maximal posterior "a" point. These lines should run parallel. The vertical distance between these lines is the "a" wave depth (Fig. 4.21). Since the "a" wave varies significantly during inspiration and expiration, this measurement should be made at the point of greatest excursion, which is usually during inspiration. Normal range is 0.2 to 0.8 cm.

e–f Slope of the Pulmonic Valve

Draw a diagonal line from the peak of the "e" point to the "f" point. Draw a horizontal line near the bottom of the tracing where it intersects the diagonal line drawn from the "e" and "f" points. From the point where the horizontal line

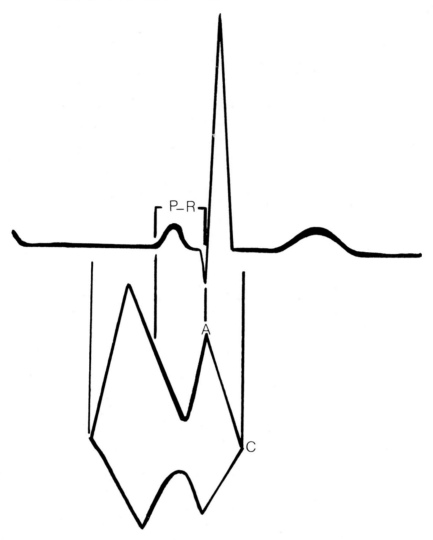

Figure 4.20. Diagrammatic representation of an echocardiogram of the mitral valve showing how to measure the P–R interval on the electrocardiogram minus the A–C interval on the echocardiogram.

intersects the diagonal, measure horizontally for one second. At that point, measure the vertical distance to the diagonal line (Fig. 4.12). The velocity is equal to the distance in mm/sec. Normal e–f slope range is 6 to 115 mm/sec.

DOPPLER FLOWMETER TECHNIQUE

Arterial or venous flow velocities have been measured using the transcutaneous Doppler flowmeter technique. The Doppler ultrasonic flowmeter telemetry system used in our studies was developed by Franklin and has been previously described

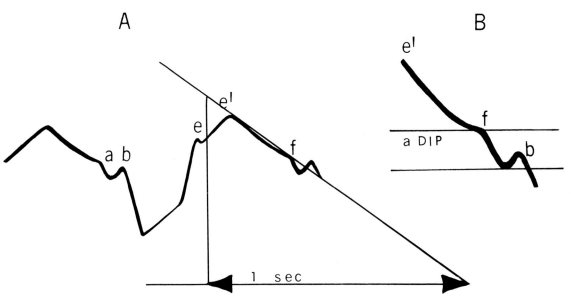

Figure 4.21. *A:* Echocardiogram showing how to measure the e–f slope of the pulmonic valve. *B:* Echocardiogram of the pulmonic valve showing how to measure the "a" dip.

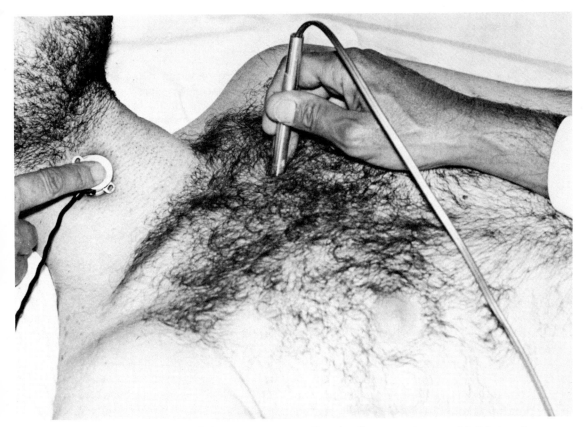

Figure 4.22. Positioning of the transcutaneous Doppler flowmeter to record left internal mammary flow velocity in normal patients and in those who have been subjected to left internal mammary artery to left anterior descending artery anastomosis.

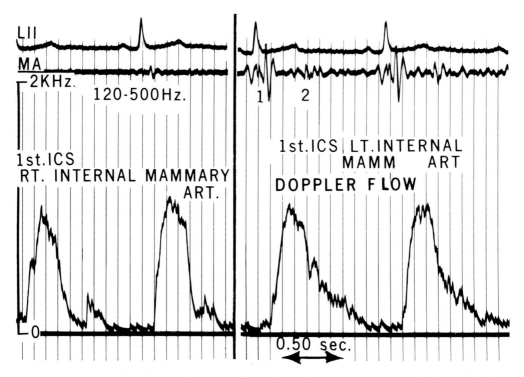

Figure 4.23. *Left:* Simultaneous recording of the electrocardiogram, mitral area (MA) phonocardiogram, and transcutaneous flow of the right internal mammary artery in a patient with coronary artery disease who had a left internal mammary to left anterior descending artery anastomosis. Flow velocity of the right internal mammary artery, which was not anastomosed, shows a rapid ascending limb near the first heart sound and very little flow during diastole. For this recording the transcutaneous probe was placed at the first intercostal space near the sternum and angulated straight toward the back. *Right:* Transcutaneous flow recording of the same patient's left internal mammary artery, which was anastomosed to the left anterior descending artery. Note the essentially identical waveform during systole, but a fairly large diastolic flow that follows the second heart sound of the phonocardiogram.

in detail. The technique utilized the Doppler shift principle. A high frequency sound (7–10 mega Hertz) is coupled to the skin by means of a piezoelectric crystal. Part of the emitted sound is backscattered and detected by a receiving crystal. The reflected signal differs in frequency from the incident signal by a quantity that is proportional to the velocity of the target, i.e., blood cells. Thus, the shift in frequency is proportional to blood velocity.

For transcutaneous measurements, the transducer containing the transmitting and receiving crystals is placed on the skin over the blood vessels being studied. The probe is positioned to obtain a maximally audible signal as heard by a loudspeaker or earphone. When a stable signal is obtained, the transducer is secured in place by means of adhesive tape or a rubber strap.

Clinical application of the transcutaneous Doppler flowmeter system is gaining increased popularity. Presently, this technique is of value in the study of venous circulation such as deep thrombophlebitis of the lower extremities, peripheral arterial occlusive disease, abnormalities of carotid artery blood velocity such as those that occur in aortic stenosis, idiopathic hypertrophic subaortic stenosis, evaluation of patency of internal mammary to left anterior descending anastomoses (Figs. 4.22 through 4.23) and the examination of jugular venous blood velocity patterns. In addition, this technique can be used to study cerebral circulation by obtaining recordings of blood velocity over the retinal arteries. This method gives a good indication of the circulation through the internal carotid arteries. Transcutaneous recordings are relatively easy to obtain and can be done by a skilled technician with proper training.

BIBLIOGRAPHY

Abelson, S.:   Reciprocal movement of the right and left heart, demonstrated by directional Doppler ultrasound. Am. Heart J., 86:651, 1973.

Benchimol, A.:   Blood flow velocity during ventricular fibrillation in man measured with the Doppler flowmeter technique. Chest, 60:265, 1971.

Benchimol, A., and Desser, K.B.:   Clinical application of the Doppler ultrasonic flowmeter. Am. J. Cardiol., 29:540, 1972.

Benchimol, A., Maia, I.G., Gartlan, J.L., Jr., and Franklin, D.:   Telemetry of arterial flow in man with a Doppler ultrasonic flowmeter. Am. J. Cardiol., 22:75, 1968.

Benchimol, A., Pedraza, A., Brener, L., Buxbaum, A., Goldstein, M.R., and Gartlan, J.:   Transcutaneous measurement of arterial flow velocity with a Doppler flowmeter in normal subjects and in patients with cardiac dysfunction. Chest, 57:69, 1970.

Benchimol, A., Stegall, H.F., and Gartlan, J.L.:   New method to measure phasic coronary blood flow velocity in man. Am. Heart J., 81:93, 1971.

Bom, N., Lancee, C.T. Jr., vanZwieten, G., Kloster, F.E., and Roelandt, J.:   Multiscan echocardiography; I. Technical description. Circulation, 48:1066, 1973.

Burggraf, G.W.:   Left ventricular volume changes after amyl nitrite and nitroglycerin in man as measured by ultrasound. Circulation, 49:136, 1974.

Edler, I.:   Atrioventricular valve motility in the living human heart recorded by ultrasound. Acta Med. Scand., 370 (Suppl.):83, 1961.

Edler, I.:   Diagnostic use of ultrasound in heart disease. Acta. Med. Scand., 308:32, 1955.

Feigenbaum, H.:   Echocardiography. 2nd ed. Philadelphia: Lea & Febiger, 1976.

Feigenbaum, H.:   Ultrasonic cardiology. Dis. Chest, 55:59, 1969.

Feigenbaum, H.:   Ultrasound as a clinical tool in valvular heart disease. Cardiovasc. Clin., 5:219, 1973.

Feigenbaum, H., Popp, R.L., Wolfe, S.B., Troy, B.L., Pombo, J.F., Haine, C.L., and Dodge, H.T.:   Ultrasound measurements of the left ventricle; a correlative study with angiocardiography. Arch. Intern. Med., 129:461, 1972.

Fortuin, M.J., Hood, W.P. Jr., Sherman, M.E., and Craige, E.:   Determination of left ventricular volumes by ultrasound. Circulation, 44:575, 1971.

Franklin, D.L.:   Technique for measurement of blood flow through intact vessels. Med. Electron. Biol. Eng., 3:27, 1965.

Franklin, D.L., Schlegel, W., and Rushmer, R.F.:   Ultrasonic Doppler shift blood flowmeter; circuitry and practical application. Proc. I.S.A. Biomed. Sci. Instrum. Symp., 1:309, 1963.

Franklin, D.L., Watson, N.W., VanCitters, R.L., and Smith, O.A.:   Blood telemetered from dogs and baboons. Fed. Proc., *23*:3030, 1964.

Goldberg, B.B.:   Suprasternal ultrasonography. J.A.M.A., *215*:245, 1971.

Goldberg, S.J., Allen, H.D., and Sahn, D.J.:   Pediatric and adolescent echocardiography: a handbook. Chicago: Year Book Medical Publishers, 1975.

Gramiak, R., and Shah, P.M.:   Detection of intracardiac blood flow by pulsed echo-ranging ultrasound. Radiology, *100*:415, 1971.

Gramiak, R., Shah, P.M., and Kramer, D.H.:   Ultrasound cardiography; contrast studies in anatomy and function. Radiology, *92*:939, 1969.

Griffith, J.M., and Henry, W.L.:   A sector scanner for real time two dimensional echocardiography. Circulation, *49*:1147, 1974.

Hirata, T., Wolfe, S.B., Popp, R.L., Helmen, C.H., and Feigenbaum, H.:   Estimation of left atrial size using ultrasound. Am. Heart J., *78*:43, 1969.

Joyner, C.R., and Reid, J.M.:   Application of ultrasound in cardiology and cardiovascular physiology. Prog. Cardiovasc. Dis., *5*:482, 1963.

King, D.L.:   Real-time cross-sectional ultrasonic imaging of the heart using a linear array multi-element transducer. J. Clin. Ultrasound, *1*:196, 1973.

Kloster, F.E., Roelandt, J., tenCate, F.J., Bom, N., and Hugenholtz, P.G.:   Multiscan echocardiography; II. Technique and initial clinical results. Circulation, *48*:1075, 1973.

Kraunz, R.F., and Kennedy, J.W.:   Ultrasonic determination of left ventricular wall motion in normal man. Am. Heart J., *79*:36, 1970.

Kraunz, R.F., and Ryan, T.J.:   Ultrasound measurements of ventricular wall motion following administration of vasoactive drugs. Am. J. Cardiol., *27*:464, 1971.

Lundstrom, N.R.:   Clinical applications of echocardiography in infants and children; I. Investigations of infants and children without heart disease. Acta Paediatr. Scand., *63*:23, 1974.

Lundstrom, N.R.:   Clinical applications of echocardiography in infants and children. II. Estimation of aortic root diameter and left atrial size: a comparison between echocardiography and angiocardiography. Acta. Paediatr. Scand., *63*:33, 1974.

Lundstrom, N., and Edler, I.:   Ultrasound in infants and children. Acta. Paediatr. Scand., *60*:116, 1971.

Maroon, J.C., Campbell, R.L., and Dyken, M.L.:   Internal carotid artery occlusion diagnosed by Doppler ultrasound. Stroke, *1*:122, 1970.

Pombo, J., Russell, R.O. Jr., Rackley, C.B., and Foster, G.L.:   Comparison of stroke volume and cardiac output determination by ultrasound and dye dilution in acute myocardial infarction. Am. J. Cardiol., *27*:630, 1971.

Roelandt, J., Kloster, F.E., tenCate, F.J., vanDorp, W.G., Honkoop, J., Bom, N., and Hugenholtz, P.G.:   Multidimensional echocardiography. An appraisal of its clinical usefulness. Br. Heart J., *36*:29, 1974.

Roper, P.A., Desser, K.B., and Benchimol, A.:   Clinical application of echocardiography. Ariz. Med., *32*:265, 1975.

Sjogren, A.L., Hytonen, I., and Frick, M.H.:   Ultrasonic measurements of left ventricular wall thickness. Chest, *58*:37, 1970.

Stegall, H.F., Rushmer, R.F., and Baker, D.W.:   A transcutaneous ultrasonic blood velocity meter. J. Appl. Physiol., *21*:707, 1966.

Strandness, D.E., McCutchen, E.P., and Rushmer, R.F.:   Application of a transcutaneous Doppler flowmeter in evaluation of occlusive arterial disease. Surg. Gynecol. Obstet., *122*:1039, 1966.

Tanaka, M.:   Ultrasonic evaluation of anatomical abnormalities of the heart in congenital and acquired heart diseases. Br. Heart J., *33*:686, 1971.

VanCitters, R.L., and Franklin, D.L.:   The Doppler ultrasonic telemetry flowmeter; application in animal experiments. Proceedings of the 20th Annual Conference on Engineering in Medicine and Biology, *27*:7, 1967.

Waltenath, C.L.:   Assessment of cardiovascular function during operation using Doppler technic. Am. Surg., *38*:352, 1972.

5

Mitral
Valvular Disease

Rheumatic fever is the most common cause of mitral valve disease, but it takes several years for patients to exhibit symptoms that require medical care. Congenital mitral stenosis (narrowing of the mitral valve) and insufficiency (leaking valve) are rare as isolated lesions, but frequently may be associated with other congenital anomalies (see Chap. 10). Mitral insufficiency may also be present in patients with disease of the coronary arteries (see Chap. 9).

MITRAL STENOSIS

Heart Sounds and Murmurs

The first heart sound has high amplitude and is analyzed best at the mitral and tricuspid areas on the logarithmic recording (Fig. 5.1). Amplitude of the first heart sound at the mitral area should be twice that of the second heart sound in patients with regular sinus rhythm. The amplitude of the first heart sound is proportional to the length of the P–R interval of the electrocardiogram; the shorter the P–R interval, the greater the amplitude. However, most adult patients with mitral stenosis have atrial fibrillation or flutter which is shown electrocardiographically by absent P waves substituted by fibrillatory (f) or flutter (F) waves and irregular R–R intervals. Therefore, amplitude of the first heart sound varies from beat to beat.

Calcification and/or thickening of the mitral valve leaflets results in decreased amplitude of the first heart sound, and is probably due to diminished motion of the mitral valve (Fig. 5.2). The second heart sound usually has two components (split second sound), as shown in Figure 5.2. The first component that represents closure of the pulmonic valve has normal amplitude. However, in patients with elevated pulmonary artery pressure above the normal level (mean above 15 mm Hg.), this sound is accentuated and recognized best in tracings recorded at the pulmonic and/or tricuspid areas. For this sound to be considered accentuated, it should exceed the amplitude of the first heart sound at the same area. Usually this accentuated sound has twice the amplitude of the first heart sound. If the second heart sound is split and there is moderate to severe pulmonary hypertension and right ventricular enlargement, the pulmonary component can usually be recorded

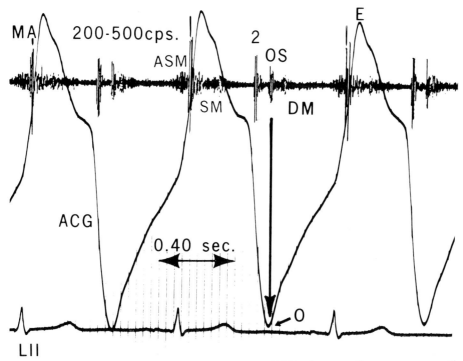

Figure 5.1. Simultaneously recorded mitral area (MA) phonocardiogram, apexcardiogram (ACG), and lead II of the electrocardiogram (LII) in a 23-year-old patient with mitral stenosis and insufficiency. Mitral stenosis was the predominant lesion. Note the accentuated first heart sound. The second heart sound is single and due to aortic valve closure. There is an opening snap which coincides with the O point of the apexcardiogram. There is a high frequency, low amplitude systolic regurgitant murmur that begins with the first heart sound and ends in midsystole. There is also the typical murmur of mitral stenosis consisting of an atrioventricular diastolic murmur that begins with the opening snap and ends before the P wave of the electrocardiogram. Following that, there is a second murmur called atriosystolic murmur that terminates with the first heart sound. The apexcardiogram is abnormal showing an absent rapid filling wave. The systolic wave is normal.

at the mitral and/or aortic areas. Therefore, it is important to obtain good recordings of heart sounds in these two areas.

In most patients with mitral stenosis, a high frequency vibration called an opening snap (Figs. 5.1 through 5.4) is recorded 0.04 to 0.14 sec after the first vibration of the second heart sound (aortic valve closure). This interval, called the second sound-opening snap interval (2–OS), is grossly proportional to the degree of severity of mitral stenosis. A very short 2–OS interval (0.03 to 0.05 sec) is usually indicative of severe mitral stenosis; an interval of 0.05 to 0.10 sec indicates moderate stenosis and 0.10 to 0.16 sec, mild stenosis. The opening snap can be confused with splitting of the second heart sound. When this is in question, a simultaneous recording of the phonocardiogram, apexcardiogram, and/or echocardiogram can be helpful. If the vibration represents splitting of the second heart sound, it should precede the O point on the apexcardiogram or the E point on the echocardiogram. If it represents the opening snap (Fig. 5.1), it should

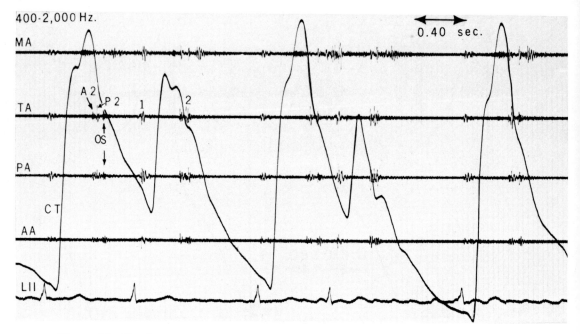

Figure 5.2. Simultaneously recorded phonocardiogram at the mitral (MA), tricuspid (TA), pulmonic (PA), and aortic areas (AA), carotid pulse tracing (CT), and lead II (LII) of the electrocardiogram in a 38-year-old patient with mitral stenosis and atrial fibrillation. The patient had a calcified mitral valve; therefore, the first heart sound is diminished. The second heart sound, well recorded at the tricuspid area, is split. The pulmonic component is accentuated because the patient has high pressure in the pulmonary arteries. There is also a very short opening snap, approximately 0.06 sec. Note the variations in amplitude of the diastolic murmur (DM) from beat to beat because of the atrial fibrillation and variation in cycle length. There is also a systolic murmur due to mild mitral insufficiency. The carotid pulse tracing is normal.

coincide with the O point of the apexcardiogram or the E point on the echocardiogram. Following surgical correction of this lesion (mitral valvulotomy, i.e., surgical incision of the mitral valve), the opening snap may disappear or decrease in amplitude and the 2–OS interval prolongs. In the presence of a heavily calcified mitral valve associated with subvalvular stenosis (fusion of the chordae that attaches the valve to the papillary muscle), amplitude of the opening snap diminishes (Fig. 5.2) or may be absent. Therefore, do not expect to record an opening snap in every patient with mitral stenosis. Another interval that can be measured in patients with mitral stenosis is the time interval from the beginning of the QRS complex of the electrocardiogram to the first high frequency vibration of the first heart sound. This interval, called the Q–T interval, shortens in proportion to the degree of stenosis, i.e., the more severe the stenosis, the shorter the Q–T interval. A Q–T interval shorter than 0.08 sec usually represents severe mitral stenosis. Extra heart sounds such as systolic ejection clicks (high frequency, early systolic sound) are seen only when there is pulmonary hypertension. A third heart sound, also called an early diastolic gallop, is not present in mitral stenosis unless

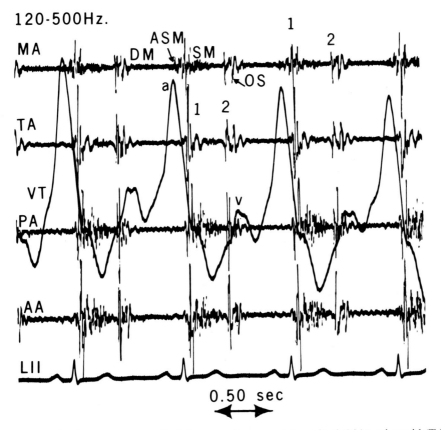

Figure 5.3. Simultaneously recorded phonocardiogram at the mitral (MA), tricuspid (TA), pulmonic (PA), and aortic areas (AA), jugular venous tracing (VT), and lead II (LII) of the electrocardiogram in a 26-year-old patient with mitral stenosis and a mild degree of aortic stenosis. The slightly accentuated first heart sound is seen best at the tricuspid area. The second heart sound is single and normal. An opening snap recorded in all precordial areas is best seen at the aortic area. The second sound–opening snap (2–OS) interval is quite short, about 0.04–0.05 sec. This type of tracing sometimes simulates splitting of the second heart sound. The 2–OS interval is short and the A wave of the jugular venous tracing is moderately accentuated due to the severe mitral stenosis with pulmonary hypertension. A high frequency, high amplitude systolic ejection murmur (SM) recorded in all precordial areas is indicative of aortic stenosis. There is also a low frequency, low amplitude diastolic murmur (DM) due to mitral stenosis, followed by an atriosystolic murmur (ASM), which coincides with the A wave of the jugular venous pulse.

there is significant pulmonary hypertension and tricuspid insufficiency. In this setting, the third heart sound most likely originates in the right ventricle. If tricuspid insufficiency is suspected, be sure to record the tracing during held inspiration and expiration; if the third heart sound originates in the right ventricle, it will increase during inspiration.

The diastolic murmur or rumble of mitral stenosis starts with mitral valve opening (Figs. 5.1, 5.2). Therefore, there is a short clear interval between the

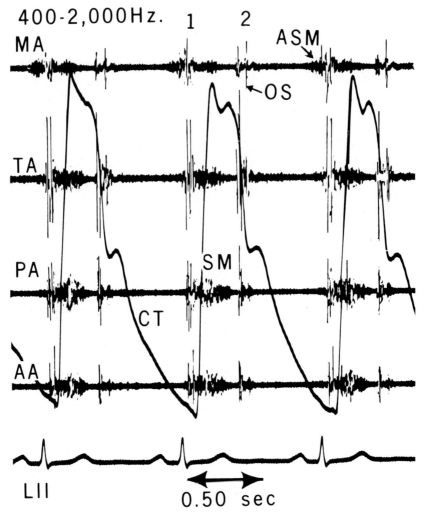

Figure 5.4. Simultaneously recorded phonocardiogram at the mitral (MA), tricuspid (TA), pulmonic (PA), and aortic areas (AA), carotid pulse tracing (CT) and lead II (LII) of the electrocardiogram of the same patient shown in Figure 5.3. The shape of the systolic murmur (SM) can be seen better because of the filter setting of 400–2,000 Hz. It is due to mild aortic stenosis. The first heart sound is slightly accentuated. The second heart sound is single. An opening snap (OS) is recorded in all precordial areas. On the carotid pulse tracing, note that the ejection time is normal. The atrioventricular diastolic murmur of mitral stenosis is not well seen but the atriosystolic component (ASM) is well recorded.

second heart sound and the beginning of the murmur. It is a low frequency murmur (50 to 500 Hz), and reaches a maximal peak in the first third of diastole. This murmur is the result of blood flow across the stenotic valve and it terminates prior to the P wave of the electrocardiogram. In patients with atrial fibrillation, it terminates 0.10 to 0.14 sec before the first heart sound (Fig. 5.2). In patients with sinus rhythm, a second, late diastolic murmur (atriosystolic murmur) due to active atrial contraction is present. It starts shortly after the P wave of the electrocardiogram and terminates with the high frequency component of the first heart sound (Fig. 5.1). The shape of this murmur usually follows the gradient across the mitral valve. The atriosystolic murmur, also known as presystolic accentuation of the diastolic murmur, is absent in patients with atrial fibrillation. Other murmurs may be present in patients with mitral stenosis. A diastolic murmur of pulmonary insufficiency is uncommon but it may be present in the late stage of this disease. This high frequency diastolic murmur (Graham–Steel murmur) is frequently confused with the murmur of aortic insufficiency because both have the same phonocardiographic characteristics. It begins with the second heart sound, diminishes during mid-diastole and terminates prior to atrial contraction. The murmur is best heard and recorded at the tricuspid and pulmonic areas with the patient in an upright or sitting position during maximal, held expiration. Recordings should be obtained at a log setting. An increase in amplitude of the murmur during inspiration favors the diagnosis of pulmonic insufficiency.

Carotid Pulse Tracing

Simultaneous recording of carotid pulse tracings with phonocardiograms helps to establish the presence of a systolic ejection click. When present, it is inscribed during the ascending limb on the carotid pulse tracing. Mitral stenosis does not cause significant abnormalities in the waveform of the carotid tracing except that ejection time may be short (Fig. 5.4).

Jugular Venous Pulse Tracing

The jugular venous pulse is normal in mild mitral stenosis and abnormal when the patient develops pulmonary hypertension or tricuspid insufficiency. When pulmonary hypertension is present, the venous tracing shows a prominent A wave (A/V ratio greater than the normal ratio of 1.5:1), as shown in Figure 5.3. Amplitude of the A wave is grossly proportional to the degree of pulmonary hypertension. If the patient develops tricuspid insufficiency, the tracing will be identical to recordings obtained in any condition which results in tricuspid insufficiency (see Chap. 7).

Apexcardiogram

The apexcardiogram recorded simultaneously with the phonocardiogram is a valuable noninvasive technique for the diagnosis of mitral stenosis. Be sure to obtain a good recording of the O point in an area where the opening snap is best appreciated. The O point coincides with, shortly precedes, or follows the opening snap of the mitral valve (Fig. 5.1). In patients with a heavily calcified mitral valve, the opening snap is absent and the 2–OS interval cannot be measured. However, through simultaneous recording of the apexcardiogram and phonocardiogram, this interval can be estimated by measuring the time from the first component of the second heart sound to the O point of the apexcardiogram. Abnormalities of the systolic wave reflect abnormal left ventricular contraction secondary to rheumatic involvement of the heart muscle. The most common abnormalities are a rapid, downward displacement in early systole followed by a late systolic bulge (late rise in the baseline reaching a peak near the second heart sound). In addition, the rapid filling and A waves are absent or quite small. It is important to obtain a technically adequate apexcardiogram (see Chap. 2) in patients with mitral stenosis, but caution should be exercised. Artifacts are recorded if proper technique is not used. We are only able to record adequate left ventricular apexcardiograms in approximately 75% of our patients with mitral stenosis. A right ventricular apex-cardiogram may be recorded in patients with mitral stenosis and pulmonary hypertension secondary to enlargement or dilatation of the right ventricle. If a good right ventricular apex tracing is obtained with the transducer placed at the fourth intercostal space or subxyphoid area, it may show an exaggerated A wave and a sustained systolic wave.

Systolic Time Intervals

Ejection time is normal in patients with mild mitral stenosis. In the setting of severe stenosis associated with moderate to severe pulmonary hypertension, ejection time is diminished. No definite data are available to determine the useful-ness of measurements of the pre-ejection period (PEP) or the pre-ejection period/left ventricular ejection time ratio unless the patient is in heart failure. In this case, these indices will be abnormal. They usually will be identical to the findings seen in patients with heart failure due to any cause.

Vectorcardiogram

Unfortunately, a large number of patients with mitral valve disease have atrial fibrillation or flutter; therefore, the P loops are not present. Their substitute is the so called f (fibrillation) or F (flutter) loops. In this situation, you have to rely on abnormalities of the QRS vectors, which show signs of right ventricular hyper-trophy in patients with mitral stenosis. This technique is superior to the electro-cardiogram and is very sensitive in detecting early signs of left atrial and/or right ventricular hypertrophy, as shown in Figures 5.5 and 5.6.

Echocardiogram

Echocardiography is an important diagnostic technique in the evaluation of pa-tients with mitral stenosis. The abnormalities include: (1) Decreased motion of the anterior leaflet of the mitral valve with a decreased E–F slope below the normal range of 35 mm/sec. In patients with atrial fibrillation, the E–F slope varies considerably from beat to beat in relation to cycle length. In order to obtain an accurate measurement of the E–F slope in patients with atrial fibrillation, at least seven consecutive cardiac cycles should be recorded. This technique is also used to determine improvement in mitral valve motion following surgery. After mitral valvulotomy, the E–F slope changes in proportion to the relief of stenosis. (2) The posterior leaflet of the mitral valve has a paradoxical motion, i.e., moving in the same direction as the anterior leaflet (anteriorly), which is the reverse of normal (Fig. 5.7). Calcification or thickening of the mitral valve results in the recording of multiple and disorganized echoes (Fig. 5.7). Gross quantitation of the degree of severity of mitral stenosis can be obtained by measuring the E–F slope. It

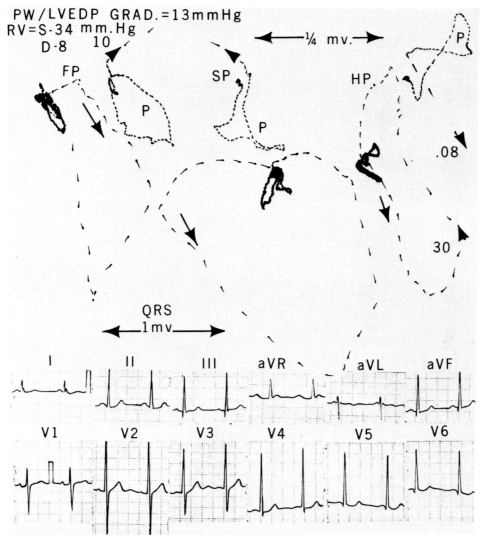

Figure 5.5. Vectorcardiogram and electrocardiogram of a 26-year-old patient with mitral stenosis. The gradient between the pulmonary "wedge" and left ventricular end-diastolic pressure (gradient across the mitral valve) was 13 mm Hg. Right ventricular systolic pressure was 34 with a diastolic pressure of 8. The frontal plane (FP) vectorcardiogram is normal. Abnormalities are seen in the horizontal plane (HP) with the forces located anterior to the O point, indicating the presence of so-called Type B right ventricular hypertrophy frequently seen in patients with mitral stenosis. This is not well seen on the electrocardiogram because of its insensitivity for detection of early signs of right ventricular hypertrophy. The P loop is located anteriorly and to the left indicative of left atrial hypertrophy. Again this is not noted on the electrocardiogram.

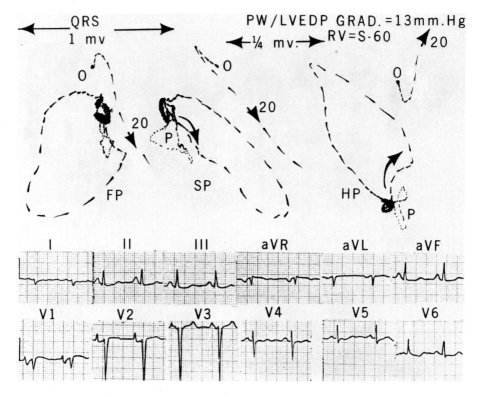

Figure 5.6. Vectorcardiogram and electrocardiogram in a patient with mitral stenosis showing Type C right ventricular hypertrophy. Most of the QRS forces in the horizontal plane (HP) are located posteriorly and to the left. The gradient between the pulmonary "wedge" and left ventricular end-diastolic pressure was 13 mm Hg., indicating moderate to severe mitral stenosis.

decreases progressively in proportion to the degree of the stenotic mitral valve lesion. In mild to moderate mitral stenosis it measures 25 to 35 mm/sec, in moderate mitral stenosis, 15 to 25 mm/sec, and in severe mitral stenosis, less than 15 mm/sec. Measurement of structure diameters frequently shows an increase in size of the left atrium above the normal range of 4 cm and of the right ventricle above 2.3 cm (Figs. 5.7, 5.8). In patients with mitral stenosis and severe pulmonary hypertension, the pulmonic valve has abnormal motion in diastole manifested by a decreased E–F slope below 6 mm/sec, a small or flat A wave or A dip and abnormal motion during systole. The valve may show a "flying W" pattern. During systole, caution must be exercised in diagnosing mitral stenosis using only abnormalities of anterior mitral valve motion. Good recordings of the posterior mitral leaflet must be obtained because other conditions, such as coronary artery disease or heart failure from any cause can result in a tracing that simulates the findings seen in mitral stenosis, such as decreased E–F slope due to low cardiac output. Some patients with calcification of the mitral valve annulus may mimic mitral stenosis because of heavy echoes behind the posterior leaflet of the mitral valve, as shown in Figure 5.8, but in the absence of mitral stenosis, the mitral leaflet has normal motion.

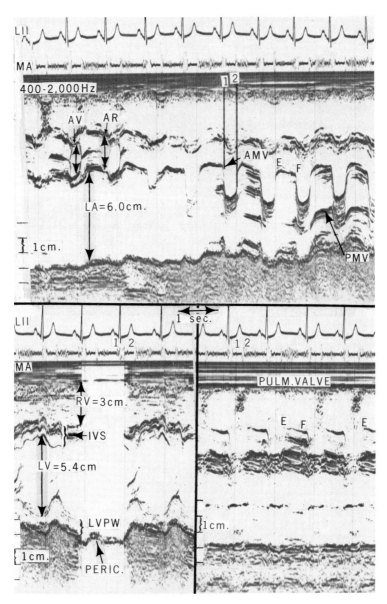

Figure 5.7. Simultaneously recorded echocardiogram, mitral area (MA) phonocardiogram, and lead II (LII) of the electrocardiogram in a 40-year-old patient with mitral stenosis. *Top*: Echocardiographic scan from the aorta to the mitral valve showing the aortic root (AR), aortic valve (AV), and an enlarged left atrium (LA) measuring 6 cm. The mitral valve shows the typical features of mitral stenosis, i.e., a decrease in the E–F slope and paradoxical anterior motion of the posterior leaflet. The heavy echoes originating from the anterior (AMV) and posterior (PMV) leaflets indicate the presence of fibrosis or calcification of the mitral valve. *Bottom Left*: The left ventricular (LV) dimension of 5.4 cm is normal, but the right ventricle (RV) is enlarged to 3 cm. *Bottom Right*: Pulmonic valve recording showing a flat E–F slope indicative of pulmonary hypertension. LVPW = left ventricular posterior wall, PERIC. = pericardium and IVS = interventricular septum.

81

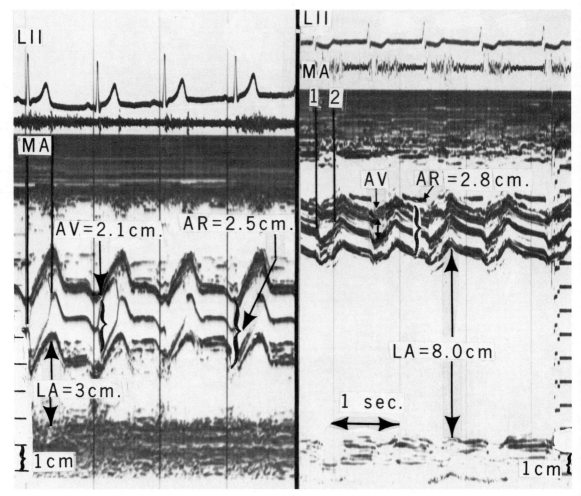

Figure 5.8. *Left*: Simultaneously recorded echocardiogram, mitral area (MA) phonocardiogram, and lead II (LII) of the electrocardiogram showing a normal left atrium (LA), aortic valve (AV), and aortic root (AR). *Right:* Simultaneously recorded echocardiogram, mitral area (MA) phonocardiogram, and lead II (LII) of the electrocardiogram. The left atrium as compared with the normal structure shown above is markedly enlarged at 8 cm. There are some heavy echoes originating from the aortic valve.

Practical Points

1. A good phonocardiogram can usually be obtained with the microphones placed at the apex area near the nipple, with the patient turned on the left side. Record the tracing with your filter turned to stetho to amplify low frequency vibrations. This will give you the best recording of diastolic murmurs present in this condition.

2. In attempting to record the diastolic murmur, do not set your amplification too high because this will introduce a number of low frequency artifacts. This is

particularly true if the patient has a hairy chest that has not been shaved in the area where the microphone is placed.

3. In order to identify the opening snap, have the patient lie on his left side with the microphone placed at the tricuspid area (third left intercostal space near the sternum) and record the phonocardiogram simultaneously with the apexcardiogram. The opening snap should coincide with, precede, or follow by a few milliseconds the O point of the apexcardiogram.

4. Frequently, patients with mitral stenosis have two components in the second heart sound, aortic and pulmonic, as well as a vibration representing the opening snap of the mitral valve. You may obtain a good recording of all three sounds by placing a microphone at the second or third intercostal space with the patient lying flat on his back. Set the bandpass filter on log and record the phonocardiogram simultaneously with the carotid pulse tracing. The aortic component precedes the dicrotic notch of the carotid pulse. The pulmonic component and opening snap of the mitral valve follow the dicrotic notch.

5. Record the jugular venous pulse tracing because many of these patients present with pulmonary hypertension and will have a prominent A wave in the neck if they are in sinus rhythm. In addition, they may present with tricuspid insufficiency, in which case large V waves are present.

6. The apexcardiogram you record may not originate in the left ventricle; it may be a right ventricular apexcardiogram. Many patients with mitral stenosis have right ventricular hypertrophy and/or enlargement, which causes the heart to rotate with the right ventricle becoming more prominent. Unfortunately, there is no way to differentiate whether it is a right or left ventricular apexcardiogram by the waveform, if the patient has right ventricular disease.

Points of Caution—Echocardiogram

1. Mitral valve motion in patients with other diseases may simulate the typical anterior mitral valve motion characteristic for mitral stenosis. Therefore, it is quite important to obtain a good recording of both the anterior and posterior leaflets of the mitral valve. Conditions that simulate abnormal anterior mitral valve motion include congestive heart failure and low cardiac output due to any condition. These patients may present with abnormal motion of the anterior leaflet, but the posterior leaflet will still have normal posterior motion and heavy echoes will not be present.

2. Most patients with mitral stenosis present with atrial fibrillation. Therefore, it is quite important to obtain a minimum of seven consecutive cardiac cycles in order for the physician to obtain a reliable mean measurement of the E–F slope. It may vary from beat to beat in patients with atrial fibrillation.

3. A good pulmonic valve recording is important, especially if the patient is in sinus rhythm. If there is a short P–R interval, the A dip cannot be accurately measured on the pulmonic valve. If the patient is in atrial fibrillation, the E–F slope is not reliable by itself for diagnosing pulmonary hypertension. Only the systolic portion is valuable if it shows systolic notching or premature closure.

4. A good aortic valve echo should be recorded to see if there is reduced flow across the valve. The left atrium should be clearly visualized beneath it.

MITRAL INSUFFICIENCY

Mitral insufficiency is commonly the result of rheumatic fever. Other etiological factors include congenital mitral insufficiency due to deformity of the mitral valve, prolapse of the mitral leaflets, mitral insufficiency due to papillary muscle dysfunction in patients with coronary artery disease, rupture of the chordae tendineae during acute myocardial infarction, or penetrating injury or trauma to the chest.

Heart Sounds and Murmurs

The first heart sound is usually diminished in mitral insufficiency. The second heart sound is normal. An early diastolic third heart sound, part of the phonocardiographic and auscultatory findings in this condition, is due to increased diastolic filling of the left ventricle (Fig. 5.9). A fourth heart sound, which follows the P wave of the electrocardiogram, is recorded in about 40% of patients with mitral insufficiency but it does not have any major clinical significance. The third heart

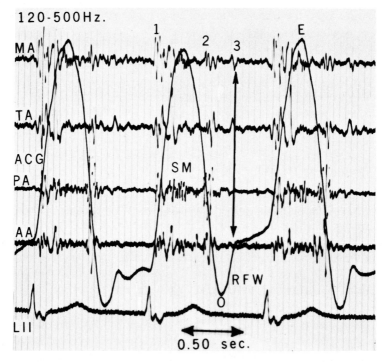

Figure 5.9. Simultaneously recorded phonocardiogram at the mitral (MA), tricuspid (TA), pulmonic (PA), and aortic areas (AA), apexcardiogram (ACG), and lead II (LII) of the electrocardiogram in a patient with mitral insufficiency. The first heart sound is slightly diminished. The second heart sound is normal. A prominent third heart sound coincides with the peak of the rapid filling wave (RFW) on the apexcardiogram. The high frequency, low amplitude systolic regurgitant murmur (SM) recorded in most precordial areas is due to mitral insufficiency. The apexcardiogram is abnormal. Due to left ventricular hypertrophy, the E point is very difficult to identify. The rapid filling wave is abnormally prominent, a feature we usually see in patients with significant mitral insufficiency.

sound coincides with the peak of the rapid filling wave (Fig. 5.9), and the fourth heart sound with the A wave of the apexcardiogram. An opening snap of the mitral valve is present in 8 to 12% of patients with pure mitral insufficiency (Fig. 5.10). The systolic murmur of mitral insufficiency has a high frequency characteristic and starts with or shortly after the first heart sound (Figs. 5.9, 5.10). The best way to recognize the beginning of the systolic murmur is by phonocardiographic recording at all precordial areas with high frequency filter settings. With logarithmic or log–log recordings, low frequency vibrations are eliminated and the beginning of the murmur may be easier to identify (Fig. 5.10). This murmur has a continuous plateau during systole and terminates with or shortly following the second heart sound. Amplitude of the murmur changes slightly during variations in cycle length in patients with atrial fibrillation or other cardiac arrhythmias (Fig. 5.11). This murmur can best be recorded when the patient is in the left lateral decubitus position (Fig. 5.12). In patients with severe mitral insufficiency, the increase in diastolic blood flow across the mitral valve may cause a soft, low amplitude mid-diastolic murmur that simulates the murmur of mitral stenosis.

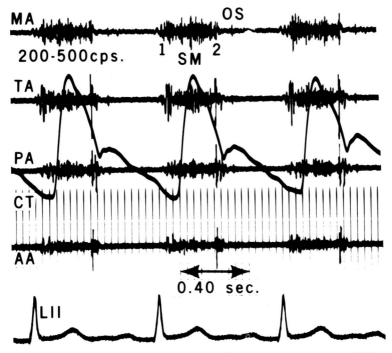

Figure 5.10. Simultaneously recorded phonocardiogram at the mitral (MA), tricuspid (TA), pulmonic (PA), and aortic areas (AA), carotid pulse tracing (CT), and lead II (LII) of the electrocardiogram in a 10-year-old patient with severe mitral insufficiency. The first heart sound is markedly diminished. The second heart sound is normal. There is an opening snap (OS), which is recorded in a small percentage of patients with mitral insufficiency without stenosis. The typical systolic regurgitant murmur (SM) of mitral insufficiency starts with the first heart sound, reaching a plateau in midsystole and terminating with the second heart sound. This murmur is well recorded at all precordial areas but is loudest at the mitral and tricuspid areas.

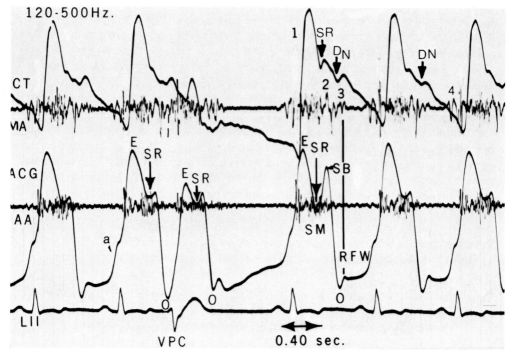

Figure 5.11. Simultaneously recorded phonocardiogram at the mitral (MA) and aortic areas (AA), carotid pulse tracing (CT), apexcardiogram (ACG), and lead II (LII) of the electrocardiogram in a 54-year-old patient with rheumatic mitral insufficiency. The first heart sound is diminished. The second heart sound is normal. There is a faint third heart sound with the regular sinus beat and this sound becomes prominent following the premature ventricular contraction. The carotid pulse tracing is abnormal. It shows a systolic retraction (SR), followed by a late systolic wave. The apexcardiogram shows a slightly prominent A wave and a midsystolic retraction, which coincides with the same event on the carotid tracing. This is usually seen in patients with mitral insufficiency and disease of the left ventricle. The ventricular premature contraction (third beat) is followed by a long pause. The beat following the premature ventricular contraction shows marked exaggeration of the late systolic bulge (SB), which follows the systolic retraction. This illustrates the importance of keeping tracings of cardiac arrhythmias for the interpreter because clinical information can be obtained from the pre- and postarrhythmia recordings. The rapid filling wave of the apexcardiogram is slightly accentuated. DN = dicrotic notch; RFW = rapid filling wave.

Carotid Pulse Tracing

The carotid pulse has little diagnostic value in mild mitral insufficiency. In patients with severe mitral insufficiency, the carotid tracing may show a rapid ascending limb, systolic retraction, diminished ejection time, a normal dicrotic notch, and a dicrotic wave (Figs. 5.11, 5.13).

Jugular Venous Pulse Tracing

The jugular venous pulse is usually normal in patients with mitral insufficiency. When there is a significant degree of pulmonary hypertension, exaggeration of the A wave may be noted.

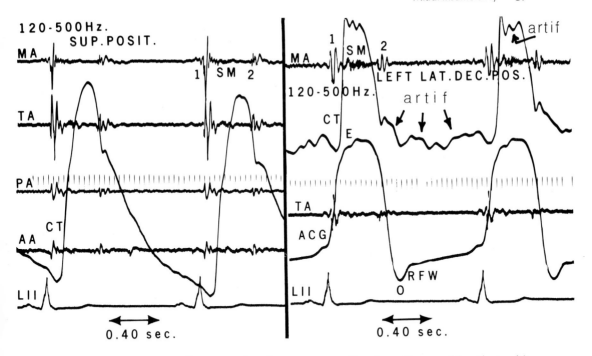

Figure 5.12. Phonocardiogram and pulse wave recording in a 61-year-old patient with rheumatic mitral insufficiency. *Left Panel*: Simultaneously recorded phonocardiogram at the mitral (MA), tricuspid (TA), pulmonic (PA), and aortic areas (AA), carotid pulse tracing (CT), and lead II (LII) of the electrocardiogram. The tracings were recorded with the patient in the supine position. The systolic murmur has very low amplitude as displayed at the mitral area. The carotid pulse tracing is normal. *Right Panel*: Simultaneously recorded phonocardiogram at the mitral and tricuspid areas, carotid pulse tracing, apexcardiogram (ACG), and lead II of the electrocardiogram on the same patient in the left lateral decubitus position. The systolic murmur is much more conspicuous because when the patient is turned to the left side the heart moves closer to the chest wall. No other abnormalities are seen on the phonocardiogram. The contour of the carotid pulse is quite different from the one in the left panel, particularly during diastole due to technical artifacts, because the transducer was not held steadily against the carotid artery. There are also some artifactual waveforms during the systolic component of the carotid pulse tracing. The apexcardiogram shows an abnormal round, systolic wave. The E point of the apexcardiogram is hard to identify because the patient has left ventricular hypertrophy.

Apexcardiogram

The apexcardiogram is abnormal, showing increased amplitude of the rapid filling wave, which reflects increased left ventricular diastolic filling (Figs. 5.9, 5.11, 5.13). The A wave may be prominent in patients with sinus rhythm. Abnormalities of the systolic wave include an early or midsystolic retraction followed by a systolic bulge or sustained and round systolic wave. They reflect abnormal left ventricular contraction or increased left ventricular wall thickness. Systolic wave abnormalities can be exaggerated if they follow an atrial or ventricular extrasystole (Fig. 5.11).

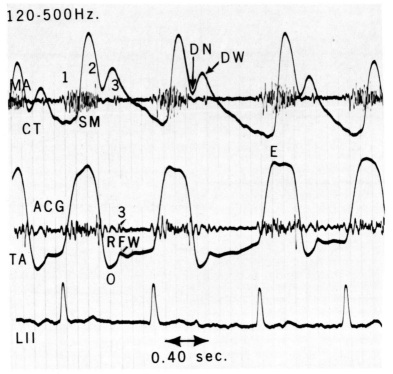

Figure 5.13. Simultaneously recorded phonocardiogram at the mitral (MA) and tricuspid areas (TA), carotid pulse tracing (CT), apexcardiogram (ACG), and lead II of the electrocardiogram in a 55-year-old patient with mitral insufficiency. The high frequency, high amplitude systolic regurgitant murmur recorded in both precordial areas is most prominent at the mitral area. This murmur starts with the first heart sound and terminates with the second heart sound. There is also a third heart sound. The carotid pulse is abnormal, showing a short ejection time and a prominent dicrotic wave (DW). This type of record is not infrequent in patients with mitral insufficiency and low cardiac output. The apexcardiogram is abnormal, showing a round systolic wave. The E point is difficult to identify due to the presence of left ventricular hypertrophy. This is part of the clinical picture of patients with mitral insufficiency. The third heart sound coincides with the peak of the rapid filling wave (RFW).

Arrhythmias, Maneuvers, and Pharmacologic Agents

Arrhythmias resulting in variations in cycle length can cause significant changes in the characteristics of heart sounds and murmurs, as shown in Figure 5.11. Squatting causes increased amplitude of the systolic murmur in patients with rheumatic mitral insufficiency. Inhalation of vasodilators (drugs such as amyl nitrite that increase blood vessel size and decrease blood pressure) cause a decrease in amplitude and shortening of the systolic murmur (Fig. 5.14). Vasopressors (drugs such as levarterenol administered intravenously that decrease blood vessel size and increase blood pressure) cause an increase in amplitude of the systolic murmur.

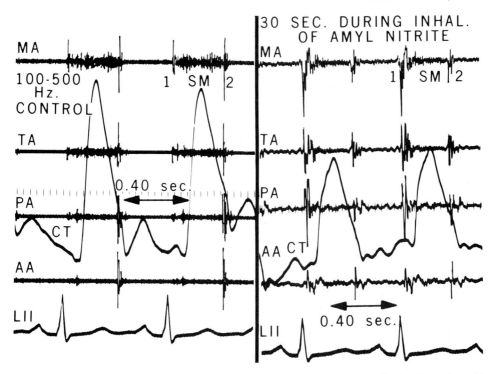

Figure 5.14. *Left*: Simultaneously recorded phonocardiogram at the mitral (MA), tricuspid (TA), pulmonic (PA), and aortic areas (AA), carotid pulse tracing (CT), and lead II (LII) of the electrocardiogram in a 19-year-old patient with a mild degree of mitral insufficiency. On the phonocardiogram, particularly at the mitral area, the first heart sound has lower amplitude than the second heart sound. The second heart sound is single and normal. A systolic murmur (SM) starts with the first heart sound, has a plateau characteristic, and terminates with the second heart sound. No extra sounds are recorded. *Right*: These tracings were recorded for 30 seconds during inhalation of amyl nitrite, a vasodilator, which decreases blood pressure and the pressure in the left ventricle, thus allowing less leakage of the mitral valve to occur. Therefore, amplitude of the systolic murmur decreases. The contour of the carotid pulse tracing is normal.

Vectorcardiogram

In patients with mitral insufficiency that is clinically significant, the left atrium and/or left ventricle are usually enlarged. Enlargement or hypertrophy of this chamber causes an increase in the QRS forces that are located posteriorly and to the left in the horizontal plane, and an increase in the magnitude of the P loop (Fig. 5.15).

Echocardiogram

Mitral insufficiency secondary to rheumatic heart disease is difficult to diagnose with the echocardiogram. Separation of the mitral leaflets during systole is technically difficult to record; therefore, the technique is of little diagnostic value. However, the mitral valve opening may be increased over 35 mm from the E point

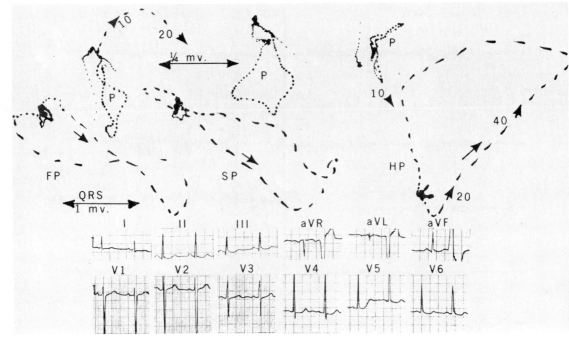

Figure 5.15. Vectorcardiogram and electrocardiogram of a 54-year-old patient with mitral insufficiency. Note an increase in voltage of the QRS forces in the frontal (FP), sagittal (SP), and particularly the horizontal (HP) plane. In the horizontal plane, most forces are located posteriorly and to the left of the O point. Analysis of the P loop shows signs of both right and left atrial hypertrophy. Observe a significant number of forces located anterior to the E point, and significant posterior and leftward forces representing left atrial hypertrophy. The electrocardiogram, recorded at one half standard, shows signs of left ventricular hypertrophy because of the tall R waves in V5, V6, and deep S waves in V1 and V2. The rhythm is sinus. Ventricular extrasystoles were recorded in leads aVR, aVL, and aVF. There are some minor abnormalities of the T waves and ST segments. The electrocardiogram does not show signs of right or left atrial hypertrophy, indicating superiority of the vectorcardiogram for diagnosis of atrial hypertrophy.

of the posterior leaflet to the E point of the anterior leaflet. Indirect signs of significant mitral insufficiency, when suspected clinically, include the presence of a large left atrium and left ventricle with hyperdynamic left ventricular wall motion (Figs. 5.16, 5.17). In addition, if pulmonary hypertension is present, an enlarged right ventricle and abnormal pulmonary valve motion during systole and diastole are seen.

Practical Points—Phonocardiogram

1. You may obtain a good recording of the systolic murmur with your bandpass filter set at log or log–log. This should allow a good recording of the systolic murmur but may introduce considerable noise interference on the tracing. Therefore, compromise the amplitude of the murmur by turning your amplitude

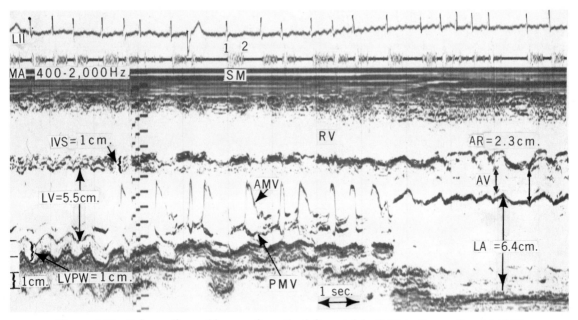

Figure 5.16. Echocardiographic scan from the left ventricle (LV) to the aortic root (AR) recorded simultaneously with a mitral area (MA) phonocardiogram and lead II (LII) of the electrocardiogram in a 62-year-old patient with rheumatic mitral insufficiency. The rhythm is atrial fibrillation. Thickness of the interventricular septum (IVS) and left ventricular posterior wall (LVPW) is normal. The left ventricular cavity measures 5.5 cm, which is at the upper limits of normal. In the midportion of the tracing a good recording of the mitral valve is shown. The anterior (AMV) and posterior (PMV) leaflets have normal motion. Variation in the configuration of the leaflets is due to the difference in cycle length, i.e., the R–R interval on the electrocardiogram varies from beat to beat due to atrial fibrillation. As the transducer is moved superiorly the aortic valve (AV), left atrium (LA) and aortic root are well seen. The aortic root and valve measurements are normal. The left atrium is enlarged to 6.4 cm. Normally, left atrial size is almost identical to aortic root size. While enlargement of the left atrium is one of the important echocardiographic features of rheumatic mitral insufficiency, some patients may present with normal left atrial size. In these patients the echocardiogram is not diagnostic, despite the fact that they may have a significant degree of mitral insufficiency.

knob slowly until the murmur shows up on the oscilloscope at an amplitude of approximately 2 cm (2cm = ¾ inch). Turn the patient to a left lateral position with the microphone placed near the apex at the area just below the nipple or apex area. Many of these patients have a moderate to markedly enlarged left ventricle and this chamber is displaced to the left and toward the back. In this situation, try to place the microphone near the area where you can palpate the apex beat.

2. Patients with mitral insufficiency usually have a prominent third heart sound. To document the presence of this sound, try to record a phonocardiogram simultaneously with an apexcardiogram with the patient on his left side. If the

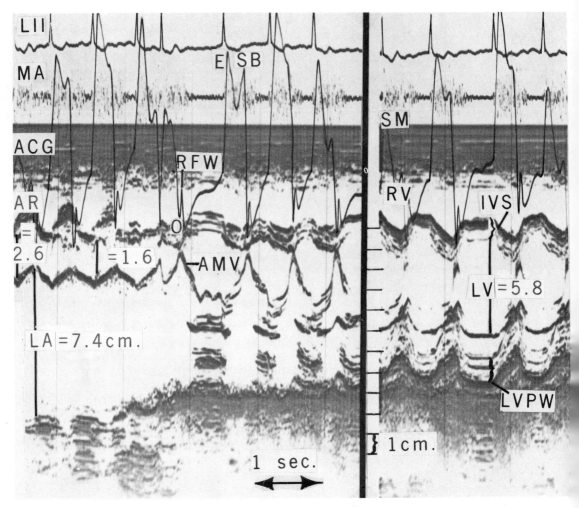

Figure 5.17. Simultaneously recorded echocardiogram, lead II (LII) of the electrocardiogram, mitral area (MA) phonocardiogram, and apexcardiogram (ACG) in a 43-year-old patient with mitral insufficiency. *Left*: This is a scan from the aorta toward the mitral valve. The aortic root (AR) and aortic valve (AV) have normal measurements. However, the left atrium (LA) is markedly enlarged, 7.4 cm. *Right*: The left ventricle is slightly enlarged, 5.8 cm. Note the presence of a systolic regurgitant murmur (SM) on the phonocardiogram.

patient has a third heart sound, it coincides with the peak of the rapid filling wave of the apexcardiogram. Set your filter on stetho so that the third heart sound will be magnified.

Points of Caution

1. When recording the apexcardiogram in patients with mitral insufficiency, *do not apply too much pressure* on the transducer over the apex. If you do so, it may create an artifactual systolic wave. Usually, these patients have a round

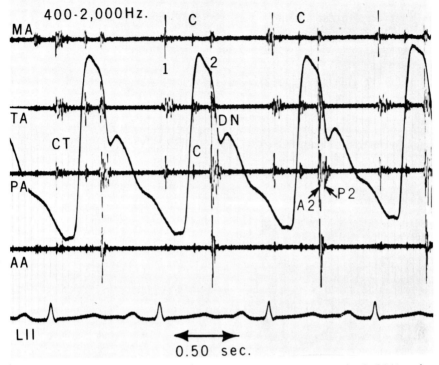

Figure 5.18. Simultaneously recorded phonocardiogram at the mitral (MA), tricuspid (TA), pulmonic (PA), and aortic areas (AA), carotid pulse tracing (CT) and lead II (LII) of the electrocardiogram in a 43-year-old patient with mitral valve prolapse. The first heart sound is normal. The second heart sound is split and both components are normal. Note the presence of a mid-to-late systolic click (C) followed by a few high frequency vibrations representing a late systolic murmur. This is a typical finding in patients with mitral valve prolapse. The carotid pulse tracing is normal.

and sustained wave throughout systole due to the presence of an enlarged or hypertrophic left ventricle. *If you apply too much pressure,* you may eliminate this important diagnostic information and the systolic wave might be considerably diminished. Hold the transducer gently with the right hand with the patient lying on his left side.

2. On the echocardiogram be sure to obtain a good recording of the aortic root, left atrium, and left ventricle for accurate determination of the left atrial size and left ventricular internal diameter. Motion of the left atrial wall is usually exaggerated in patients with mitral insufficiency.

PROLAPSE OF THE MITRAL VALVE

Prolapse of the mitral valve is a syndrome that has been recognized with increasing frequency for the past few years. It is clinically manifested by the presence of a mid-to-late systolic click followed by a late systolic murmur (Barlow syndrome). In this condition, there is redundancy of the tissue of the mitral leaflets with elongation of the chordae. Therefore, when the left ventricle contracts during systole the valve prolapses back into the left atrium simulating what is called "parachuting" mitral valve. Several patients present with a significant degree of mitral insufficiency, which is manifested on the phonocardiogram by the late systolic murmur.

Heart Sounds and Murmurs

The first and second heart sounds have normal characteristics. If mitral insufficiency is severe, the second heart sound is split due to early closure of the aortic

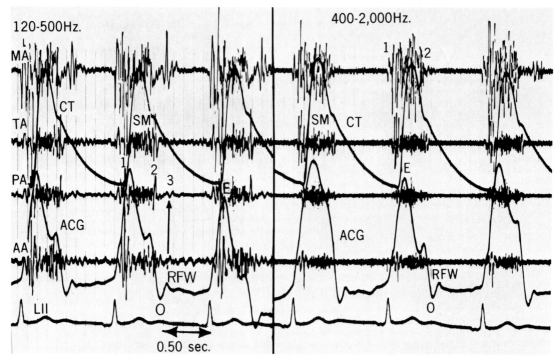

Figure 5.19. Simultaneously recorded phonocardiogram at the mitral (MA), tricuspid (TA), pulmonic (PA), and aortic areas (AA), carotid pulse tracing (CT), apexcardiogram (ACG), and lead II (LII) of the electrocardiogram in a 61-year-old patient with severe prolapse of the mitral valve. The tracings were recorded at bandpass filter settings of 120–500 Hz. (*left*) and 400–2,000 Hz. (*right*). *Left*: There is a slight decrease in amplitude of the first (1) heart sound. The second (2) heart sound is sharp, and normal. A third (3) heart sound occurs approximately 0.14 sec after the second heart sound. A high frequency, high amplitude systolic regurgitant murmur (SM) occupies most of systole. The usual midsystolic click seen in this condition is not well recognized, probably because the degree of mitral insufficiency was so severe that the ejection click moved toward the first heart sound. There is a high frequency, high amplitude systolic regurgitant murmur recorded in all precordial areas. The contour of the carotid pulse tracing is normal. The apexcardiogram shows a sharp E point followed by a downward deflection and a small systolic retraction. There is also a short, conspicuous rapid filling wave (RFW) and its peak coincides with the third heart sound. *Right*: The effect of filtering on the systolic murmur and third heart sound is shown. At this setting the systolic murmur becomes clearly identifiable although the amplitude is lower as compared with the left panel. The third heart sound is absent because of the filter setting.

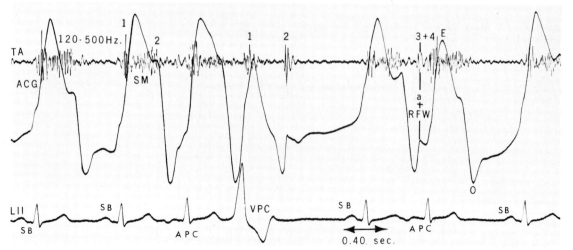

Figure 5.20. Simultaneously recorded tricuspid area (TA) phonocardiogram, apexcardiogram (ACG), and lead II (LII) of the electrocardiogram in a 58-year-old patient with mitral valve prolapse and mitral insufficiency. During this recording, the patient was having atrial (APC) and ventricular premature contractions (VPC). The first and second heart sounds are normal. A high frequency, high amplitude systolic regurgitant murmur (SM) starts with the first heart sound and terminates with the second heart sound. It is due to mitral insufficiency. During atrial premature contractions, the systolic murmur is less prominent. This is followed by a ventricular premature contraction with a long compensatory pause. Following the pause, the sinus beat shows slightly diminished amplitude of the systolic murmur, which is common in patients with mitral insufficiency. There are also third and fourth heart sounds that fuse together and correspond to the peak of the A and rapid filling waves of the apexcardiogram.

valve. Single or multiple early, mid-, or late systolic clicks (high frequency sounds) are the characteristic findings (Fig. 5.18). In general, location of the click during systole is related to the severity of mitral insufficiency. The greater the degree of insufficiency, the earlier the onset of the click. The presence of multiple systolic clicks has no relationship to the degree of mitral insufficiency. Third heart sounds may be present if mitral insufficiency is hemodynamically important (Fig. 5.19).

The murmur of prolapse of the mitral valve characteristically starts in midsystole following the click. There is a progressive increase in amplitude in late systole and it terminates with the second heart sound. It is a high frequency murmur, musical at times, with varying intensity. If the posterior leaflet is involved, the murmur transmits anteriorly toward the sternum. As the degree of mitral insufficiency increases, the murmur and click move toward the first heart sound. In some patients, the systolic click may be inscribed during midsystole, and at times it is preceded by a short systolic murmur. Diastolic murmurs are not present in this condition unless mitral insufficiency is very severe. In this case, a third heart sound is present, followed by a low frequency, mid-diastolic murmur due to increased diastolic blood flow across the mitral valve.

Maneuvers and Pharmacologic Agents

Maneuvers such as Valsalva, squatting, exercise, and the use of vasodilators such as amyl nitrite, or vasopressors increase the degree of mitral insufficiency resulting in early onset of the click–murmur.

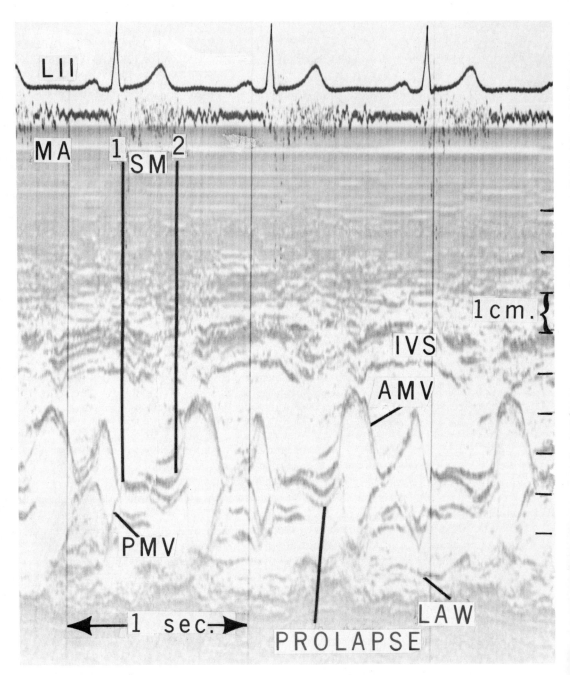

Figure 5.21. Simultaneously recorded echocardiogram with lead II (LII) of the electrocardiogram and mitral area (MA) phonocardiogram in a 48-year-old patient with prolapse of the mitral valve. Note that the anterior (AMV) and posterior (PMV) leaflets of the mitral valve are prolapsed during systole between the first and second heart sound. There is also a very prominent systolic regurgitant murmur (SM) recorded at the mitral area. IVS = interventricular septum and LAW = left atrial wall.

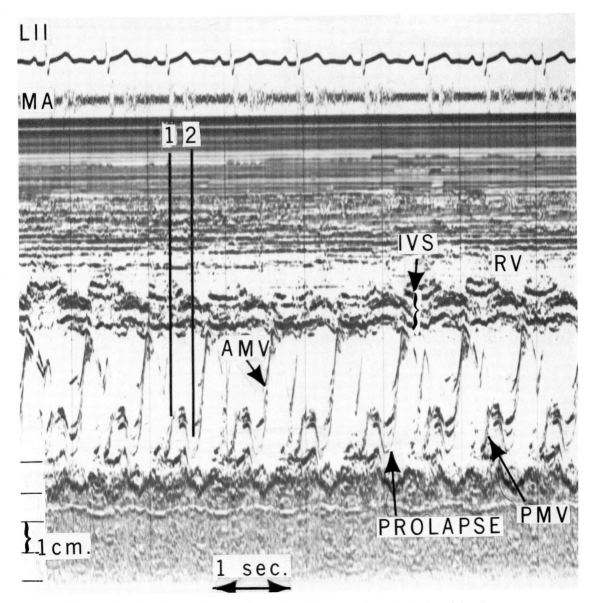

Figure 5.22. Simultaneously recorded echocardiogram with lead II (LII) of the electrocardiogram and mitral area (MA) phonocardiogram in a 23-year-old patient with marked prolapse of the anterior (AMV) and posterior (PMV) leaflets of the mitral valve. IVS = interventricular septum and RV = right ventricle.

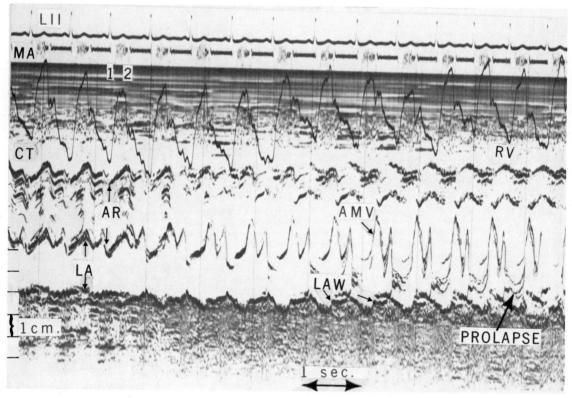

Figure 5.23. Echocardiographic scan from the aortic root (AR) to the mitral valve in a 43-year-old patient with aortic valvular stenosis and mitral valve prolapse recorded simultaneously with the carotid pulse tracing (CT), mitral area (MA) phonocardiogram, and lead II (LII) of the electrocardiogram. The aortic root measures 3.3 cm and the left atrium (LA) measures 2.4 cm. Note heavy and disorganized echoes within the walls of the aorta and aortic valve on the left side. In many patients with significant aortic valvular stenosis, the presence of heavy calcification of the valve makes identification of the aortic cusp quite difficult. As the transducer is moved inferiorly toward the left ventricular cavity, the mitral valve is well seen. The anterior mitral valve (AMV) has normal motion in diastole. However, in systole the valve moves posteriorly toward the left atrial posterior wall, which is indicative of prolapse. In the middle section of the recording, left atrial wall motion is seen. This is characterized by anterior movement during diastole and posterior motion during systole.

Carotid Pulse Tracing

The carotid pulse tracing can be useful in the evaluation of patients with prolapse of the mitral valve. The tracing shows a rapid ascending limb and systolic retraction followed by a late systolic bulge. The tracings sometimes simulate those seen in idiopathic hypertrophic subaortic stenosis and other hyperdynamic circulatory disease states.

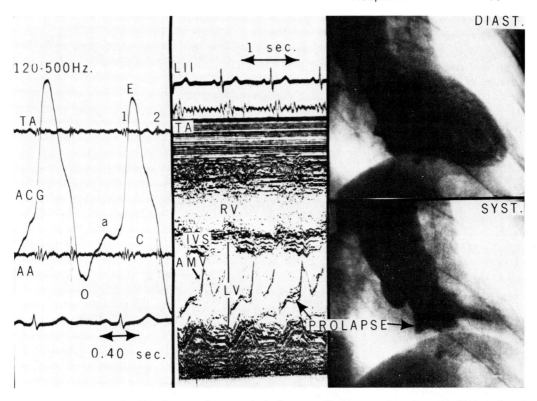

Figure 5.24. *Left*: Simultaneously recorded phonocardiogram at the tricuspid (TA) and aortic areas (AA), apexcardiogram (ACG), and lead II (LII) of the electrocardiogram in a 50-year-old patient with mitral valve prolapse. The first and second heart sounds are normal. There is a very low amplitude click (C) in the first part of systole. The apexcardiogram is normal. *Middle:* Simultaneously recorded echocardiogram with lead II (LII) of the electrocardiogram and tricuspid area (TA) phonocardiogram in the same patient showing mitral valve prolapse during systole. *Right:* Left ventricular angiogram with contrast agent injected into the left ventricle with the patient in a right anterior oblique projection. The top view is during diastole and the bottom view is during systole. Note the areas where the mitral valve prolapse is seen.

Jugular Venous Tracing

The jugular venous tracing has no diagnostic value in this disease state.

Apexcardiogram

The apexcardiogram shows a sharp E point and abnormal systolic retraction, which coincides with onset of the midsystolic click. A late systolic rise inscribed at the time of the late crescendo systolic murmur follows the click. These changes reflect abnormal left ventricular contraction and sometimes are more apparent following extrasystoles (Fig. 5.20). The rapid filling wave is exaggerated only if mitral regurgitant flow is physiologically important.

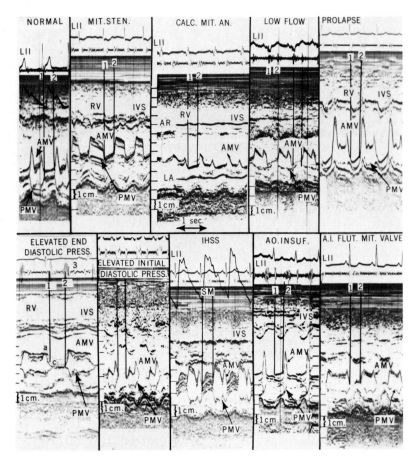

Figure 5.25. This illustration shows a normal echocardiogram and several abnormalities involving the mitral valve. The normal mitral valve recording (*upper left*) shows a brisk upward ascent in early diastole to the maximal anterior peak called the E point, followed by a rapid descent in mid-diastole where the valve remains in a semiclosed position called the F point. The valve then moves anteriorly again with the P wave of the electrocardiogram. This is known as the A point. After the A point, the valve moves posteriorly to the C or closure point. Observe normal motion of the posterior leaflet (PMV). During diastole, it moves in the opposite direction of the anterior leaflet (AMV), i.e., posteriorly. The motion of the posterior leaflet has somewhat identical characteristics to the anterior leaflet except that it has slightly reduced motion. During systole, both leaflets remain together and move parallel to each other, remaining horizontal or drifting slightly anterior to the D or opening point of the next cycle. *Mitral Stenosis*: The typical abnormalities are shown. The flat motion results in reduced excursion of the anterior leaflet (AMV) with heavy echoes suggesting fibrosis or calcification of the valve. In addition, the posterior mitral valve (PMV) has abnormal anterior motion, which is one of the important echocardiographic features of mitral stenosis. The time of inscription of the first (1) and second (2) heart sounds is illustrated. *Calcified Mitral Annulus*: On this echocardiogram, you can identify the anterior leaflet of the mitral valve (AMV), which has normal motion. However, heavy echoes are located behind the posterior leaflet indicating the presence of a calcified mitral annulus. This was documented by cinefluoroscopy and cardiac catheterization. *Low Flow*: This tracing illustrates the echocardiographic features in patients with heart failure from any cause who have reduced flow across the mitral valve. Note the reduced excursion of

100

Systolic Time Intervals

Ejection time is normal or shortened slightly.

Vectorcardiogram

In patients with prolapsed mitral valves, the vectorcardiogram is of no value in establishing the diagnosis unless the patient has a severe degree of mitral insufficiency, and this is a rare situation.

Echocardiogram

The echocardiogram is a very valuable noninvasive technique in the diagnosis of prolapse of the mitral valve leaflets. Several patterns on the echocardiogram have been described by investigators. They all reflect abnormal mitral valve motion and show late or holosystolic posterior motion of 2 mm or more in systole of one or both leaflets. Increased mitral valve opening may be seen in both the anterior and posterior leaflets. Various types of abnormalities seen on echocardiograms in this condition are shown in Figures 5.21 through 5.25.

Practical Points

1. Careful examination of the mitral valve with the transducer perpendicular to the chest is necessary. If the transducer is placed too high, for example, at the

---

the anterior leaflet (AMV) as compared with the normal valve. The posterior leaflet (PMV) moves normally, i.e., posteriorly with reduced excursion. *Prolapse*: The anterior (AMV) and posterior (PMV) mitral leaflets move normally during diastole with the exception of an increased E–F slope. However, during systole note the backward posterior motion of the leaflets. This is a characteristic finding in patients with prolapse of the mitral valve. *Elevated End-Diastolic Pressure*: The opening of the mitral valve in patients with elevated left ventricular end-diastolic pressure is normal. The closing of the valve is prolonged, which is reflected by a prolonged A–C interval. When the A–C interval is subtracted from the P–R interval of the electrocardiogram, it should be greater than 0.06 sec. In this case, it is shorter due to the elevated pressure. *Elevated Initial Left Ventricular Diastolic Pressure*: In this recording of the mitral valve in a patient with increased initial diastolic pressure, the A wave exceeds the E point as seen on the anterior leaflet (AMV) of the valve. *Idiopathic Hypertrophic Subaortic Stenosis*: Patients with this pathological condition exhibit abnormal motion of the mitral valve. Observe that in early diastole the E point is inscribed quite close to the interventricular septum. In addition, during systole, note a marked anterior displacement of the mitral leaflets as they move toward the interventricular septum, almost obliterating the left ventricular cavity, known as systolic anterior motion (SAM) of the mitral valve. *Aortic Insufficiency*: Patients with severe aortic insufficiency may show premature closure of the mitral valve with a brisk opening to the E point and then a fast descent to the F point. The mid-to-end diastolic portion of the mitral valve is almost closed. *Aortic Insufficiency With Fluttering of the Mitral Valve*: Patients with aortic insufficiency may exhibit what is called "flutter" of the mitral valve. This is manifested by high frequency vibrations of the valve during diastole, particularly well seen at the anterior mitral valve (AMV). AR = aortic root; RV = right ventricle; IVS = interventricular septum.

second intercostal space, and if the transducer is aiming inferior to record the mitral leaflets, a false positive prolapse may result. This is due to the annulus moving anteriorly in diastole and posteriorly in systole.

2. Ideally, both leaflets of the mitral valve should be recorded simultaneously with a clear closing point (C point) and a clear opening point (D point). The transducer needs to be placed high enough on the chest so that the mitral valve is not buried in the left atrial or ventricular walls. Most prolapses are recorded best with the left atrial wall beneath the mitral valve.

3. Very careful examination of the mitral valve is necessary because often the maximum prolapsing echo is faint and can be missed frequently.

4. If a prolapse is suspected and there is a systolic click and murmur and the mitral valve appears normal, the tricuspid valve should be studied for prolapse, or provocative maneuvers should be used.

5. The tricuspid valve should routinely be examined for prolapse in the presence of mitral prolapse because a great number of patients have prolapse of both valves.

6. Prolapse in the presence of a significant pericardial effusion is probably due to the pericardial effusion itself and abnormal cardiac motion.

BIBLIOGRAPHY

Aronow, W.S., Kaplan, M.A., and Ellestad, M.:   Prediction of left ventricular contractility in mitral valve disease by EICT and LVET/EICT measurements (abstract). Clin. Res., *17*:226, 1969.

Aykent, Y., Thurmann, M., and Bussmann, B.W.:   Continuous murmur in mitral stenosis. Am. J. Cardiol., *15*:715, 1965.

Barlow, J.B., and Bosman, C.K.:   Aneurysmal protrusion of the posterior leaflet of the mitral valve. An auscultatory–electrocardiographic syndrome. Am. Heart J., *71*:166, 1966.

Benchimol, A., Dimond, E.G., Waxman, D., and Shen, Y.:   Diastolic movement of the precordium in mitral stenosis and regurgitation. Am. Heart J., *60*:417, 1960.

Benchimol, A., Harris, C.L., and Desser, K.B.:   Midsystolic carotid pulse wave retraction in subjects with prolapsed mitral valve leaflets. Chest, *62*:614, 1972.

Bridgen, W., and Leatham, A.:   Mitral insufficiency. Br. Heart J., *15*:55, 1953.

Craige, E.:   Phonocardiographic studies in mitral stenosis. N. Engl. J. Med., *257*:650, 1957.

DeMaria, A.N., King, V.F., Bogren, H.G., Lies, J.E., and Mason, D.T.:   The variable spectrum of echocardiographic manifestations of the mitral valve prolapse syndrome. Circulation, *50*:33, 1974.

Dock, W.:   Production mode of systolic clicks due to mitral cusp prolapse. Arch. Intern. Med., *132*:118, 1972.

Edler, I.:   Ultrasound cardiogram in mitral valve disease. Acta Chir. Scand., *111*:230, 1956.

Edler, I., and Gustafson, A.:   Ultrasonic cardiogram in mitral stenosis. Acta Med. Scand., *159*:85, 1957.

Effert, S.:   Pre- and postoperative evaluation of mitral stenosis by ultrasound. Am. J. Cardiol., *19*:59, 1967.

Fleming, H.A., and Wood, P.:   The myocardial factor in mitral valve disease. Br. Heart J., *21*:117, 1959.

Friedman, N.J.:   Echocardiographic studies of mitral valve motion: Genesis of opening snap in mitral stenosis. Am. Heart J., *80*:177, 1970.

Gustafson, A.:   Correlation between ultrasoundcardiography, hemodynamics and surgical findings in mitral stenosis. Am. J. Cardiol., *19*:32, 1967.

Hancock, E.W., and Cohn, K.:   The syndrome associated with midsystolic click and late systolic murmur. Am. J. Med., *41*:183, 1966.

Hultgren, H.N., and Leo, T.F.:   The tricuspid component of the first heart sound in mitral stenosis. Circulation, *18*:1012, 1958.

Joyner, C.R., Dyrda, I., Barrett, J.S., and Reid, J.M.:   Preoperative determination of the functional anatomy of the mitral valve. Circulation, *32*:110, 1965.

Kelly, J.J., Jr.:   Diagnostic value of phonocardiography in mitral stenosis. Am. J. Med., *19*:862, 1955.

Leo, T., and Hultgren, H.:   Phonocardiographic characteristics of tight mitral stenosis. Medicine, *38*:85, 1959.

Mercer, J.L.:   Presystolic murmur in mitral stenosis. Lancet, *2*:765, 1972.

Mounsey, P., Bridgen, W.:   The apical systolic murmur in mitral stenosis. Br. Heart J., *16*:255, 1954.

Nixon, P.G.F., and Wooler, G.H.:   Phases of diastole in various syndromes of mitral valvular disease. Br. Heart J., *25*:393, 1963.

Nixon, P.G.F., Wooler, G.H., and Radigan, L.R.:   The opening snap in mitral incompetence. Br. Heart J., *22*:395, 1960.

Oreshkov, V.I.:   Isovolumic contraction time and isovolumic contraction time index in mitral stenosis. Study on basis of polygraphic tracing (apex cardiogram, phonocardiogram, and carotid tracing). Br. Heart J., *34*:533, 1972.

Popp, R.L.:   Echocardiographic abnormalities in the mitral valve prolapse syndrome. Circulation, *49*:428, 1974.

Proctor, M. H., Walker, R.C., Hancock, E.W., and Abelmann, W.H.:   The phonocardiogram in mitral valvular disease. Am. J. Med., *24*:861, 1958.

Sasse, L.:   Echocardiography of mitral valve prolapse. Circulation, *49*:595, 1974.

Segal, B.L., Likoff, W., and Kingsley, B.:   Echocardiography: clinical application in mitral stenosis. J.A.M.A., *193*:161, 1956.

Weissler, A.M., Leonard, J.J., and Warren, J.V.:   Observations in delayed first heart sound in mitral stenosis and hypertension. Circulation, *18*:165, 1958.

Wells, B.G.:   The assessment of mitral stenosis by phonocardiography. Br. Heart J., *16*:261, 1954.

Wharton, C.F.P., Bescos, L.L.:   Mitral valve movement: a study using an ultrasound technique. Br. Heart J., *16*:261, 1954.

Wood, P.:   An appreciation of mitral stenosis. Br. Med. J., *1*:1051, 1954.

6

Aortic
Valvular Disease

Aortic valvular disease is most frequently due to rheumatic heart disease or calcification of the aortic valve in older subjects with diffuse atherosclerosis. It can also result from a congenital deformity wherein the aortic valve may have two cusps (bicuspid aortic valve) instead of three and tends to calcify later in life and become stenotic. Aortic valve disease is also seen with Paget's disease, Marfan's syndrome, rheumatoid arthritis, and other diseases of the connective tissue. In this chapter, noninvasive diagnosis of aortic valvular disease, idiopathic hypertrophic subaortic stenosis, subvalvular and supravalvular diseases will be discussed.

AORTIC VALVULAR STENOSIS

Heart Sounds and Murmurs

The first heart sound has normal amplitude in patients with aortic valvular disease (Figs. 6.1 and 6.2). The second heart sound may be normal in mild forms of aortic stenosis (Fig. 6.2). With moderate to severe disease, there is decreased mobility of the aortic cusps. They become fused and calcified, resulting in impairment of valve motion. Therefore, the aortic component of the second heart sound decreases in amplitude (Figs. 6.1 and 6.3). In very severe aortic valvular stenosis, the second heart sound may show paradoxical or reverse splitting (Fig. 6.3), i.e., the pulmonic component will precede the aortic component. Normally, the aortic component of the second heart sound precedes the pulmonic component.

Phonocardiographic recordings should be obtained during expiration and inspiration simultaneously with the carotid pulse tracing. If reverse splitting is present, the A2–P2 interval shortens during inspiration or it becomes single (reverse of normal). If the second heart sound is single, both components of the second heart sound will precede the dicrotic notch of the carotid pulse tracing (Fig. 6.3). A systolic ejection click, common in young patients with valvular or subvalvular aortic stenosis (Fig. 6.2), may be the result of the rapid impact of high velocity blood flow from the left ventricle into a dilated aorta. A third heart sound recorded on the phonocardiogram of young patients with congenital aortic valvular stenosis has no diagnostic value unless it is associated with other signs of congestive heart

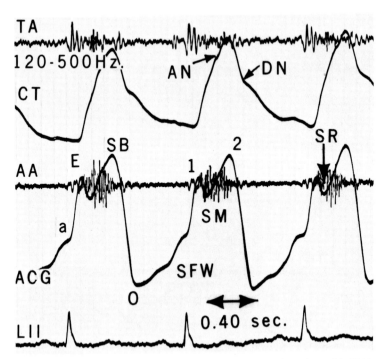

Figure 6.1. Simultaneously recorded phonocardiogram at the tricuspid (TA) and aortic areas (AA), carotid pulse tracing (CT), apexcardiogram (ACG), and lead II (LII) of the electrocardiogram in a 62-year-old patient with aortic valvular stenosis. The first heart sound is normal. The second heart sound is diminished due to calcification of the aortic valve, which makes it immobile. There is a high frequency, high amplitude systolic ejection murmur (SM) recorded best at the aortic area, with a midsystolic peak. There are no diastolic murmurs. The undulation of the baseline at the tricuspid area represents a low frequency artifact. The abnormal carotid pulse tracing shows a very slow ascending limb and a high placed anacrotic notch (AN). The dicrotic notch (DN), marking closure of the aortic valve, is very conspicuous. Ejection time is prolonged. The apexcardiogram is abnormal. There is a large A wave, and a normal E point followed by a systolic retraction (SR) and a late systolic bulge (SB). This type of apexcardiogram is seen in patients with disease of the left ventricular myocardium.

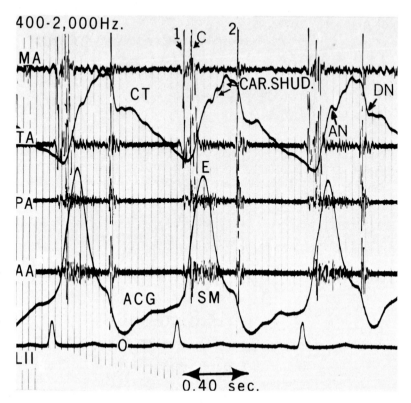

Figure 6.2. Simultaneously recorded phonocardiogram at the mitral (MA), tricuspid (TA), pulmonic (PA), and aortic areas (AA), carotid pulse tracing (CT), apexcardiogram (ACG), and lead II (LII) of the electrocardiogram in a 17-year-old patient with aortic valvular stenosis. The normal first heart sound is followed by a sharp, high frequency vibration, which is a systolic ejection click (C). The single second heart sound has normal amplitude. No diastolic murmurs are present. The carotid pulse tracing is typical for a patient with aortic valvular stenosis. There is a slow rise in the ascending limb and a high placed anacrotic notch (AN). The systolic ejection click occurs during the ascending limb. Following the anacrotic notch there is a high frequency vibration representing carotid shudder (CAR. SHUD.). After the second heart sound the dicrotic notch (DN) is seen, but it is not well defined due to decreased mobility of the aortic valve. The apexcardiogram is normal.

106

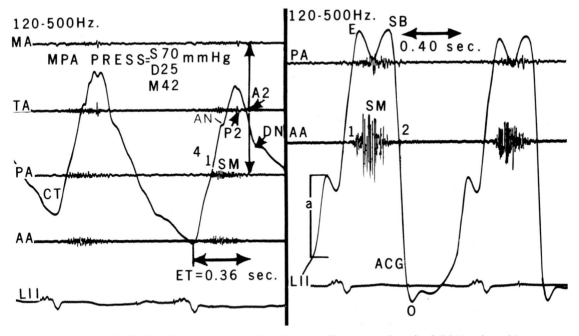

Figure 6.3. *Left*: Simultaneously recorded phonocardiogram at the mitral (MA), tricuspid (TA), pulmonic (PA), and aortic areas (AA), carotid pulse tracing (CT), and lead II (LII) of the electrocardiogram in a 71-year-old patient with aortic valvular stenosis and pulmonary hypertension secondary to left heart failure. Pulmonary artery pressure is elevated to 70 systolic and 25 diastolic with a mean of 42 mm Hg. The first and second heart sounds are diminished. Both components of the second sound precede the dicrotic notch (DN) on the carotid tracing, which indicates regurgitant splitting of the second heart sound, i.e., the pulmonic component precedes the aortic, which is the reverse of normal. There is a faint fourth heart sound, and a high frequency, high amplitude systolic ejection murmur (SM) which is recorded best at the tricuspid, pulmonic, and aortic areas. The carotid pulse tracing is markedly abnormal showing a very slow, but high anacrotic notch (AN) and a very slow ascending limb. The peak of the carotid pulse is reached near the second heart sound. The dicrotic notch is very inconspicuous and ejection time is prolonged. *Right*: Simultaneously recorded phonocardiogram at the pulmonic and aortic areas, apexcardiogram, and lead II of the electrocardiogram on the same patient. On this recording amplitude at the aortic area is much higher and the systolic murmur is better delineated. The apexcardiogram is markedly abnormal, showing a prominent A wave and E point followed by a systolic retraction and a late systolic bulge (SB). Compare with Figure 6.1.

107

failure. However, this third heart sound has important clinical implications in subjects over age 30–40 where it may suggest decreased left ventricular contractions (Fig. 6.4). This sound is also called an early, protodiastolic gallop or ventricular gallop. A fourth heart sound, also called atrial sound or atrial gallop, is one of the phonocardiographic features in adult patients with this type of valvular heart disease but it does not necessarily indicate the degree of severity of the stenotic lesion or the presence of heart failure (Fig. 6.4). If one or both of these conditions are noted, the fourth heart sound is always present if the patient is in

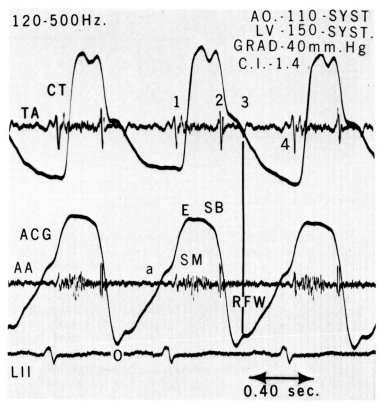

Figure 6.4. Simultaneously recorded phonocardiogram at the tricuspid (TA) and aortic areas (AA), carotid pulse tracing (CT), apexcardiogram (ACG), and lead II (LII) of the electrocardiogram in a 47-year-old patient with aortic valvular stenosis. The gradient across the aortic valve was 40 mm Hg and the cardiac index was 1.4 L/Min/M². The first and second heart sounds are not remarkable. There is a third heart sound that is not normal for this condition, particularly in patients past age 30. It coincides with the peak of the rapid filling wave (RFW) on the apexcardiogram. A fourth heart sound is recorded at the tricuspid area. There is a high frequency, high amplitude systolic ejection murmur (SM) recorded best at the aortic area with a maximal peak during systole that terminates prior to the second heart sound. The carotid pulse tracing shows a somewhat rapid ascending limb with a systolic retraction. The dicrotic notch is inconspicuous. The normal ejection time is an abnormal finding in patients with aortic stenosis and usually suggests heart failure. The apexcardiogram is typical for left ventricular hypertrophy. It shows an exaggerated A wave and an E point that is difficult to identify because it is followed by a round systolic wave.

sinus rhythm. This sound may be caused by sudden deceleration of blood into the ventricular cavity due to forceful atrial contraction.

Systolic murmurs of rheumatic aortic valvular stenosis, congenital bicuspid aortic stenosis, or membranous aortic stenosis have similar characteristics. The murmur has a characteristic diamond shape and begins with a high frequency sound called a systolic ejection click shortly after the first heart sound (Figs. 6.1 through 6.8). The maximum peak of this murmur, reached in the first half of systole, corresponds to the period of maximum rapid left ventricular ejection (Figs. 6.1 and 6.3 through 6.9). It decreases in amplitude during late systole, terminating at, or shortly before the second heart sound. It is recorded best at the mitral, tricuspid, and aortic areas. In many subjects with aortic stenosis, the murmur is recorded best at the mitral area and may, therefore, be confused with

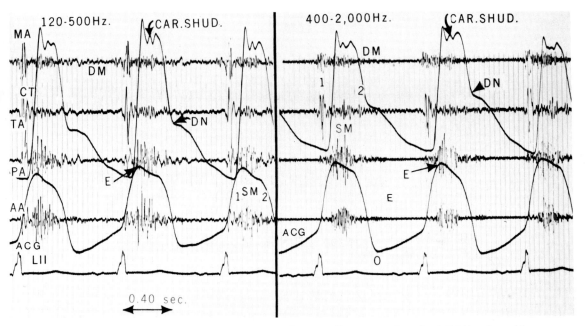

Figure 6.5. *Left*: Simultaneously recorded phonocardiogram at the mitral (MA), tricuspid (TA), pulmonic (PA), and aortic areas (AA), carotid pulse tracing (CT), apexcardiogram (ACG), and lead II (LII) of the electrocardiogram in a 42-year-old patient with aortic stenosis and insufficiency. The filter setting is 120–500 Hz. The first and second heart sounds and systolic murmur (SM) have the same characteristics described previously. There is a high frequency, low amplitude arterial diastolic murmur of aortic insufficiency. An important finding on the carotid pulse tracing is the presence of high frequency vibrations, seen best on the second beat, which represents carotid shudder (CAR. SHUD.). It is due to turbulent flow around the carotid arteries from the stenotic aortic valve. The dicrotic notch (DN) is inconspicuous and ejection time is prolonged. On the apexcardiogram the E point is difficult to identify and is followed by a round systolic wave. These findings are typical in left ventricular hypertrophy. The rapid filling wave is absent. *Right*: Recording with the filter setting at 400–2,000 Hz, pointing out the importance of different filter settings. In this tracing the third and fourth heart sounds are eliminated and the characteristics of the systolic ejection murmur are more prominent.

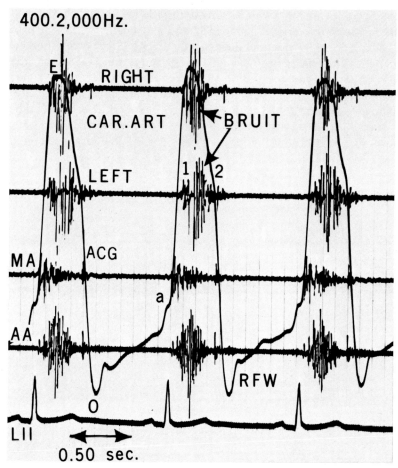

Figure 6.6. Simultaneously recorded phonocardiogram at the mitral and aortic areas (AA), with two other microphones placed over the right and left carotid arteries, apexcardiogram (ACG), and lead II (LII) of the electrocardiogram in a 25-year-old patient with aortic valvular stenosis. The first heart sound is normal. The second heart sound is diminished at the mitral and aortic areas. A high frequency, high amplitude systolic ejection murmur (SM) is recorded in both precordial areas. The amplitude of this murmur is most prominent in the tracing recorded over the left carotid artery. The apexcardiogram is not remarkable. It shows a small A wave and a normal rapid filling wave (RFW).

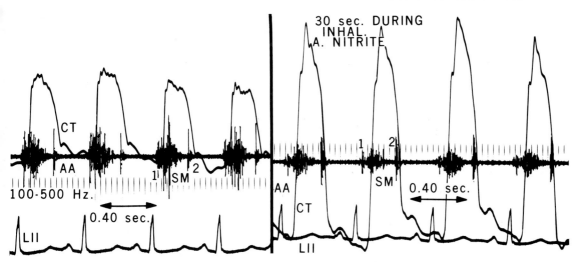

Figure 6.7. *Left*: Simultaneously recorded phonocardiogram at the aortic area (AA), carotid pulse tracing (CT), and lead II (LII) of the electrocardiogram in an 11-year-old patient with aortic valvular stenosis. There is a high frequency, high amplitude systolic ejection murmur (SM). The second heart sound is single and normal. *Right*: In this tracing recorded during inhalation of amyl nitrite, there is a marked decrease in amplitude of the systolic murmur due to a decrease in blood pressure and a decrease in the gradient across the aortic valve.

the murmur of mitral insufficiency. However, the characteristic ejection and noisy qualities of the murmur of aortic stenosis are helpful in differential diagnosis, as are abnormalities of the carotid pulse tracing. This murmur radiates well to both carotid arteries (Fig. 6.6), but is transmitted best to the right carotid artery. Therefore, placing a microphone over the patient's right carotid artery while recording the phonocardiogram may be helpful. Amplitude of this murmur varies with cycle length during cardiac arrhythmias, as shown in Figures 6.8 through 6.10. If the patient is in atrial fibrillation or has atrial, junctional, or ventricular ectopic beats, it is important to record the phonocardiogram during and after the ectopic beats.

Maneuvers and Pharmacologic Agents

Exercise causes an increase in amplitude of the systolic murmur. Inhalation of vasodilators such as amyl nitrite results in a significant decrease in amplitude of this murmur, probably as a result of a decrease in arterial blood pressure and a decreased gradient across the stenotic aortic valve (Fig. 6.7). The effect of administration of vasopressor agents is just the opposite, i.e., an increase in amplitude of the ejection murmur.

Carotid Pulse Tracing

Abnormalities of the carotid pulse tracing have diagnostic value in the assessment of patients with aortic valvular disease. Typical features of the arterial pulse wave

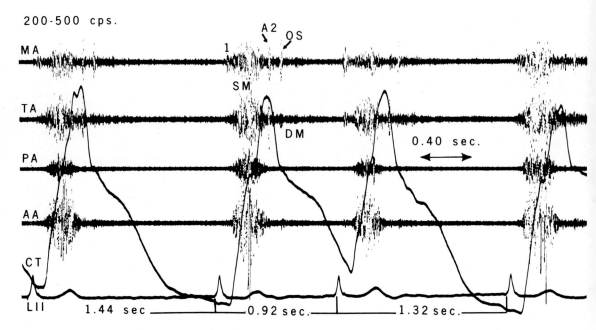

Figure 6.8. Simultaneously recorded phonocardiogram at the mitral (MA), tricuspid (TA), pulmonic (PA), and aortic areas (AA), carotid pulse tracing (CT), and lead II (LII) of the electrocardiogram in a 55-year-old patient with aortic stenosis and insufficiency, mitral stenosis, and atrial fibrillation. The first heart sound is slightly diminished. The second heart sound is normal. There is a high frequency, low amplitude, arterial diastolic murmur of aortic insufficiency. There is a high frequency vibration following aortic valve closure, which is the opening snap (OS) of the mitral valve. There is a high frequency, high amplitude systolic ejection murmur (SM) that exhibits the characteristics previously described. Of interest are the beats preceded by a long cycle length. Amplitude of the systolic murmur is more prominent in the last beat with a long cycle length of 1.32 sec as compared with the beat shown in the center, which has a cycle length of 0.92 sec. The carotid pulse tracing shows the typical features described for patients with aortic valvular stenosis.

form in this condition are a slow rise in upstroke time ("U" time), which is measured from its beginning until the tracing reaches a peak. This measurement may be difficult to obtain because in many patients the peak of the carotid tracing may not be well delineated. A prominent anacrotic notch is recorded on the ascending limb of the carotid pulse tracing (Figs. 6.1 through 6.3). An inconspicuous dicrotic notch is frequently present but at times is difficult to identify, making accurate measurements of ejection time difficult (Figs. 6.1 through 6.3, 6.5 and 6.8). There also may be high frequency vibrations called carotid shudder, which are most conspicuous on the carotid tracing as compared with other peripheral artery tracings (Figs. 6.2, 6.7, and 6.11). Ejection time is prolonged due to increased duration of left ventricular systole.

Jugular Venous Pulse Tracing

The jugular venous pulse tracing is not helpful in the diagnosis of aortic valvular stenosis (Fig. 6.12) unless the patient has pulmonary hypertension secondary to

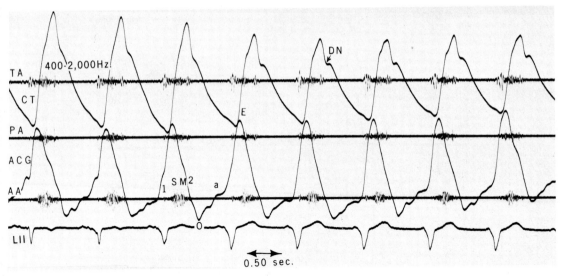

Figure 6.9. Simultaneously recorded phonocardiogram at the pulmonic (PA), tricuspid (TA), and aortic areas (AA), carotid pulse tracing (CT), apexcardiogram (ACG), and lead II (LII) of the electrocardiogram in a 50-year-old patient with aortic stenosis and insufficiency and atrioventricular dissociation by interference. The first heart sound is normal. The second heart sound is diminished. There is a high frequency, systolic ejection murmur (SM), which changes amplitude depending upon the relationship of the P wave to the QRS complex on the electrocardiogram. This type of arrhythmia is called atrioventricular dissociation by interference. The basic rhythm is junctional. When the P wave is inscribed several msec before the QRS complex, amplitude of the systolic murmur increases significantly as seen in the beats with the labeled P wave. When the P wave comes too close to the QRS complex, the murmur begins to decrease in amplitude, and finally becomes very small as seen in the last two beats where P waves are not seen. Also note the changes in amplitude on the carotid pulse tracing when the beats are preceded by a P wave. Amplitude of the carotid pulse tracing and ejection time are increased slightly as the P wave merges with the QRS complexes. This tracing emphasizes the importance of recordings during cardiac arrhythmias and the significance of the atrial contribution to ventricular filling. The A wave on the apexcardiogram is well appreciated in the first five beats and progressively disappears in the last three beats. DN = dicrotic notch.

left ventricular failure, at which time the A wave becomes quite prominent (Fig. 6.13).

Apexcardiogram

The apexcardiogram is very useful in evaluating patients with aortic valvular stenosis. Amplitude of the A wave is increased, representing forceful left atrial contraction against a nondistensible left ventricle (Figs. 6.1 and 6.3). The E point, which represents opening of the aortic valve, is difficult to identify because the systolic phase of the apexcardiogram is round and, therefore, the E point is in direct continuation with the remaining segment of the systolic wave (Figs. 6.4, 6.5 and 6.12). The O point is normal and is followed by a small or absent rapid filling wave. If a third heart sound is present in patients with heart failure, the rapid

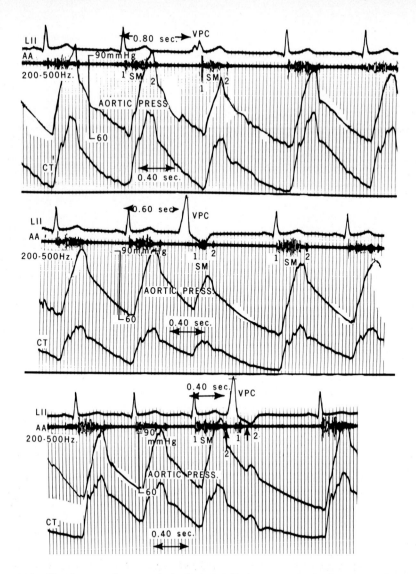

Figure 6.10. Simultaneously recorded phonocardiogram at the aortic area (AA), lead II (LII) of the electrocardiogram, aortic pulse pressure curve, and carotid pulse tracing (CT) in a 40-year-old patient with aortic stenosis and ventricular premature contractions. *Top*: Note the ventricular premature contraction (VPC) with a coupling interval (time interval) in relation to the QRS complex of 0.80 sec. There is very little change in the amplitude of the systolic ejection murmur (SM) in relation to the previous two beats. The somewhat identical configuration of the carotid pulse tracing as compared with the aortic pressure curve shows that the carotid tracing is a good indicator of aortic pressure contour. *Middle*: Recording of the same patient with a ventricular premature contraction. The cycle length is short and the systolic murmur has less amplitude as compared with the upper panel. *Bottom*: In this recording, the patient has a premature ventricular contraction at the beginning and the sinus beat is 0.40 sec, which is quite short. In this case, the systolic murmur practically disappears after a long compensatory pause. Following the ventricular premature contraction, the systolic ejection murmur increases markedly in amplitude as compared with the pre-extrasystolic beats. On all three tracings, the amplitude of both the aortic and carotid pulse pressures decreases progressively as the coupling interval decreases.

114

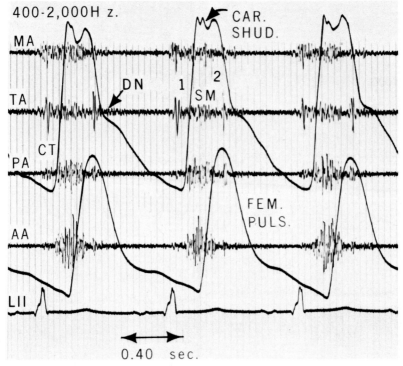

Figure 6.11. Simultaneously recorded phonocardiogram at the mitral (MA), tricuspid (TA), pulmonic (PA), and aortic areas (AA), carotid pulse tracing (CT), transcutaneous femoral pulse tracing (FEM PULS), and lead II (LII) of the electrocardiogram in a 42-year-old patient with aortic stenosis and insufficiency. The configuration of the first and second heart sounds and the systolic murmur (SM) are essentially identical to the ones described previously. This illustration is to demonstrate the carotid shudder (CAR SHUD) best appreciated on the carotid pulse tracing and not recognizable in the tracings taken over the transcutaneous femoral pulse. This is of great importance in demonstrating abnormalities of aortic stenosis. DN = dicrotic notch.

filling wave becomes prominent and its peak coincides with the time of inscription of the third heart sound (Figs. 6.4 and 6.13). In most cases, the rapid filling wave is small, resembling the ones seen in patients with mitral stenosis (Figs. 6.5 and 6.14). At times one may detect the presence of pulsus alternans on the apexcardiogram and carotid pulse tracing (Fig. 6.14).

Systolic Time Intervals

Left ventricular ejection time and total left ventricular systole are prolonged (Figs. 6.1 through 6.3, 6.8, 6.10 and 6.12). Prolongation of left ventricular ejection time is grossly proportional to the degree of severity of aortic valvular stenosis. The pre-ejection period is slightly decreased, and the combination of prolonged left ventricular ejection time (LVET) and pre-ejection period (PEP) results in a PEP/LVET ratio lower than normal.

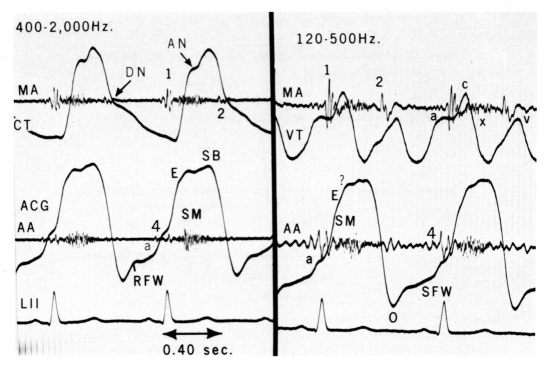

Figure 6.12. *Left*: Simultaneously recorded phonocardiogram at the mitral (MA), and aortic areas (AA), carotid pulse tracing (CT), apexcardiogram (ACG), and lead II (LII) of the electrocardiogram in a 41-year-old patient with aortic stenosis. The first heart sound is normal. The second heart sound is diminished. The systolic murmur (SM) has the typical characteristics seen in patients with aortic stenosis. The carotid pulse tracing has a slow ascending limb, anacrotic notch (AN), late systolic peak, an inconspicuous dicrotic notch (DN), and prolonged ejection time. The apexcardiogram shows a slightly inconspicuous A wave and a late systolic bulge (SB). The rapid filling wave (RFW) is normal. *Right*: Simultaneously recorded phonocardiogram at the mitral and aortic areas, jugular venous pulse tracing (VT), apexcardiogram, and lead II of the electrocardiogram. This patient was not in heart failure; therefore, the jugular venous tracing is normal. There is an artifactually high C wave on this record. The A wave has normal amplitude in relation to the V wave. The apexcardiogram shows an inconspicuous E point. SFW = slow filling wave.

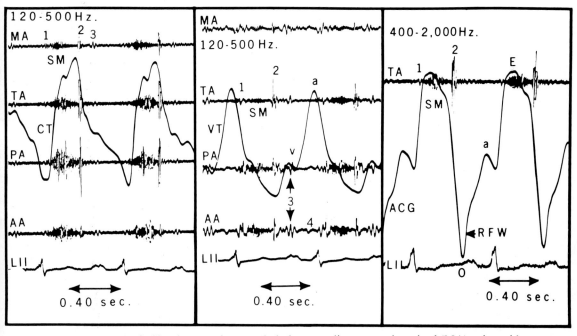

Figure 6.13. *Left*: Simultaneously recorded phonocardiogram at the mitral (MA), tricuspid (TA), pulmonic (PA), and aortic areas (AA), carotid pulse tracing (CT), and lead II (LII) of the electrocardiogram in a 68-year-old patient with aortic valvular stenosis. The patient is in heart failure. The first and second heart sounds are normal. There is a high frequency, high amplitude systolic ejection murmur (SM) recorded best at the pulmonic and aortic areas. There is also a third heart sound, which is an abnormal finding in patients with aortic stenosis, particularly in this age group. It is transmitted well to all areas including the aortic area. *Middle*: This tracing shows the value of the jugular venous pulse (VT) in recognizing the presence of heart failure or increased right sided pressures secondary to left ventricular failure. There is a prominent A wave that coincides with a fourth heart sound, well seen at the aortic area. The V wave is small. *Right*: Simultaneously recorded phonocardiogram at the tricuspid area, apexcardiogram, and lead II of the electrocardiogram showing markedly exaggerated A and rapid filling waves (RFW) of the type seen in patients with aortic stenosis and heart failure. The systolic wave is round, indicating left ventricular hypertrophy or dysfunction.

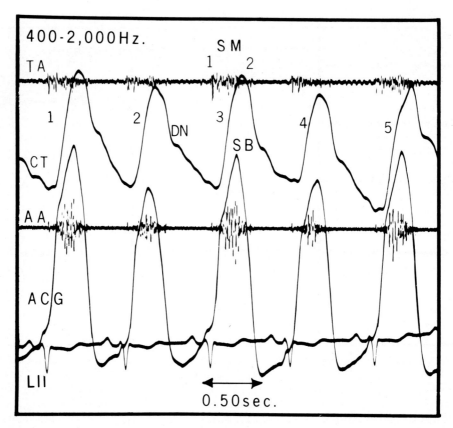

Figure 6.14. Simultaneously recorded phonocardiogram at the tricuspid (TA), and aortic areas (AA), carotid pulse tracing (CT), apexcardiogram (ACG), and lead II (LII) of the electrocardiogram in a 73-year-old patient with severe aortic stenosis, congestive heart failure, pulsus alternans and murmur alternans. Beats one and three are the weaker beats and two and four are the stronger beats. Amplitude of the systolic murmur (SM) in beats one and three is weak as compared with beats two and four. This is associated with lower amplitude of the pulse waves on the carotid pulse tracing and apexcardiogram in the weaker beats, as compared with a stronger configuration in beats two and four. Due to the late, terminal stage of congestive heart failure where there is significant disease of the heart muscle, a lot of blood is left in the left ventricle when ejection terminates. However, in the following beats the fiber shortening is much stronger, allowing more blood to be ejected from the left ventricle into the aorta and carotid arteries. The mechanism of pulsus alternans is still controversial, but appears to be due to alternation in the rate of shortening of the myocardial fibers.

A shortening of the systolic left ventricular ejection time, mechanical systole and pre-ejection period, usually seen in patients subjected to successful aortic valve surgery, represents improvement in cardiac function.

Vectorcardiogram

The vectorcardiogram is quite helpful in the noninvasive evaluation of patients with aortic valve disease to detect signs of left ventricular hypertrophy. A good recording of the QRS loop usually shows a maximal deflection vector exceeding 2.2 mv in the horizontal plane and 1.8 mv in the frontal plane (Figs. 6.15 and 6.16). In addition, it is quite important to obtain good magnification of the initial 10–20

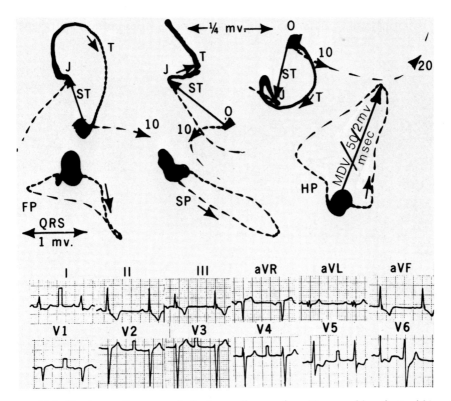

Figure 6.15. Vectorcardiogram and electrocardiogram in a 49-year-old patient with aortic stenosis. The electrocardiogram shows sinus rhythm; the P wave is followed by a QRS complex. The precordial leads recorded at half standard show signs of left ventricular hypertrophy. One ventricular extrasystole was recorded in lead V6. Note the normal T waves and ST segments usually seen in patients with myocardial ischemia, left ventricular strain, or drug effect. The vectorcardiogram in the horizontal plane shows increased amplitude of the QRS forces, which exceeds the maximal upper limit of 2.2 mv as measured from the O point to maximal excursion. There is significant displacement of the ST segment and T loop, which opposes the QRS complex. This is measured from the O to the J point on the horizontal loop and shows left ventricular strain involving the anterior wall. There is also abnormal repolarization of the heart as seen on the frontal plane and in leads I, II, III and aVF of the electrocardiogram.

msec QRS vectors (Fig. 6.16). In many patients, the electrocardiogram may show loss of the R wave in V1, V2, and V3, which makes it very difficult to rule out the diagnosis of a myocardial infarction involving the anterior wall of the left ventricle. If the 10 and/or 20 msec vectors are located in front of the O point, the diagnosis of an anteroseptal myocardial infarction could be excluded with a moderate degree of confidence. In addition, record a good, magnified P loop in the horizontal plane. Many patients with significant aortic valve disease, either stenosis or insufficiency, might present with hypertrophy, dilatation or fibrosis of the left ventricle. In this situation, left ventricular end-diastolic pressure is elevated. This will require a more powerful atrial contraction against a nondistensible left ventricle and, therefore, create overloading in the left atrium. This overloading can be expressed on the vectorcardiogram by an increase in amplitude of the P loop particularly well seen in the horizontal plane (Fig. 6.16). The vectorcardiogram is not helpful in differentiating aortic stenosis from aortic insufficiency.

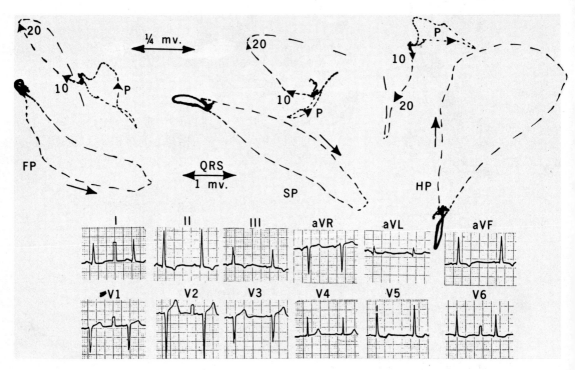

Figure 6.16. Vectorcardiogram and electrocardiogram in a 30-year-old patient with aortic stenosis and insufficiency, left ventricular hypertrophy and strain, and normal coronary arteries. The rhythm is sinus on the electrocardiogram and vectorcardiogram. The only difference on this illustration as compared with Figure 6.15 is that despite the marked increase in voltage of the QRS complex, indicating left ventricular strain, the loop rotates clockwise in both the sagittal and horizontal planes. This is definitely an abnormal finding in this age group. Normally, rotation of the QRS loop should be counterclockwise. In approximately 10–15% of patients with aortic stenosis and severe left ventricular hypertrophy, the loop rotates clockwise and this is usually indicative of myocardial infarction. However, this patient had normal coronary arteriograms.

Echocardiogram

Echocardiography is a useful noninvasive technique to evaluate patients with aortic valvular stenosis (Figs. 6.17 through 6.19). Calcification of the aortic annulus may be seen in Figure 6.20. Angling the transducer to position 4 (pointing toward the base of the heart) usually produces good aortic valve echoes, particularly in patients with aortic valvular stenosis. It is important to record multiple cardiac cycles and a scan from the base of the heart to the apex for proper identification of the cardiac structures. Simultaneous recording of the phonocardiogram and/or carotid pulse tracing is helpful to identify the beginning and end of ventricular systole. The normal range of aortic valve opening is 1.7 to 2.6 cm, with an average of 1.9 cm. Echoes derived from the aortic valve seem to represent motion of the right and noncoronary cusps. However, this is controversial and it appears that it is better to refer to anterior and posterior aortic cusp motion. Aortic valvular lesions can be detected by a decrease in the size of the aortic valve opening, and this measurement should be compared with the size of the aortic root. This structure is frequently dilated, especially in patients with severe aortic

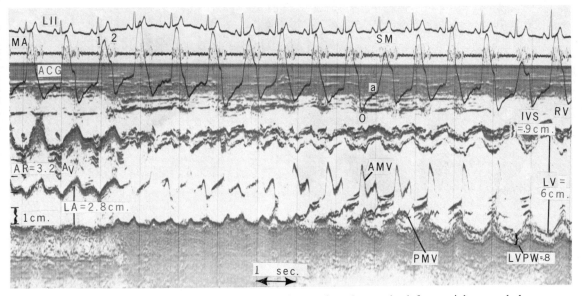

Figure 6.17. Echocardiographic scan from the aortic valve to the left ventricle recorded simultaneously with the phonocardiogram at the mitral area (MA), apexcardiogram (ACG), and lead II (LII) of the electrocardiogram in an 18-year-old patient with mild to moderate aortic stenosis and a minimal degree of aortic insufficiency. On the left side of the scan a recording of the aortic valve (AV) and aortic root (AR) shows multiple diastolic echoes indicating a mild degree of aortic valvular stenosis. The aortic root size is 3.2 cm, which is within the normal range. The left atrial (LA) size of 2.8 cm also is normal. As the transducer is moved toward the mitral valve and left ventricle, one sees that the left ventricle is enlarged to 6 cm. Thickness of the interventricular septum (IVS) and the left ventricular posterior wall (LVPW) is normal and so is the ratio. Movement of the mitral valve is normal. The apexcardiogram has a normal configuration. AMV = anterior mitral valve, PMV = posterior mitral valve, RV = right ventricle, SM = systolic murmur.

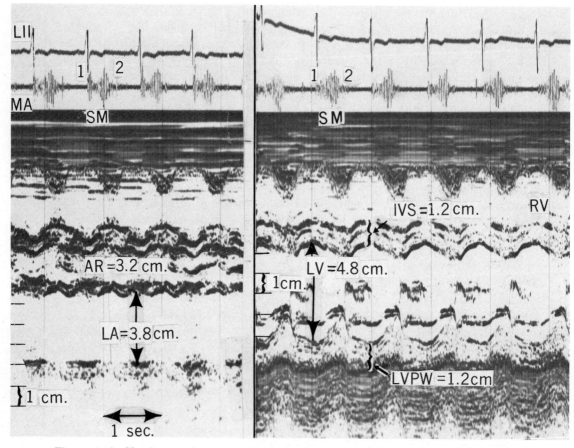

Figure 6.18. Simultaneously recorded echocardiogram, mitral area (MA) phonocardiogram, and lead II (LII) of the electrocardiogram in a patient with aortic stenosis and insufficiency. *Left*: Echocardiogram of the aortic root (AR) and left atrium (LA). Left atrial size is normal but there are very heavy and disorganized echoes within the aortic root. The leaflets of the aortic cusp are not well seen due to calcification of the valve. At cardiac catheterization and fluoroscopy, this patient had a marked degree of calcification around the aortic root and cusps. The simultaneously recorded phonocardiogram shows the presence of a prominent systolic murmur (SM), which is typical for this condition. The diastolic murmur of aortic insufficiency is not well recorded. *Right*: Recording of the mitral valve, interventricular septum (IVS), and left ventricular posterior wall (LVPW). The interventricular septum and left ventricular posterior wall have slightly increased thickness, but septal motion is normal. The left ventricular (LV) cavity size is within normal range; however, note the fine fluttering motion of the mitral leaflets due to aortic insufficiency. RV = right ventricle.

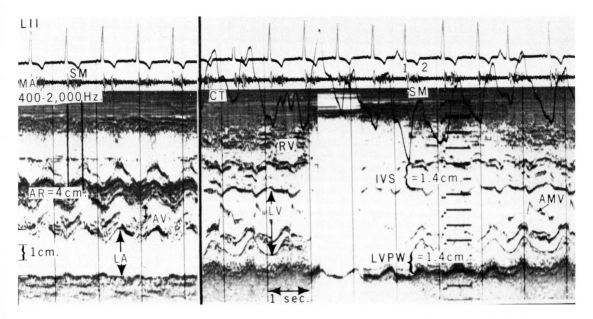

Figure 6.19. Echocardiogram, mitral area (MA) phonocardiogram, lead II (LII) of the electrocardiogram, and carotid pulse tracing (CT) in a 51-year-old patient with aortic stenosis and concentric left ventricular hypertrophy. *Left*: The aortic valve (AV) opening is smaller than normal. The left atrium (LA) is not enlarged. *Right*: Thickness of the interventricular septum (IVS) and left ventricular posterior wall (LVPW) are at the upper limits of normal at 1.4 cm, indicating concentric ventricular hypertrophy. Recording of the mitral valve shows normal motion. AR = aortic root, SM = systolic murmur, AMV = anterior mitral valve, RV = right ventricle.

stenosis. A decrease in size of the aortic valve opening may be seen in other cardiac diseases, such as heart failure from any cause, resulting in decreased blood flow across a normal aortic valve. Echocardiography is also useful for measurements of left atrial and left ventricular internal diameters that may be above normal limits in patients with moderate to severe aortic stenosis with or without heart failure. A good recording of the interventricular septum and posterior wall of the left ventricle for determination of structure thickness helps to determine the degree of left ventricular involvment in this disease state (concentric left ventricular hypertrophy).

Careful examination of the aortic valve in patients with aortic stenosis is critical, especially in severely calcified valves where a technically good aortic valve opening is hard to find. Heavy echoes in the aortic root may be recorded and, usually, the more echoes present, the more severe is the stenosis or calcification. By incorrect angulation, the aortic valve may appear to be more calcified than it actually is. Some leaflet motion must be detected to make certain that the transducer is not directed eccentrically through the aorta. In addition to a good recording of the aortic valve try to obtain a good recording of the mitral valve because this may detect a prolonged mitral valve closure if the diastolic pressure in the left ventricle is elevated.

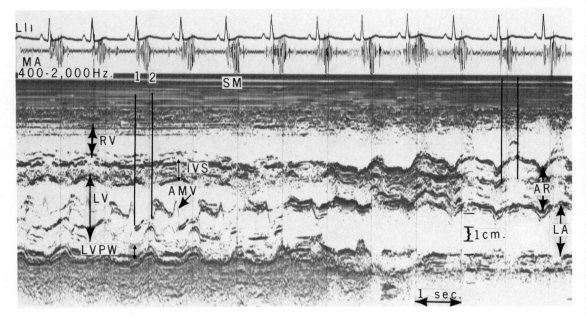

Figure 6.20. Echocardiographic scan from the mitral valve toward the aortic valve recorded simultaneously with lead II (LII) of the electrocardiogram and mitral area (MA) phonocardiogram in a 61-year-old patient with aortic stenosis and calcified aortic annulus. Multiple heavy and disorganized echoes originate in the aortic root. There are also heavy echoes located anteriorly and posteriorly in the left ventricular outflow tract representing the calcified aortic annulus.

In children with congenital aortic stenosis where the valve is not calcified and only minimally fibrotic, it may appear to be normal due to doming of the valve leaflets. In this situation, the left ventricular wall thickness and volume measurements are more diagnostic.

Points of Caution and Importance

1. The two most important phonocardiographic aspects in patients with aortic stenosis are a good recording of the systolic ejection murmur and the second heart sound. For a good recording of the systolic ejection murmur, set your bandpass filter to log or log–log to record a murmur that will be approximately 2 cm in amplitude with the microphone placed at the aortic, mitral, or tricuspid areas. The patient should be lying flat. Record during quiet, held expiration or you will amplify the baseline noise. It is recommended that the area where the microphone is placed be shaved on male patients so that you will have good contact of the microphone with the patient's skin.

2. The carotid pulse tracing is the second most important recording to obtain. Try not to apply too much pressure over the carotid arteries with your transducer because many of these patients have a sensitive carotid sinus and this may cause marked slowing of the heart rate. This can be quite dangerous in patients

with aortic stenosis. The carotid pulse tracing should be recorded simultaneously with a logarithmic recording of the phonocardiogram.

3. In all patients with aortic stenosis, be sure to record a tracing during inspiration and expiration at a paper speed of 50 mm/sec with $\frac{1}{10}$ sec time lines. This will allow documentation of normal splitting of the second heart sound and so-called paradoxical splitting, in which the pulmonic valve closure sound precedes the aortic closure sound. If the patient has paradoxical splitting, during inspiration this sound becomes single and during expiration the components are separated, which is the opposite of normal.

4. A good recording of the apexcardiogram is quite helpful in the diagnosis of this condition. It should show a prominent A wave. In many patients, the E point cannot be clearly identified (Fig. 6.21). This is not an artifact. It is due to a moderate to severe degree of left ventricular hypertrophy.

5. Try to obtain a good recording of the diastolic phase of the apexcardiogram. Many patients with aortic stenosis will show a diminished or absent rapid filling wave due to lack of distensibility of the left ventricle. During the diastolic phase of the apexcardiogram the tracing simulates the ones seen in patients with mitral stenosis.

6. When recording the jugular venous pulse, look for the A wave. This recording is of value only to identify the presence of increased pulmonary artery pressure, which occurs in the late natural history of this disease and is indicated by a very large A wave.

7. In recording the echocardiogram be sure that you get the correct damping setting to identify properly the presence of fibrosis or calcification of the aortic valve, which is characterized by disorganized echoes within the aortic root structure.

8. A decrease in the aortic valve excursion is not always diagnostic of aortic stenosis. Any condition associated with decreased cardiac output, such as congestive heart failure or primary myocardial disease, can cause this.

AORTIC SUBVALVULAR STENOSIS AND BICUSPID AORTIC VALVE

The auscultatory, phonocardiographic, pulse wave, and systolic time interval abnormalities in patients with subvalvular aortic stenosis or bicuspid aortic valve do not differ significantly from those in patients with aortic valvular stenosis (Fig. 6.21).

Echocardiogram

The echocardiogram in patients with membranous aortic stenosis usually shows an early, partial closure of the aortic valve during the first third of systole followed by a secondary opening during the remaining phases (Figs. 6.22 through 6.25).

A good scan from the aortic to the mitral valve is important to show narrowing of the outflow tract if it is present. Also obtain a good recording of the aortic valve from the beginning to the end of systole to determine midsystolic closure of the valve.

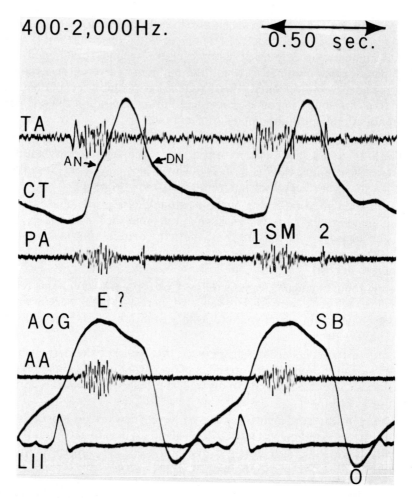

Figure 6.21. Simultaneously recorded phonocardiogram at the tricuspid (TA), pulmonic (PA), and aortic areas (AA), carotid pulse tracing (CT), apexcardiogram (ACG), and lead II (LII) of the electrocardiogram in a 43-year-old patient with aortic valvular stenosis. The first heart sound is normal. The second heart sound is diminished. There is a high frequency, high amplitude systolic ejection murmur (SM), which is typical for aortic valvular stenosis. The carotid tracing shows a slow ascending limb, low placed anacrotic notch (AN), and an inconspicuous dicrotic notch (DN). The ejection time is prolonged. On the apexcardiogram it is very difficult to identify the E point because of a round systolic wave. This type of tracing, seen in patients with severe left ventricular hypertrophy, demonstrates that the apexcardiogram cannot be used to identify the beginning of ventricular systole. In this case, the carotid pulse tracing is more valuable because one can clearly see the beginning of the rise of the ascending limb. SB = systolic bulge.

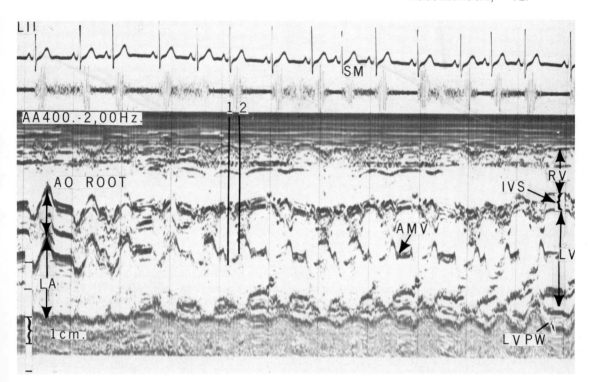

Figure 6.22. Echocardiographic scan from the aortic root (AO ROOT) into the left ventricular cavity recorded simultaneously with lead II (LII) of the electrocardiogram and aortic area (AA) phonocardiogram in a 5-year-old patient with subvalvular aortic stenosis. The echoes within the left ventricular outflow tract probably originated in the membrane located below the aortic valve. The aortic valve opening is within the normal range. Mitral valve motion is normal. The left ventricular (LV) internal dimension is within the normal range. SM = systolic murmur, IVS = interventricular septum, AMV = anterior mitral valve, LVPW = left ventricular posterior wall.

SUPRAVALVULAR AORTIC STENOSIS

In patients with congenital supravalvular stenosis, the findings are nearly identical to those in aortic valvular stenosis. The systolic ejection click is usually absent. A systolic ejection murmur is frequently radiated to the left carotid artery with poor transmission to the right carotid artery. The right carotid pulse tracing will show the characteristic findings described for aortic valvular stenosis.

AORTIC INSUFFICIENCY

The most common type of aortic insufficiency or regurgitation is due to rheumatic heart disease. Other disease states associated with aortic insufficiency are dissecting aortic aneurysm, rheumatoid arthritis, and diseases of the collagen system (connective tissue disorder such as Marfan's syndrome). In the majority of cases,

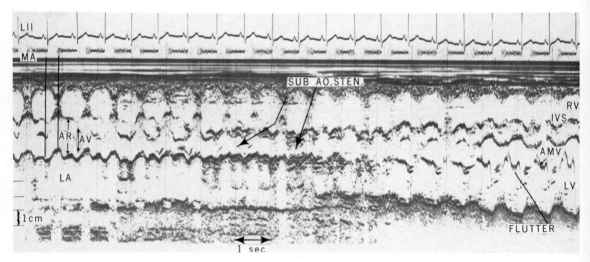

Figure 6.23. Echocardiographic scan from the aortic root (AR) into the left ventricular cavity recorded simultaneously with a mitral area (MA) phonocardiogram and lead II (LII) of the electrocardiogram in a patient with subaortic stenosis. The aortic valve (AV) has a normal excursion. Areas of heavy echoes derived from the subvalvular membrane are indicated. The interventricular septum (IVS) and posterior wall thickness are within normal range. This patient also has some degree of aortic insufficiency that causes fluttering of the mitral valve. LA = left atrium, LV = left ventricle, AMV = anterior mitral valve, RV = right ventricle.

the auscultatory, phonocardiographic, and pulse wave abnormalities are alike. The characteristic murmur of aortic insufficiency is seen in most of these conditions. The murmur is musical in patients with rupture of the aortic cusps or rheumatoid arthritis.

Heart Sounds and Murmurs

The first heart sound is normal or slightly accentuated. A systolic ejection click is present in 30 to 40% of patients with aortic insufficiency due to dilatation of the ascending aorta. The second heart sound is single and accentuated due to increased intensity of the aortic valve closure sound secondary to increased aortic pulse pressure. It is best recorded at the aortic and tricuspid areas (Fig. 6.26). A third heart sound, frequently recorded on the phonocardiogram in patients with aortic insufficiency, is due to increased diastolic blood volume of the left ventricle secondary to the regurgitation. A fourth heart sound (atrial gallop) is present but should not be considered a sign of heart failure.

A typical, noisy, high frequency arterial diastolic murmur is heard and best recorded at the tricuspid, aortic, and mitral areas, particularly with the patient sitting or standing. It begins with the aortic component of the second heart sound, which is the point of maximum intensity of the diastolic murmur (Fig. 6.27). It is best recorded with a bandpass filter setting in the range of 500–2,000 Hz. This murmur peaks in mid-diastole and terminates prior to atrial contraction, before the

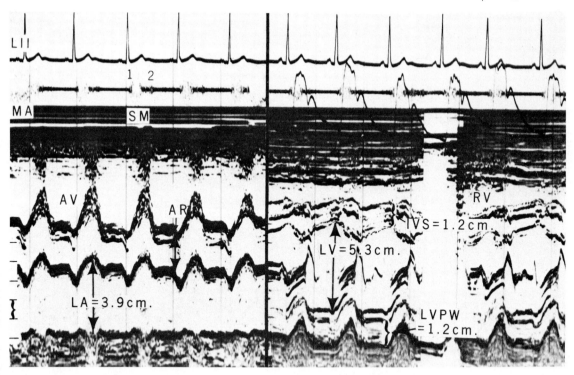

Figure 6.24. Echocardiogram, mitral area (MA) phonocardiogram, and lead II (LII) of the electrocardiogram in a patient with a bicuspid aortic valve. *Left*: Note the eccentric location of the aortic valve (AV) during diastole, which is one of the important echocardiographic signs of a bicuspid aortic valve. *Right*: Recording on the same patient for measurement of left ventricular dimensions. The thickness of the interventricular septum (IVS) and left ventricular posterior wall (LVPW) is slightly increased. Motion of the mitral valve and the interventricular septum is within normal range. RV = right ventricle, SM = systolic murmur, AR = aortic root, LA = left atrium, LV = left ventricle.

P wave of the electrocardiogram. A systolic ejection murmur is frequently heard and recorded but does not necessarily indicate the presence of significant aortic valvular stenosis. This murmur is the result of increased blood flow across a nonstenotic aortic valve. A short, low frequency mid-diastolic murmur called the Austin–Flint murmur may also be heard in patients with aortic insufficiency. It is recorded best at the mitral area. This murmur may be confused with the murmur of mitral stenosis because at times it has a presystolic accentuation. It seems to be related to turbulent regurgitant aortic flow against the mitral valve.

Carotid Pulse Tracing

Abnormalities on the carotid pulse tracing include the presence of a rapid ascending limb followed by a rapid midsystolic retraction, a late systolic bulge (pulsus bisferiens) and prolonged ejection time (Fig. 6.26). The dicrotic notch, located near the baseline, is quite conspicuous (Fig. 6.26).

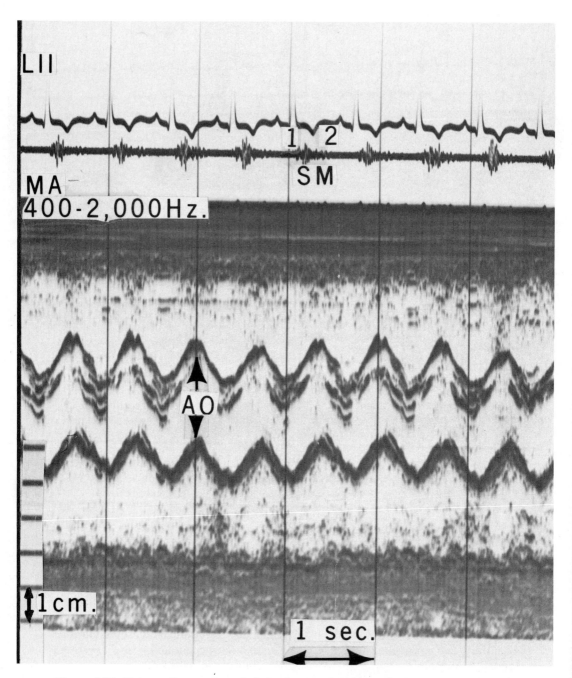

Figure 6.25. Echocardiogram recorded simultaneously with a mitral area (MA) phonocardiogram and lead II (LII) of the electrocardiogram. The echocardiogram shows the eccentric position of the aortic valve (AV) in diastole indicating a bicuspid aortic valve. The aortic root size is normal. SM = systolic murmur.

130

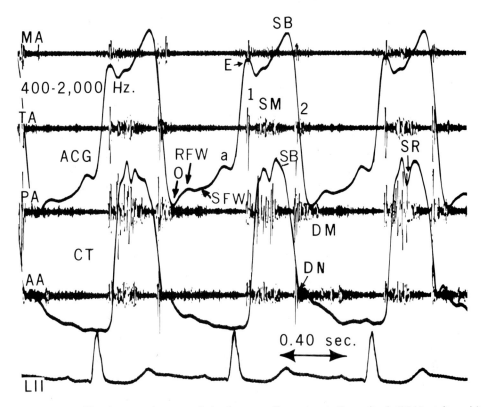

Figure 6.26. Simultaneously recorded phonocardiogram at the mitral (MA), tricuspid (TA), pulmonic (PA), and aortic areas (AA), apexcardiogram (ACG), carotid pulse tracing (CT), and lead II (LII) of the electrocardiogram in a 36-year-old patient with rheumatic aortic stenosis and insufficiency. The first heart sound is normal. The second heart sound is single and accentuated and best defined at the aortic area. There is a high frequency, medium amplitude systolic ejection murmur (SM) recorded best at the tricuspid, pulmonic, and aortic areas. A high frequency, high amplitude decrescendo arterial diastolic murmur (DM), best recorded at the pulmonic area, starts with the second heart sound, reaching maximal intensity in early diastole. The apexcardiogram shows an abnormal configuration. There is a prominent A wave. Following the E point, which marks the beginning of ventricular ejection, there is a downward deflection, but the tracing quickly begins to rise again in mid- and late systole, reaching its maximal peak near the second heart sound. This is characteristic of the systolic bulge (SB) seen in patients with ventricular hypertrophy or left ventricular dyskinesis. The O point is inscribed after the beginning of the diastolic murmur indicating that it is an arterial and not an atrioventricular diastolic murmur, which is seen in patients with mitral or tricuspid stenosis. The murmur of mitral stenosis would start after the O point of the apexcardiogram. This is a good example of why the apexcardiogram is a good reference tracing to differentiate between these two types of murmurs. Following the O point, there is a small rapid filling wave of the type seen in patients with ventricular hypertrophy. After the rapid filling wave (RFW), there is a slow filling wave (SFW), which is normal. The carotid pulse tracing also has abnormal characteristics. It shows a rapid rise of the ascending limb. At the top of the tracing, there are several notches representing carotid shudder. On the third beat, a clearly defined systolic retraction (SR) is present followed by a late systolic bulge. Following this, the tracing quickly moves toward the baseline where the dicrotic notch (DN) is inscribed. The configuration of the carotid pulse tracing suggests that aortic insufficiency may be the dominant lesion. This was confirmed by cardiac catheterization and angiography.

131

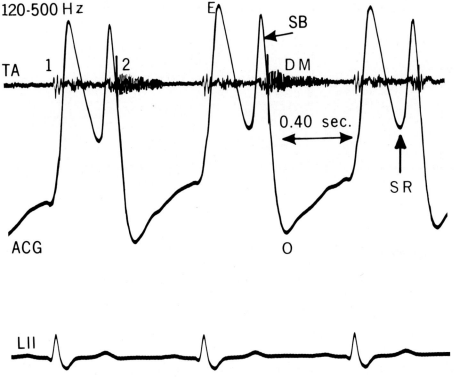

Figure 6.27. Simultaneously recorded tricuspid area (TA) phonocardiogram, apexcardiogram (ACG), and lead II (LII) of the electrocardiogram in a 41-year-old patient with aortic insufficiency. The first heart sound is normal. The second heart sound is accentuated. There is a high frequency, low amplitude systolic ejection murmur. Immediately following the second heart sound there is a high frequency, high amplitude arterial diastolic murmur (DM) that terminates in mid-diastole. The apexcardiogram is abnormal. It shows a midsystolic retraction (SR) followed by a late systolic bulge (SB). This is the type of apexcardiogram that is usually seen in patients with aortic insufficiency.

Systolic Time Intervals

Patients with aortic insufficiency have prolonged left ventricular ejection time. The pre-ejection period is reduced. The PEP/LVET ratio is decreased. As described for patients with aortic valvular stenosis, the presence of congestive heart failure will normalize the systolic time intervals.

Jugular Venous Pulse Tracing

The jugular venous pulse waveform is normal in this condition. If the patient develops heart failure and pulmonary hypertension, the A wave becomes prominent.

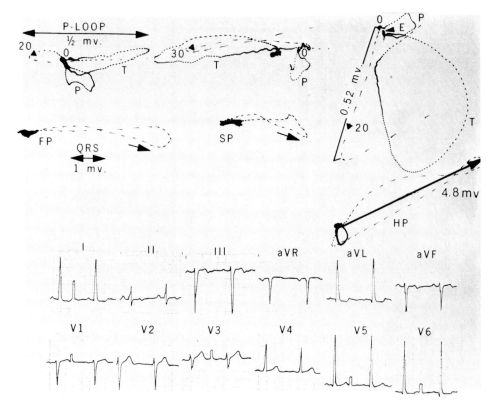

Figure 6.28. Vectorcardiogram and electrocardiogram in a 49-year-old patient with aortic insufficiency. The electrocardiogram shows sinus rhythm, left axis deviation, left ventricular hypertrophy and strain. On the vectorcardiogram there are large initial forces especially in the horizontal plane going rightward and anteriorly from the O point to the maximal distance from the O point, which measures 0.52 mv., and exceeds the normal limit of 0.18 mv. This is a sign of septal hypertrophy and is sometimes seen in patients with myocardial infarction involving the lateral wall of the left ventricle. In this case, it is septal hypertrophy that is commonly seen in patients with aortic stenosis or insufficiency. In addition, there is a marked increase in the forces going posteriorly and to the left, which is the area where the left ventricle is located, indicating the presence of left ventricular hypertrophy. The maximal force again exceeds 2.2 mv and is a typical sign of left ventricular hypertrophy.

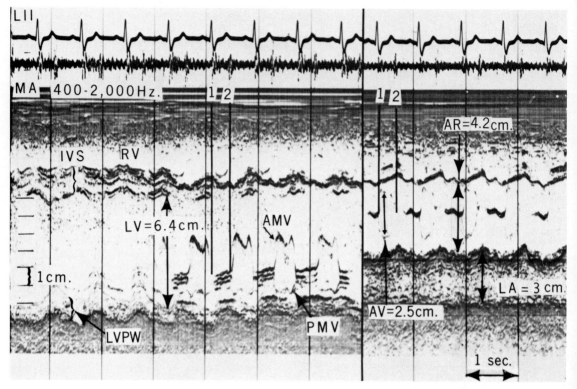

Figure 6.29. Simultaneously recorded echocardiogram, mitral area (MA) phonocardiogram, and lead II (LII) of the electrocardiogram in a 38-year-old patient with aortic insufficiency. *Left*: Echocardiographic recording of the mitral valve, interventricular septum
(IVS), and left ventricular posterior wall (LVPW) showing a large left ventricle (6.4cm) and
concentric left ventricular hypertrophy, with increased thickness of the interventricular
septum (1.3cm). The left ventricular posterior wall measures 1.3 cm. *Right*: Echocardiogram of the aortic root (AR) and aortic valve (AV) showing a dilated aortic root (4.2cm) and
a normal sized left atrium (LA), 3cm. RV = right ventricle, LV = left ventricle, PMV =
posterior mitral valve.

Apexcardiogram

The apexcardiogram shows a prominent A wave, a sustained or bifid systolic wave
(Fig. 6.26), and an accentuated rapid filling wave. In patients with severe left
ventricular hypertrophy, the systolic wave is round and the E point is difficult to
identify.

Maneuvers and Pharmacologic Agents

Cardiac arrhythmias can cause significant changes in the configuration and maximal time amplitude of the murmur of aortic insufficiency.

Administration of vasopressor agents resulting in an increase in systemic arterial pressure causes an increase in the diastolic regurgitant flow and accentuation

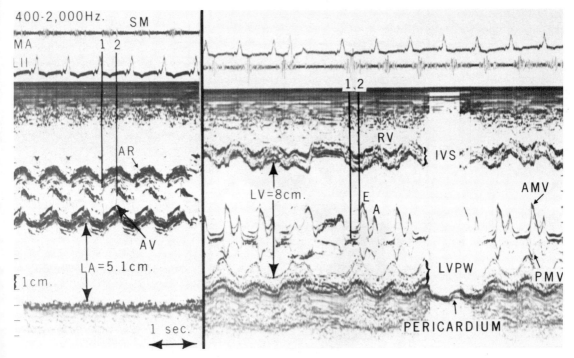

Figure 6.30. *Left*: Echocardiogram, mitral area (MA) phonocardiogram, and lead II (LII) of the electrocardiogram in a patient with aortic insufficiency and a mild degree of aortic stenosis. Note heavy echoes originating around the aortic valve (AV) and aortic root (AR) suggesting fibrosis and calcification of the aortic valve. The left atrial size (LA) is increased to 5.1 cm. *Right*: Echocardiogram recorded simultaneously with the phonocardiogram and lead II of the electrocardiogram showing increased left ventricular (LV) internal dimension to 8 cm. SM = systolic murmur, RV = right ventricle, LVPW = left ventricular posterior wall, AMV = anterior mitral valve, PMV = posterior mitral valve, IVS = interventricular septum.

of the diastolic murmur of aortic insufficiency. Administration of vasodilators such as inhalation of amyl nitrite causes a decrease in amplitude of the diastolic murmur of aortic insufficiency and a slight increase in amplitude of the systolic ejection murmur.

Vectorcardiogram

The vectorcardiogram shows signs of left ventricular hypertrophy and strain as well as septal hypertrophy. These forces are located anterior and rightward for septal hypertrophy and posterior and to the left of the O point for left ventricular hypertrophy (Fig. 6.28).

Echocardiogram

The echocardiogram is useful in studying patients with aortic insufficiency. The most common findings are a dilated aortic root with or without thickening or

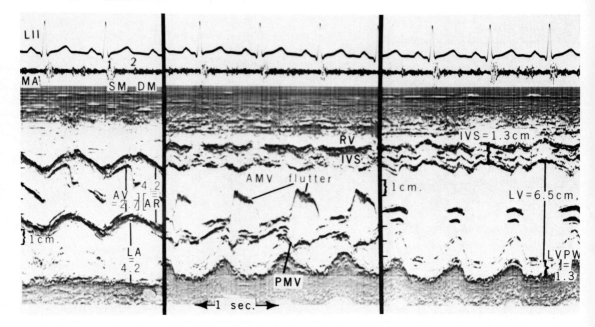

Figure 6.31. Echocardiogram, mitral area (MA) phonocardiogram, and lead II (LII) of the electrocardiogram in a patient with aortic insufficiency. *Left*: Recording of the aortic valve (AV) showing a slightly dilated aortic root (AR) that measures 4.2 cm. The left atrial (LA) size is normal. *Middle*: Recording of the mitral valve showing fluttering of the valve. The patient is in sinus rhythm. A different kind of flutter is seen in patients with atrial fibrillation. *Right*: Recording of the left ventricle showing an increase in left ventricular size to 6.5 cm and concentric left ventricular hypertrophy with an increase in the interventricular septum and posterior wall thickness to 1.3 cm, which makes a ratio of 1:1.

calcification of the aortic valve, multiple diastolic echoes (Fig. 6.29), and incomplete closure of the valve during systole. Increased motion of the interventricular septum and an increase in left ventricular and/or left atrial diameters should be seen (Figs. 6.29 through 6.31), as these are the echocardiographic features of patients with aortic insufficiency. Abnormal motion of the leaflets of the mitral valve is usually seen, such as the presence of "flutter" of the valve during diastole. It is a fine fluttering as compared with coarse fluttering seen in patients with atrial fibrillation (Fig. 6.31) without aortic insufficiency. However, if the patient has associated mitral valve disease with thickening or calcification of the mitral valve, fluttering may not be detected. An additional important echocardiographic sign in very severe aortic insufficiency is premature closure of the mitral valve (Fig. 6.32). The valve loses its double diamond appearance and only has one diamond representing an opening point or E point followed by an F point where the valve appears to close; the A wave is lost. The mitral valve closes before the QRS complex of the electrocardiogram. For patients with vegetation in the aortic valve, as seen in cases of subacute bacterial endocarditis, one may be able to record these vegetations, as shown in Figure 6.33.

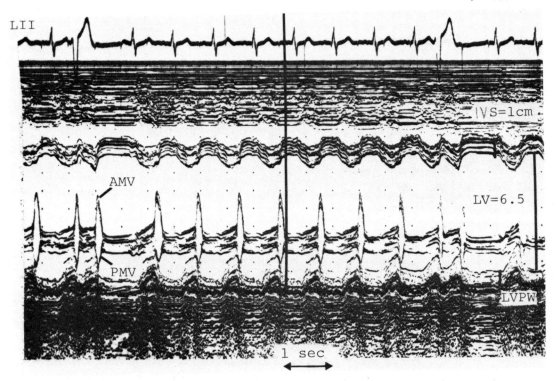

Figure 6.32. *Left*: Echocardiogram of the mitral valve with lead II of the electrocardiogram in a patient with severe aortic insufficiency. Note the very premature closure of the mitral valve, which is usually a sign of severe aortic insufficiency. *Right*: Recording of the left ventricle reveals an increase in the left ventricular cavity size to 6.5 cm. Note the ventricular extrasystoles recorded on the electrocardiogram in both panels. AMV = anterior mitral valve, PMV = posterior mitral valve, LVPW = left ventricular posterior wall, IVS = interventricular septum.

Points of Importance and Caution

1. Patients with aortic insufficiency present with a high frequency, diastolic murmur that is best recorded on logarithmic or log–log recording. At this setting the baseline noise is amplified. Therefore, you have to compensate for the gain in the amplifier so that you do not record artifacts. The best area to place the microphone is at the third or fourth intercostal space near the sternum. Record the tracings during quiet, held expiration. At times, the recording is best obtained with the patient in a sitting position. Record the phonocardiogram simultaneously with a carotid pulse tracing. Be sure not to apply too much pressure over the carotid artery because you may eliminate one of the most important abnormalities of the carotid pulse tracing, called pulsus bisferiens (double peaking during systole).

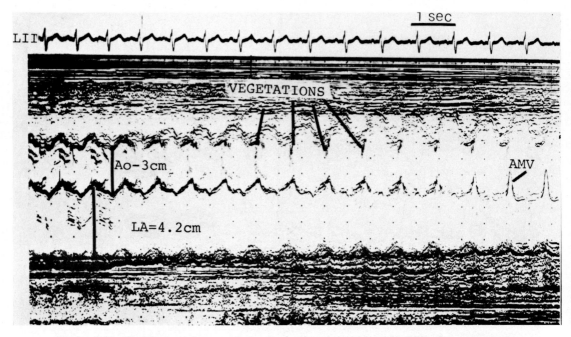

Figure 6.33. Simultaneously recorded echocardiogram and lead II (LII) of the electrocardiogram in a 24-year-old patient with severe aortic insufficiency and subacute bacterial endocarditis. On this scan from the aorta (AO) to the mitral valve (AMV), there are some echoes originating near the valve, which probably represent the vegetation of bacterial endocarditis. The left atrial (LA) internal dimension is increased and the aortic root is normal.

2. Turn the patient in a left lateral position, place the microphone at the mitral area, and set the amplifier for stethoscopic recording. A phonocardiogram recorded from this area simultaneously with the apexcardiogram helps to detect the presence of low frequency diastolic murmurs seen in this condition (Austin–Flint murmur).

3. Try to obtain a good recording of the apexcardiogram, which usually shows a round systolic wave and a prominent rapid filling wave. Do not apply too much pressure on the transducer over the apex.

4. In recording the echocardiogram, be sure to obtain a good tracing of the left ventricular cavity, mitral and aortic valves. Patients with aortic insufficiency present with a dilated aortic root and flutter of the mitral valve.

5. Do not rely on fluttering of the mitral valve for the diagnosis of aortic insufficiency. Flutter may occur in patients without aortic insufficiency. It is seen with atrial fibrillation and if the recording unit has sixty-cycle interference. In very severe aortic insufficiency, the mitral valve may close early and the A wave is lost. A separation of the valve leaflets in diastole is an unreliable sign in aortic insufficiency. The size of the aortic root and left ventricle are more conclusive. They should be dilated.

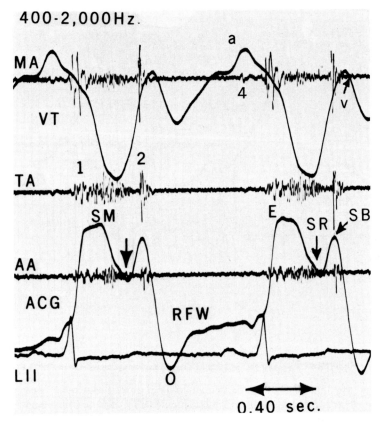

Figure 6.34. Simultaneously recorded phonocardiogram at the mitral (MA), tricuspid (TA), and aortic areas (AA), jugular venous tracing (VT), apexcardiogram (ACG), and lead II (LII) of the electrocardiogram in a 77-year-old patient with idiopathic hypertrophic subaortic stenosis. Note the presence of a fourth heart sound at the mitral area followed by normal first and second heart sounds. There is a high frequency, high amplitude systolic ejection murmur (SM) recorded in all precordial areas. The jugular venous tracing has normal contour. The patient was not in heart failure; therefore, the jugular venous tracing has no value in the diagnosis of idiopathic hypertrophic subaortic stenosis. The apexcardiogram shows an E point followed by a downward slope, systolic retraction (SR), and a late systolic bulge (SB). RFW = rapid filling wave.

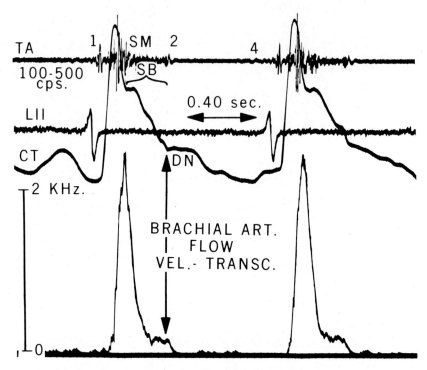

Figure 6.35. Simultaneously recorded phonocardiogram at the tricuspid area (TA), lead II (LII) of the electrocardiogram, carotid pulse tracing (CT), and the transcutaneous brachial artery flow velocity curve recorded with Doppler flowmeter technique. The first and second heart sounds are normal. There is a fourth heart sound. There is a high frequency, systolic ejection murmur (SM) recorded at the tricuspid area. The carotid pulse tracing shows the typical features of idiopathic hypertrophic subaortic stenosis including a rapid ascending limb followed by a rapid downward slope and a late systolic bulge (SB). The dicrotic notch (DN) is normal. Ejection time is prolonged. The rapid ejection at the beginning of systole is due to emptying of blood from the left ventricular cavity, which is unobstructed. The second bulge is the so-called secondary ejection of blood through the obstructed segment of the left ventricle. The brachial artery contour on the flow velocity curve shows that most of the ejection of blood is occurring in the first part of systole.

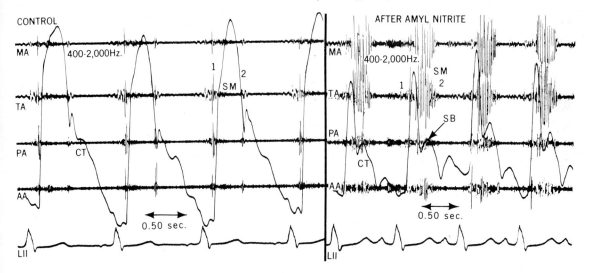

Figure 6.36. *Left*: Simultaneously recorded phonocardiogram at the mitral (MA), tricuspid (TA), pulmonic (PA), and aortic areas (AA), carotid pulse tracing (CT), and lead II (LII) of the electrocardiogram in a 52-year-old patient with idiopathic hypertrophic subaortic stenosis. The first and second heart sounds are normal. There is a high frequency, low amplitude systolic ejection murmur (SM) recorded best at the tricuspid area. Interestingly, the contour of the carotid pulse tracing is normal. This is not unusual in some patients with idiopathic hypertrophic subaortic stenosis. However, the use of maneuvers such as Valsalva, inhalation of amyl nitrite, exercise, etc. can precipitate changes in the contour of the carotid pulse wave. *Right*: Response of a patient with idiopathic hypertrophic subaortic stenosis after inhalation of amyl nitrite. There is a marked increase in amplitude of the systolic murmur, an increase in the heart rate, and the carotid tracing assumes the characteristic features of idiopathic hypertrophic subaortic stenosis as seen in Figure 6.35.

IDIOPATHIC HYPERTROPHIC SUBAORTIC STENOSIS

Idiopathic hypertrophic subaortic stenosis (IHSS) is a disease of unknown etiology in which there is asymmetric septal hypertrophy, or ASH phenomenon, causing obstruction of ventricular ejection.

Heart Sounds and Murmurs

The first heart sound is normal. The second heart sound shows normal amplitude of the aortic valve closure sound, which helps to differentiate IHSS from aortic valvular stenosis. Reverse splitting of the second heart sound (pulmonary closure sound preceding the aortic closure sound) is frequently seen, particularly in patients with a significant gradient at rest. Systolic ejection clicks, infrequent in this condition, are seen in less than 10% of patients. Prominent fourth heart sounds are quite common (Figs. 6.34 and 6.35). Third heart sounds are not heard unless the patient develops heart failure.

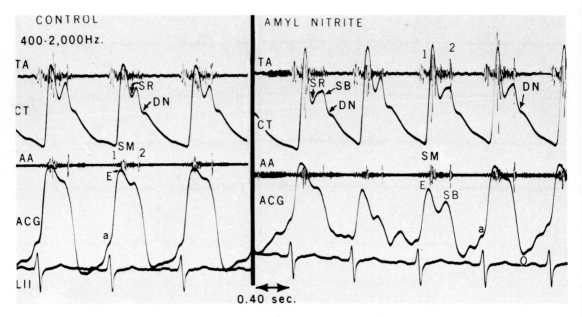

Figure 6.37. Simultaneously recorded phonocardiogram at the tricuspid (TA), and aortic areas (AA), carotid pulse tracing (CT), apexcardiogram (ACG), and lead II (LII) of the electrocardiogram in a patient with idiopathic hypertrophic subaortic stenosis. *Left*: The phonocardiographic features are the same as described previously. Of interest on this tracing is that the carotid pulse tracing does show the features of idiopathic hypertrophic subaortic stenosis. *Right*: The systolic retraction (SR) and the late systolic bulge (SB) become markedly exaggerated during inhalation of amyl nitrite. DN = dicrotic notch, SM = systolic murmur.

High frequency, high amplitude systolic ejection murmurs are common. They are recorded at the aortic and/or mitral areas and may radiate to both carotid arteries. This murmur probably represents turbulent flow across the midcavity obstruction and it usually has noisy characteristics (Figs. 6.34 and 6.35). It will increase in amplitude during maneuvers such as Valsalva and administration of isoproterenol, inhalation of amyl nitrite (Figs. 6.36 and 6.37), squatting, and in cardiac cycles following an atrial, junctional, or ventricular premature contraction or postural changes.

The murmur of aortic insufficiency has been described in this condition, although it is quite rare.

Carotid Pulse Tracing

The carotid pulse tracing is very useful in the diagnosis of idiopathic hypertrophic subaortic stenosis. The usual features include a rapid upstroke time followed by a rapid systolic retraction and a late systolic bulge, which is usually inscribed in the last third of ventricular systole. The dicrotic notch is normal and an anacrotic notch is not present (Figs. 6.36 and 6.37). If the carotid pulse tracing has a normal contour at rest, the pressure gradient across the midcavity of the left ventricle is

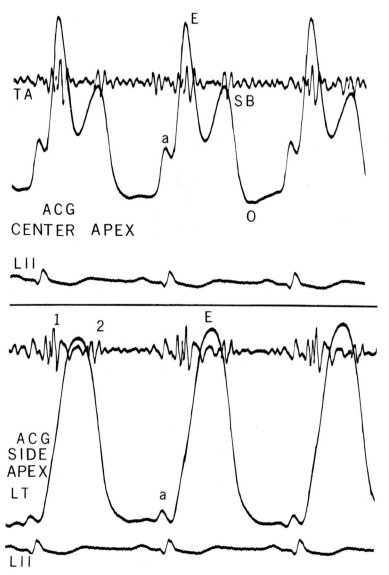

Figure 6.38. Simultaneously recorded phonocardiogram at the tricuspid area (TA), apex-cardiogram (ACG), and lead II (LII) of the electrocardiogram in a patient with idiopathic hypertrophic subaortic stenosis. The first and second heart sounds are normal. Note the low frequency vibratory artifacts seen during diastole on the phonocardiogram. The systolic murmur is not well recorded. *Top*: The apexcardiogram was recorded with the transducer placed exactly at the center of maximal apical impulse. It shows the typical features of idiopathic hypertrophic subaortic stenosis, including a prominent A wave, sharp E point followed by a downward slope and a late systolic bulge (SB). The rapid and slow filling waves are normal. *Bottom*: The transducer was located near the side of the apex and probably near the lateral aspect of the left ventricle. The recording now shows a small A wave and a systolic wave completely different from the one seen above. Both tracings are valid although the one on the top is more representative of this condition. The bottom tracing most likely represents hypertrophy of the left ventricle because there is a sustained systolic impulse throughout systole. The systolic retraction is not recorded.

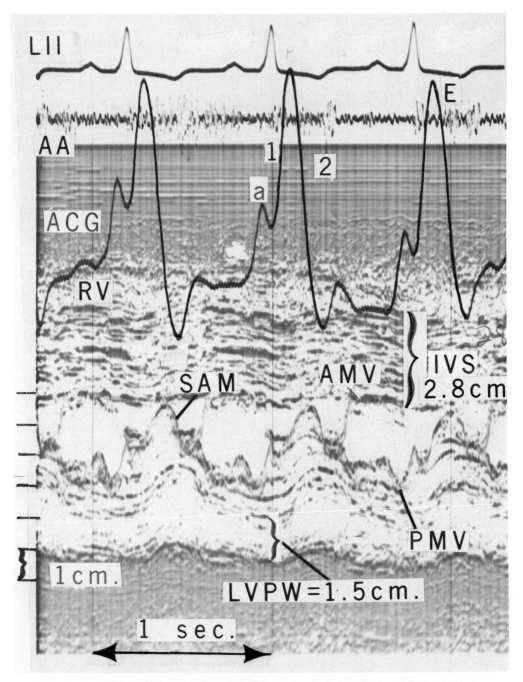

Figure 6.39. Echocardiogram of the mitral valve recorded simultaneously with aortic area (AA) phonocardiogram, apexcardiogram (ACG), and lead II (LII) of the electrocardiogram. In patients with idiopathic hypertrophic subaortic stenosis, the anterior mitral valve (AMV) bulges anteriorly causing a systolic anterior motion (SAM) of the valve. The valve almost touches the interventricular septum (IVS). Note the disproportional increase in thickness of the interventricular septum, which measures 2.8 cm with the left ventricular posterior wall (LVPW) measuring 1.5 cm indicating eccentric or asymmetric septal hypertrophy. PMV = posterior mitral valve, RV = right ventricle.

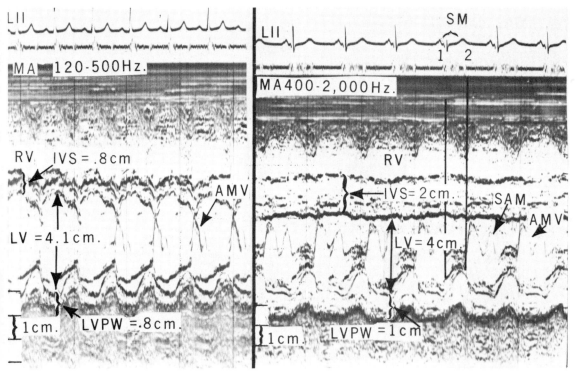

Figure 6.40. *Left*: Simultaneously recorded echocardiogram, mitral area (MA) phonocardiogram, and lead II (LII) of the electrocardiogram showing normal interventricular septal (IVS) motion and thickness. Right (RV) and left ventricular (LV) cavity size and left ventricular posterior wall (LVPW) thicknesses are normal. The septal/posterior wall ratio of 1:1 is normal. *Right*: Simultaneously recorded echocardiogram, mitral area (MA) phonocardiogram, and lead II (LII) of the electrocardiogram in a patient with idiopathic hypertrophic subaortic stenosis. Interventricular septal thickness is increased to 2 cm and left ventricular posterior wall thickness is normal at 1 cm. An important feature in this condition is that septal thickness exceeds that of the left ventricular posterior wall and the ratio is usually greater than 1.3:1. In this patient, the ratio is 2:1. Increased septal thickness, known as asymmetric septal hypertrophy, is seen primarily in idiopathic hypertrophic subaortic stenosis, but may be found in other conditions. In contrast, patients with aortic valvular stenosis or other forms of left ventricular hypertrophy exhibit increased thickness of these structures in identical degrees (concentric hypertrophy). In this patient, right and left ventricular dimensions are normal. The mitral valve has normal diastolic motion, but there is systolic anterior motion (SAM), which is also an important feature in the diagnosis of idiopathic hypertrophic subaortic stenosis.

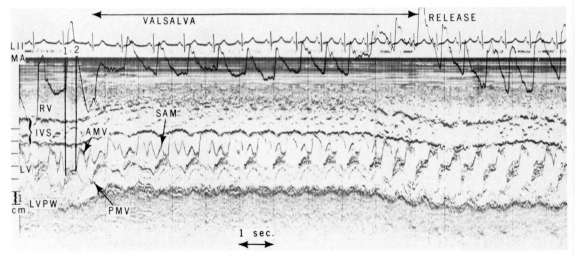

Figure 6.41. Simultaneous echocardiogram, mitral area (MA) phonocardiogram, carotid pulse tracing, and lead II (LII) of the electrocardiogram recorded prior to, during and after the Valsalva maneuver in a 41-year-old patient with idiopathic hypertrophic subaortic stenosis. Note the abnormal motion of the mitral valve during systole where it bulges anteriorly (SAM). During the Valsalva maneuver it is more accentuated and becomes less conspicuous after the maneuver. There is also asymmetric septal hypertrophy with the interventricular septum (IVS) being thicker than the left ventricular posterior wall (LVPW). PMV = posterior mitral valve, AMV = anterior mitral valve, RV = right ventricle, LV = left ventricle.

usually small. If the features described above are not present and this diagnosis is suspected clinically, administration of amyl nitrite (Figs. 6.36 and 6.37), isoproterenol, and the Valsalva maneuver usually induce the features described above.

Jugular Venous Pulse Tracing

The jugular venous pulse usually is not helpful in the diagnosis of this disease (Fig. 6.34). At times, one may detect a large A wave, which probably represents a marked degree of asymmetric septal hypertrophy that would impair normal right ventricular contraction. However, it must be emphasized that cases of idiopathic hypertrophy of the outflow tract of the right ventricle have been described simulating the findings seen in idiopathic hypertrophic subaortic stenosis.

Apexcardiogram

The apexcardiogram shows a prominent A wave, probably due to decreased left ventricular distensibility (Fig. 6.38). The E point is usually sharp and well recognized and is followed by a midsystolic retraction. For this retraction to be significant, the maximal downward systolic deflection should reach approximately one third of the total amplitude of the apexcardiogram as measured from the E to the O point. After the systolic retraction, there is a late systolic bulge that has a

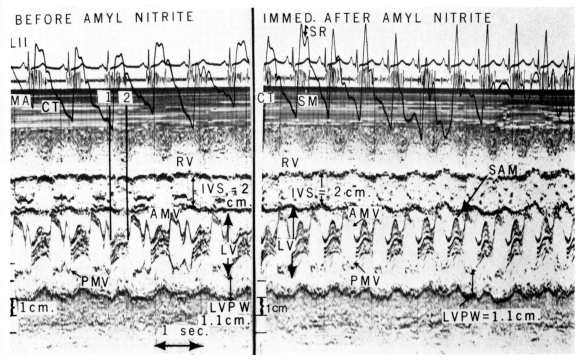

Figure 6.42. *Left*: Simultaneously recorded echocardiogram, mitral area (MA) phonocardiogram, carotid pulse tracing (CT), and lead II (LII) of the electrocardiogram in a 41-year-old patient with idiopathic hypertrophic subaortic stenosis. This shows the typical features of idiopathic hypertrophic subaortic stenosis, including systolic anterior motion (SAM) of the mitral valve, and increased thickness of the interventricular septum (IVS) in relation to the posterior wall of the left ventricle (LVPW). *Right*: Inhalation of amyl nitrite exaggerates the systolic anterior motion of the mitral valve and causes tachycardia and more conspicuous abnormalities on the carotid pulse tracing as compared with the left panel. PMV = posterior mitral valve, AMV = anterior mitral valve, SR = systolic retraction, SM = systolic murmur, RV = right ventricle, LV = left ventricle.

maximal peak near the second heart sound (Figs. 6.34 and 6.37). Occasionally, a round systolic wave of the type seen in patients with severe left ventricular hypertrophy from any cause is seen. The rapid filling wave is usually small and the transition between this wave and the slow filling wave is inconspicuous. As described for heart murmurs and the carotid pulse tracing, some of these changes, if not present at rest, may be induced by exercise, Valsalva maneuver, administration of drugs, extrasystoles, etc.

Systolic Time Intervals

Ejection time is prolonged in patients with idiopathic hypertrophic subaortic stenosis who have significant outflow tract obstruction. Valsalva maneuver, exercise, postextrasystolic beats, administration of vasopressor agents and inhalation of amyl nitrite will increase the gradient across the outflow tract of the left ventricle, therefore prolonging the ejection time.

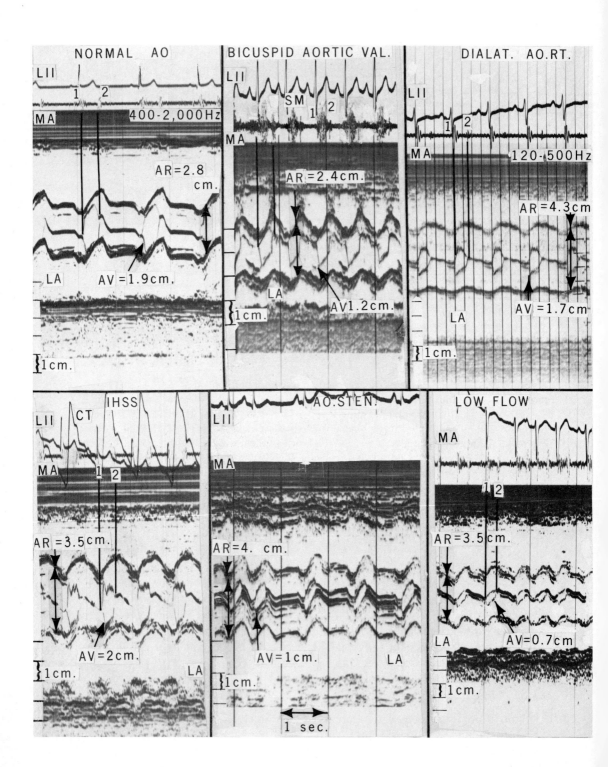

148

Vectorcardiogram

The vectorcardiogram may be normal if the patient has a mild degree of idiopathic hypertrophic subaortic stenosis. However, in more severe states, it will show signs of left ventricular hypertrophy and strain and in some patients may mimic myocardial infarction pattern.

Echocardiogram

It must be emphasized that the pathophysiology of this disease is still not fully understood. However, echocardiography is a very important noninvasive technique in the diagnosis of idiopathic hypertrophic subaortic stenosis (Figs. 6.39 through 6.43). It is also useful for follow-up to determine if the degree of obstruction is increasing. A common finding in patients with idiopathic hypertrophic subaortic stenosis, with or without gradient, is increased thickness of the interventricular septum in relation to left ventricular posterior wall thickness, also called asymmetric septal hypertrophy. In most patients the ratio of the interventricular septum to the left ventricular posterior wall is greater than the normal ratio of 1.3:1 (Figs. 6.39, 6.40, and 6.42). Echocardiographic findings also include abnormal systolic anterior motion of the mitral valve, which may contribute to the midcavity obstruction (Figs. 6.39 through 6.42). In some patients, the degree of systolic anterior motion or SAM of the anterior mitral valve may be so exaggerated that it will touch the interventricular septum. However, caution must be exercised in interpreting this finding. If the ultrasonic beam is pointed superiorly at the point where the mitral valve leaflet is seen, echoes from the mitral annulus are recorded and this structure may actually move anteriorly during ventricular contraction. False positive findings may, therefore, be encountered in normal individuals. An index for the degree of obstruction developed by several investigators takes into consideration the abnormal anterior mitral valve motion, separation of the anterior mitral leaflet, and the interventricular septum. It must be emphasized that the interventricular septum to posterior wall thickness ratio may be abnormal in children with congenital heart disease and associated right ventricular hypertrophy, such as tetralogy of Fallot, transposition of the great vessels, and other congenital abnormalities. Abnormal motion of the aortic valve is seen in

---

Figure 6.43. This is a composite figure showing the most common echocardiographic abnormalities of the aortic valve. *Top Left*: Recording of a normal aortic valve and left atrium. *Top Middle*: A bicuspid aortic valve showing eccentric motion of the valve in diastole. *Top Right*: Recording of a patient with low cardiac output and a dilated aortic root. The aortic valve seems quite small in relation to the aortic root. However, it has a normal opening excursion. *Bottom Left*: Recording of a patient with idiopathic hypertrophic subaortic stenosis showing a relatively normal aortic valve opening but exhibiting systolic notching. *Bottom Middle*: Recording of the aortic valve in a patient with aortic stenosis showing a very small aortic opening excursion. The aortic root size is at the upper limits of normal. The aortic valve opening is 1 cm. Heavy echoes originating in the valve indicate calcification and fibrosis. *Bottom Right*: Recording of the aortic valve in a patient with congestive heart failure from unknown cause. The low cardiac output causes a small rate of excursion of the valve that seems to be stenotic when in reality it is not. The valve excursion is small because of the small stroke volume.

many patients with idiopathic hypertrophic subaortic stenosis, particularly those who have significant gradients at rest. In these patients, premature systolic closure of the aortic valve is seen. It probably is due to the fact that most of the left ventricular stroke output is ejected into the aorta in the first third of mechanical systole with the valve subsequently moving to a semiclosed position and then reopening during late ventricular systole.

Maneuvers and Pharmacologic Agents

The Valsalva maneuver is important in the recognition of hypertrophic subaortic stenosis. It causes a decrease in left ventricular volume, which greatly increases the obstruction. Therefore, during the Valsalva maneuver, intensity of the systolic ejection murmur is markedly increased. Pharmacologic agents such as amyl nitrite provoke an increase in the gradient across the outflow tract of the left ventricle and are, therefore, useful in the diagnosis of this condition. As shown in Figure 6.42, inhalation of amyl nitrite results in an exaggeration of abnormalities on the echocardiogram as described above.

Points of Caution and Importance—Echocardiogram

1. If all the criteria for this condition are not present, such as asymmetric septal hypertrophy with midsystolic closure of the aortic valve and systolic anterior motion of the mitral valve, provocative maneuvers should be used.
2. Asymmetric septal hypertrophy should be determined at the mitral level. Look for systolic anterior motion when the mitral leaflets are recorded simultaneously.
3. Make sure that tricuspid valve echoes superimposed on the septum do not falsely create the impression of asymmetric septal hypertrophy.

BIBLIOGRAPHY

Abelmann, W.H.:   Aortic stenosis in older patients. N. Engl. J. Med., *281*:1305, 1969.

Bache, R.J., Wang, Y., and Greenfield, J.C., Jr.:   Left ventricular ejection time in valvular aortic stenosis. Circulation, *47*:527, 1973.

Benchimol, A.:   Non-invasive diagnostic techniques in cardiology. Baltimore: Williams & Wilkins, 1977.

Benchimol, A., and Matsuo, S.:   Ejection time before and after aortic valve replacement. Am. J. Cardiol., *27*:244, 1971.

Boiteau, G.M., Libanoff, A.J., and Allenstein, B.J.:   Upstroke time ratio in valvular aortic insufficiency. Am. J. Cardiol., *14*:162, 1964.

Bonner, A.J., Jr., Sacks, H.N., and Tavel, M.E.:   Assessing the severity of aortic stenosis by phonocardiography and external carotid pulse recordings. Circulation, *48*:247, 1973.

Braunwald, E., Lambrew, C.T., Rockoff, S.D., Ross, J. Jr., and Morrow, A.G.:   Idiopathic hypertrophic subaortic stenosis. I. A description of the disease based upon an analysis of 64 patients. Circulation, *30*(4):3, 1964.

Caulfield, W.H., deLeon, A.C. Jr., Perloff, J.K., and Steelman, R.B.:   The clinical significance of the fourth heart sound in aortic stenosis. Am. J. Cardiol., *28*:179, 1971.

Cohn, K.E., Flamm, M.D., and Hancock, E.W.:   Amyl nitrite inhalation as a screening test for hypertrophic subaortic stenosis. Am. J. Cardiol., *21*:681, 1968.

Cohn, K.E., Sandler, H., and Hancock, E.W.:   Mechanisms of pulsus alternans. Circulation, *36*:372, 1967.

Dressler, W., and Rubin, R.:   Complex shape and variability of the diastolic murmur of aortic regurgitation. Am. J. Cardiol., *18*:616, 1966.

Eddleman, E.E. Jr., Bancroft, W.H. Jr., and Swatzell, R.H. Jr.:   A contour study of the carotid pulse in normal subjects, aortic valvular disease, and hypertrophic subaortic stenosis. Comput. Biomed. Res., *3*:274, 1970.

Epstein, E.J., Coulshed, N., Brown, A.K., and Doukas, N.G.:   The "A" wave of the apex cardiogram in aortic valve disease and cardiomyopathy. Br. Heart J., *30*:591, 1968.

Fearon, R.E., Cohen, L.S., O'Hara, J.M., and Goodyer, A.V.N.:   Diastolic murmurs due to two sequelae of atherosclerotic coronary artery disease: ventricular aneurysm and coronary artery stenosis. Am. Heart J., *76*:252, 1968.

Feizi, O., Symons, C., and Yacoub, M.:   Echocardiography of the aortic valve. I. Studies of normal aortic valve, aortic stenosis, aortic regurgitation, and mixed aortic valve disease. Br. Heart J., *36*:341, 1974.

Feizi, O., Symons, C., and Yacoub, M.:   Echocardiography of normal and diseased aortic valve. Br. Heart J., *35*:560, 1973.

Finegan, R.E., Gianelly, R.E., and Harrison, D.C.:   Aortic stenosis in the elderly. Relevance of age to diagnosis and treatment. N. Engl. J. Med., *281*:1261, 1969.

Fishleder, B.L.:   Exploración cardiovascular y fonomecano-cardiografía clinica. Mexico, D.F.: La Prensa Medica Mexicana, 1966.

Frank, S., and Braunwald, E.:   Idiopathic hypertrophic subaortic stenosis. Clinical analysis of 126 patients with emphasis on the natural history. Circulation, *37*:759, 1968.

Giles, T.D., Martinez, E.C., and Burch, G.E.:   Gallavardin phenomenon in aortic stenosis. A possible mechanism. Arch. Intern. Med., *134*:747, 1974.

Gramiak, R., Shah, P.M.:   Echocardiography of the aortic root. Invest. Radiol., *3*:356, 1968.

Hancock, E.W., and Eldridge, F.:   Muscular subaortic stenosis. Reversibility with varying cardiac cycle length. Am. J. Cardiol., *18*:515, 1966.

Henry, W.L., Clark, C.E., and Epstein, S.E.:   Asymmetric septal hypertrophy. Echocardiographic identification of the pathognomonic anatomic abnormality of IHSS. Circulation, *47*:225, 1973.

Hernberg, J., Weiss, B., and Keegan, A.:   The ultrasonic recording of aortic valve motion. Radiology, *94*:361, 1970.

Joyner, C.R., Harrison, F.S., and Gruber, J.W.:   Diagnosis of hypertrophic subaortic stenosis with a Doppler velocity flow detector. Ann. Intern. Med., *74*:692, 1971.

Judge, T.P., and Kennedy, J.W.:   Estimation of aortic regurgitation by diastolic pulse wave analysis. Circulation, *41*:659, 1970.

Lillehei, C.W., Bonnabeau, R.C. Jr., and Sellers, R.D.:   Subaortic stenosis: Diagnostic criteria, surgical approach, and late follow-up in 25 patients. J. Thorac. Cardiovasc. Surg., *55*:94, 1968.

Lyle, D.P., Bancroft, W.H. Jr., Tucker, M., and Eddleman, E.E. Jr.:   Slopes of the carotid pulse wave in normal subjects, aortic valvular disease and hypertrophic subaortic stenosis. Circulation, *43*:374, 1971.

Macieira-Coelho, E., Faleiro, L.L., and Santos, A.L.: Evaluation of aortic stenosis by noninvasive techniques. Acta. Cardiol., (Brux) *27*:680, 1972.

Marcus, F.I., and Jones, R.C.: The use of the Valsalva maneuver to differentiate fixed-orifice aortic stenosis from muscular subaortic stenosis. Am. Heart J., *69*:473, 1965.

Marcus, F.I., Perloff, J.K., and DeLeon, A.C.: The use of amyl nitrite in the hemodynamic assessment of aortic valvular and muscular subaortic stenosis. Am. Heart J., *68*:468, 1964.

Mason, D.T., Braunwald, E., and Ross, J. Jr.: Effects of changes in body position on the severity of obstruction to left ventricular outflow in idiopathic hypertrophic subaortic stenosis. Circulation, *33*:374, 1966.

Moreyra, E., Klein, J.J., Shimada, H., and Segal, B.L.: Idiopathic hypertrophic subaortic stenosis diagnosed by reflected ultrasound. Am. J. Cardiol., *23*:32, 1969.

Morrow, A.G., Fort, L. III, Roberts, W.C., and Braunwald, E.: Discrete subaortic stenosis complicated by aortic valvular regurgitation; clinical, hemodynamic, and pathologic studies and the results of operative treatment. Circulation, *31*:163, 1965.

Moskowitz, R.L., and Wechsler, B.M.: Left ventricular ejection time in aortic and mitral valve disease. Am. J. Cardiol., *15*:809, 1965.

Nanda, N.C., Gramiak, R., Manning, J., Mahoney, E.B., Lipchik, E.O., and DeWeese, J.A.: Echocardiographic recognition of the congenital bicuspid aortic valve. Circulation, *49*:870, 1974.

Nanda, N.C., Gramiak, R., Shah, P.M., Stewart, S., and DeWeese, J.A.: Echocardiography in the diagnosis of idiopathic hypertrophic subaortic stenosis co-existing with aortic valve disease. Circulation, *50*:752, 1974.

Nasser, W., Tavel, M.E., Feigenbaum, H., and Fisch, C.: Austin–Flint murmur versus the murmur of organic mitral stenosis. N. Engl. J. Med., *275*:1007, 1966.

Parisi, A.F., Salzman, S.H., and Schechter, E.: Systolic time intervals in severe aortic valve disease; changes with surgery and hemodynamic correlations. Circulation, *44*:539, 1971.

Park, S.C., Steinfeld, L., and Dimich, I.: Systolic time intervals in infants with congestive heart failure. Circulation, *47*:1281, 1973.

Parker, E., Craige, E., and Hood, W.P. Jr.: The Austin–Flint murmur and the a wave of the apexcardiogram in aortic regurgitation. Circulation, *43*:349, 1971.

Pasyk, S., and Dubiel, J.: The external carotid pulse wave in aortic stenosis. Cor Vasa, *9*:48, 1967.

Perloff, J.K.: Clinical recognition of aortic stenosis. The physical signs and differential diagnosis of the various forms of obstruction to left ventricular outflow. Prog. Cardiovasc. Dis., *10*:323, 1967.

Popp, R.L., and Harrison, D.C.: Ultrasound in the diagnosis and evaluation of therapy of idiopathic hypertrophic subaortic stenosis. Circulation, *40*:905, 1969.

Pridie, R.B., Benham, R., and Oakley, C.M.: Echocardiography of the mitral valve in aortic valve disease. Br. Heart J., *33*:296, 1971.

Rich, L.L., and Tavel, M.E.: Arterial "triple hump" of idiopathic hypertrophic subaortic stenosis. Chest, *60*:595, 1971.

Roberts, W.C., Perloff, J.K., and Costantino, T.: Severe valvular aortic stenosis in patients over 65 years of age: a clinicopathologic study. Am. J. Cardiol., *27*:497, 1971.

Rothbaum, D.A., DeJoseph, R.L., and Tavel, M.: Diastolic heart sound produced by mid-diastolic closure of the mitral valve. Am. J. Cardiol., *34*:367, 1974.

Sainani, G.S., Luisada, A.A., and Gupta, P.: Mapping of the precordium; II. Murmurs and abnormal sounds. Acta. Cardiol., (Brux) *23*:152, 1968.

Sarewitz, A.B., and Muehsam, G.E.:   Aortic insufficiency simulating combined aortic stenosis and insufficiency. Dis. Chest, *48*:291, 1965.

Schlant, R.C.:   Calcific aortic stenosis. Am. J. Cardiol., *27*:581, 1971.

Schwab, R.H., and Killough, J.H.:   The phonocardiographic differentiation of pulmonic and aortic insufficiency. Circulation, *32*:352, 1965.

Shah, P.M., Gramiak, R., Adelman, A.G., and Wigle, E.D.:   Echocardiographic assessment of the effects of surgery and propranolol on the dynamics of outflow obstruction in hypertrophic subaortic stenosis. Circulation, *45*:516, 1972.

Shah, P.M., Gramiak, R., Adelman, A.G., and Wigle, E.D.:   Role of echocardiography in diagnostic and hemodynamic assessment of hypertrophic subaortic stenosis. Circulation, *44*:891, 1971.

Shibuya, M.:   Auscultatory findings of heart sounds and murmurs in congenital heart anomalies and acquired valvular diseases. Special reference to the determination of the severity of the condition on the basis of phonocardiography. Jap. J. Thorac. Surg., *18*:1008, 1965.

Starr, I., Ambrosi, C., Manchester, J.H., and Shelburne, J.C.:   Diagnosis of aortic stenosis from the carotid pulse and its derivative. Br. Heart J., *35*:1062, 1973.

Stefadouros, M.A., and Witham, A.C.:   Systolic time intervals by echocardiography. Circulation, *51* (1):114, 1975.

Stein, P.D., and Munter, W.A.:   New functional concept of valvular mechanics in normal and diseased aortic valves. Circulation, *44*:101, 1971.

Tafur, E., Cohen, L.S., and Levine, H.D.:   The apex cardiogram in left ventricular outflow tract obstruction. Circulation, *30*:392, 1964.

Tajik, A.J., Gau, G.T., Ritter, D.G., and Schattenberg, T.T.:   Illustrative echocardiograms: mitral valve motion in severe aortic regurgitation. Chest, *63*:271, 1973.

Tavel, M.E.:   Clinical phonocardiography. Reversed (paradoxic) splitting of the second heart sound in aortic stenosis. Dis. Chest, *54*:55, 1968.

Tavel, M.E., and Nasser, W.K.:   Murmur alternans in aortic stenosis. Chest, *57*:176, 1970.

Usher, B.W., Goulden, D., and Murgo, J.P.:   Echocardiographic detection of supravalvular aortic stenosis. Circulation, *49*:1257, 1974.

Vogel, J.H.K., and Blount, S.G. Jr.:   Clinical evaluation in localizing level of obstruction to outflow from left ventricle; importance of early systolic ejection click. Am. J. Cardiol., *15*:782, 1965.

Vogelpole, L., Nellen, M., Beck, W., and Schrire, V.:   The value of squatting in the diagnosis of mild aortic regurgitation. Am. Heart J., *77*:709, 1969.

Wigle, E.D., Auger, P., and Marquis, Y.:   Muscular subaortic stenosis; the direct relation between the intraventricular pressure difference and the left ventricular ejection time. Circulation, *36*:36, 1967.

Winsberg, F., Gabor, G.E., Hernberg, J.G., and Weiss, B.:   Fluttering of the mitral valve in aortic insufficiency. Circulation, *41*:225, 1970.

Yeh, H. D., Winsberg, F., and Mercer, E. N.:   Echographic aortic valve orifice dimension: its use in evaluating aortic stenosis and cardiac output. J. Clin. Ultrasound, *1*:182, 1973.

7
Tricuspid
Valvular Disease

Primary organic involvement of the tricuspid valve, either stenosis or insufficiency, is rare, and when present is usually due to rheumatic heart disease in the adult population or congenital heart disease in children. Tricuspid insufficiency, however, is relatively common in the late stage of other valvular lesions such as with mitral stenosis or insufficiency, myocardial disease, coronary artery disease, or any other conditions associated with heart failure. The development of high pressure in the pulmonary circulation causes dilation of the right ventricle and, as a secondary event, the tricuspid annulus dilates and allows insufficiency to occur.

The auscultatory and phonocardiographic findings in tricuspid stenosis or insufficiency grossly simulate the ones seen in mitral valvular disease as described in Chapter 5.

TRICUSPID STENOSIS

Heart Sounds and Murmurs

The first heart sound is usually accentuated and best recorded at the tricuspid area. With progressive thickening or calcification of the tricuspid valve, amplitude of the first heart sound decreases proportionally due to a diminished mobility of the valve (Fig. 7.1). The second heart sound is usually normal. Third or fourth heart sounds originating in the right ventricle are not present unless there is associated tricuspid insufficiency. A high frequency, early diastolic vibration occurring 0.06–0.14 sec after the second heart sound is usually due to the opening snap of the tricuspid valve, and has phonocardiographic characteristics similar to the opening snap of the mitral valve as seen in patients with mitral stenosis. The second sound-opening snap interval should be measured from the pulmonary component of the second heart sound to the opening snap and not from the aortic component of the second heart sound. However, this is not always possible since many of these patients have a single second heart sound and, therefore, this interval cannot be measured accurately.

The murmur of tricuspid stenosis has a low frequency characteristic and is best recorded on the stethoscopic setting (50–500 Hz). This murmur starts shortly after the second heart sound or after the opening snap, if present; it reaches a maximal peak in mid-diastole, coinciding with the maximal velocity of flow across the

154

stenotic tricuspid valve (Fig. 7.1). Subsequently, the murmur diminishes in amplitude at the end of diastole and terminates prior to atrial contraction. With the onset of atrial contraction, a second diastolic murmur can be recorded if the patient is in regular sinus rhythm (Fig. 7.1). This atrial systolic murmur, also called presystolic accentuation of the diastolic murmur, has the same characteristics as those described for the murmur of mitral stenosis, with the maximal peak at the time of inscription of the P wave of the electrocardiogram. It terminates with the first heart sound. The mid-diastolic rumble or murmur and atrial systolic murmur increase during inspiration because during that phase of the respiratory cycle there is increased return of blood flow across the stenotic tricuspid valve, creating more turbulent blood flow across the tricuspid valve.

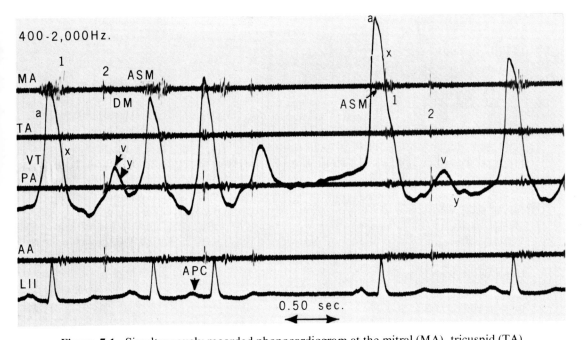

Figure 7.1. Simultaneously recorded phonocardiogram at the mitral (MA), tricuspid (TA), pulmonic (PA), and aortic areas (AA), jugular venous tracing (VT), and lead II (LII) of the electrocardiogram in a patient with tricuspid stenosis due to rheumatic heart disease. The first two heart beats are sinus beats. The third beat is an atrial premature contraction (APC), which is followed by a compensatory pause. In the regular sinus beat the A wave is quite prominent. The first heart sound is diminished. The second heart sound is of normal amplitude. There is a medium frequency, high amplitude mid-diastolic murmur that starts shortly after the second heart sound. It decreases in amplitude in midsystole and increases again during atrial contraction when the atriosystolic murmur is recorded. The jugular venous tracing shows the typical abnormalities seen in patients with tricuspid stenosis, including a quite prominent A wave followed by a normal X descent and a V wave that is followed by a very slow Y descent. This is particularly well seen in the third beat, which is an atrial premature contraction followed by a long compensatory pause. Following the premature atrial contraction, amplitude of the A wave increases markedly due to augmentation of blood in the right atrium, which elevates pressure load in that chamber.

Carotid Pulse Tracing

The contour of the carotid pulse tracing is normal. If the patient is in congestive heart failure, the ejection time shortens and the pre-ejection period is prolonged.

Jugular Venous Pulse Tracing

It is very important to obtain a technically good jugular venous tracing. This is one of the most important pulse waves for the diagnosis of tricuspid stenosis, particularly if the patient is in sinus rhythm. A large A wave is frequently present due to forceful right atrial contraction against the stenotic tricuspid valve (Fig. 7.1). In some cases, the A–V wave ratio may be as high as 5:1. Following the A wave, the X descent is recorded during systole and has normal characteristics. The V wave has a normal configuration and amplitude and its peak coincides with, precedes, or follows the opening snap of the tricuspid valve if this vibration is present. After the V wave, the Y descent is inscribed. It is characterized by a slow downslope due to the decreased rate of emptying of the right atrium into the right ventricle (Fig. 7.1).

Apexcardiogram

The apexcardiogram of the left ventricle is normal and may be very difficult to record because most of the precordial vibrations are caused by right atrial and right ventricular motion. However, in some patients, a right ventricular apexcardiogram may be recorded. A technically satisfactory tracing is difficult to obtain and requires a great deal of patience from the technician. A good recording should show a small A wave, sharp E point, and rapid systolic retraction, and the O point of the right ventricular apexcardiogram should coincide with the opening snap of the tricuspid valve. The rapid filling wave is absent or shallow and the transition between the rapid filling wave and the slow filling wave is inconspicuous. Measurement of these intervals does not contribute significantly to the diagnosis of this condition.

Vectorcardiogram

The vectorcardiogram is usually helpful by showing signs of right atrial or right ventricular hypertrophy in which case a good recording of the P loop, especially in the horizontal plane, shows most forces in front of the O point. The QRS loop is also oriented anteriorly and to the right or left of the O point, which is indicative of right ventricular hypertrophy (Fig. 7.2).

Echocardiogram

We have recorded very few echocardiograms of the tricuspid valve in patients with tricuspid stenosis. The normal echocardiographic pattern of tricuspid valve motion is shown in Figure 7.3. The waveform configuration of the tricuspid valve is very similar to normal mitral valve motion on the echocardiogram (see Chap. 5). Abnormalities of tricuspid valve motion in tricuspid stenosis are similar to those described for patients with mitral stenosis, i.e., decrease in the E–F slope of the

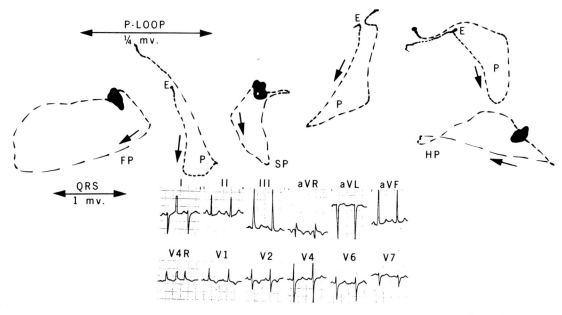

Figure 7.2. Simultaneously recorded vectorcardiogram and electrocardiogram in a nine-year-old patient with tetralogy of Fallot, characterized by a ventricular septal defect, pulmonary stenosis, the aorta overriding the interventricular septum, and right ventricular hypertrophy. This patient also has some degree of tricuspid insufficiency. The electrocardiogram shows sinus rhythm, right axis deviation, and prominent R waves in V4R and V1 indicating right ventricular hypertrophy. The important feature on the vectorcardiogram is marked displacement of the P loop to the front of the E point, indicating right atrial hypertrophy. There is also anterior displacement of the QRS forces in the horizontal plane indicating right ventricular hypertrophy.

anterior leaflet and paradoxical anterior motion of the posterior leaflet. Unfortunately, good recordings of the posterior leaflet are not always possible to obtain. Multiple and disorganized echoes derived from this valvular structure indicate calcification or thickening of the tricuspid valve. Elevation of right ventricular end-diastolic pressure is usually indicative of poor, late right ventricular end-diastolic compliance, resulting in prolongation of the A–C interval. Measurements of the P–R interval on the electrocardiogram minus the A–C interval on the echocardiogram are shortened considerably. Closure of the tricuspid valve may also be interrupted by a deflection occurring shortly after the P wave of the electrocardiogram or at the beginning of the QRS complex.

TRICUSPID INSUFFICIENCY

Heart Sounds and Murmurs

The first sound is diminished because the velocity of motion of the tricuspid leaflets is decreased (Figs. 7.4 through 7.8). The second heart sound is normal or has increased amplitude (Figs. 7.4, 7.6, 7.7). If the second heart sound is split and

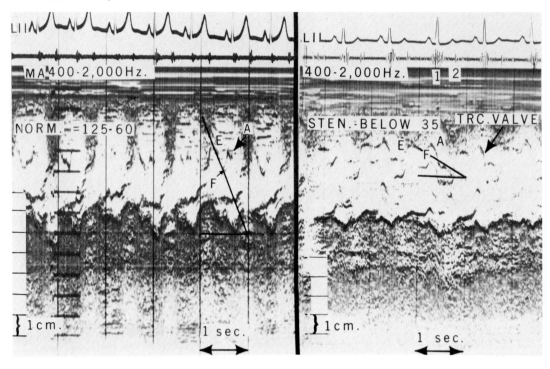

Figure 7.3. *Left:* Simultaneously recorded echocardiogram, mitral area (MA) phonocardiogram, and lead II (LII) of the electrocardiogram revealing a normal tricuspid valve and showing how to measure the E–F slope. *Right:* Simultaneously recorded echocardiogram, mitral area phonocardiogram, and lead II of the electrocardiogram of a patient with tricuspid stenosis showing a marked decrease in the E–F slope below 35 mm/sec. Note the paradoxical anterior motion of the posterior leaflet of the tricuspid valve.

both the aortic and pulmonic components are clearly identified, the pulmonary valve closure sound may be accentuated, indicating pulmonary hypertension. If pulmonary hypertension is very severe, exceeding ±60 mm Hg, the pulmonary valve closure sound is well transmitted to the mitral and aortic areas. Therefore, it is important to obtain phonocardiographic recordings at the mitral and aortic areas in patients with tricuspid valvular disease. Systolic ejection clicks, recorded in approximately 20% of patients with tricuspid insufficiency, are due to marked dilatation of the pulmonary arteries. A third heart sound, also called proto- or early diastolic gallop, is part of the auscultatory and phonocardiographic findings in tricuspid insufficiency (Figs. 7.6, 7.8). It reflects augmented right ventricular filling due to a large volume of blood crossing the insufficient tricuspid valve in early diastole. This is not necessarily a sign of congestive heart failure. A fourth heart sound may also be recorded if the patient is in sinus rhythm (Figs. 7.6, 7.8).

The systolic murmur of tricuspid insufficiency starts during the period of isovolumic contraction, i.e., with or shortly after the first heart sound. This regurgitant murmur is best recorded with a logarithmic setting and has a maximum peak in early systole, reaching a plateau in midsystole, and terminating prior to or

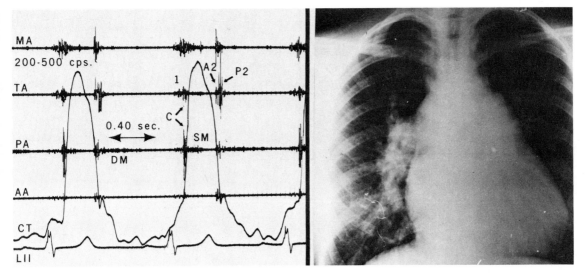

Figure 7.4. *Left:* Simultaneously recorded phonocardiogram at the mitral (MA), tricuspid (TA), pulmonic (PA), and aortic areas (AA), carotid pulse tracing (CT), and lead II (LII) of the electrocardiogram in a 23-year-old patient with a ventricular septal defect, severe pulmonary hypertension, and tricuspid insufficiency. The first heart sound is diminished. The second heart sound is slightly split and the pulmonic component is markedly accentuated. There is also a systolic ejection click due to a dilated pulmonary artery, and a high frequency, high amplitude systolic regurgitant murmur that reaches a peak in early systole. This murmur is most likely due to tricuspid insufficiency, although some component of this murmur is due to the ventricular septal defect. *Right:* Chest X-ray of the same patient in the PA position showing marked enlargement of the heart with prominence of the main and right pulmonary arteries, as well as enlargement of the cardiac chambers. (From A. Benchimol: Non-Invasive Diagnostic Techniques in Cardiology. Copyright 1977 by The Williams & Wilkins Company, Baltimore. Used by permission.)

with the second heart sound (Figs. 7.4, 7.5, 7.7). This murmur is recorded best at the tricuspid area and transmits well to the right side of the precordium and spine. In patients with severe tricuspid insufficiency a low frequency, short, mid-diastolic rumbling murmur is present, representing diastolic augmentation of flow across the tricuspid valve, similar to the murmur in patients with mitral stenosis (Fig. 7.5). The murmur of tricuspid insufficiency characteristically increases in the early phase of inspiration (Carvallo's sign). Therefore, it is important to record the tracing during expiration and inspiration. Arterial diastolic murmurs sometimes heard in patients with tricuspid insufficiency represent either aortic or pulmonic insufficiencies and the differentiation between the two is difficult to make by auscultation or phonocardiography.

Carotid Pulse Tracing

The carotid pulse tracing has a normal configuration in tricuspid insufficiency.

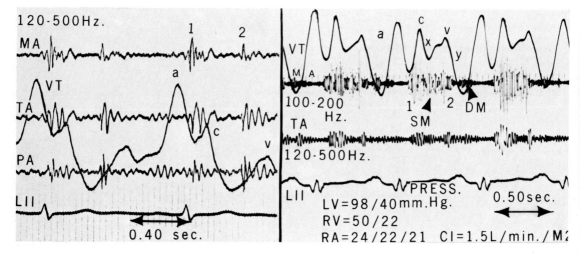

Figure 7.5. *Left:* Simultaneously recorded phonocardiogram at the mitral (MA), tricuspid (TA), and pulmonic areas (PA), jugular venous pulse tracing (VT), and lead II (LII) of the electrocardiogram in a normal subject. The first and second heart sounds are normal. The oscillations at the baseline in diastole are artifacts. The jugular venous tracing shows a normal configuration. Compare with right panel. *Right:* Simultaneously recorded phonocardiogram at the mitral (MA) and tricuspid areas (TA), jugular venous pulse tracing, and lead II (LII) of the electrocardiogram in a patient with primary myocardial disease and tricuspid insufficiency. The first heart sound is markedly diminished. The second heart sound is accentuated. There is a high frequency, high amplitude systolic regurgitant murmur (SM) that occupies all of systole, and a mid-diastolic murmur (DM) that is due to increased flow across the tricuspid valve. This is best appreciated at the mitral area. The jugular venous pulse tracing is markedly abnormal showing a very prominent A wave, small X descent, and a prominent V wave followed by a rapid Y descent. Right ventricular and right atrial pressures at the time of cardiac catheterization were markedly elevated and the cardiac index was decreased to 1.5 L/min/M² (normal 2.2). (From A. Benchimol: Non-Invasive Diagnostic Techniques in Cardiology. Copyright 1977 by The Williams & Wilkins Company, Baltimore. Used by permission.)

Jugular Venous and Hepatic Pulse Tracing

Recording the jugular venous pulse tracing (Figs. 7.5 through 7.8) and pulsations over the liver (Fig. 7.8) is quite helpful in recognizing tricuspid insufficiency. If this diagnosis is suspected, try to obtain a good hepatic pulse tracing. The technique is essentially identical to the one used to record jugular venous tracings. Place the transducer at the right epigastric area (below the sternum or slightly to the right) over the liver and hold firmly. If the patient is in sinus rhythm, the A wave of the jugular venous pulse or the liver pulsations will have increased amplitude (Fig. 7.5), but not to the degree seen in tricuspid stenosis. The X descent is small and a sustained systolic wave is present (Figs. 7.5 through 7.8). This systolic plateau or wave terminates at the time of inscription of the second heart sound and is followed by the peak of a prominent V wave which in many situations is not clearly identified (Fig. 7.6).

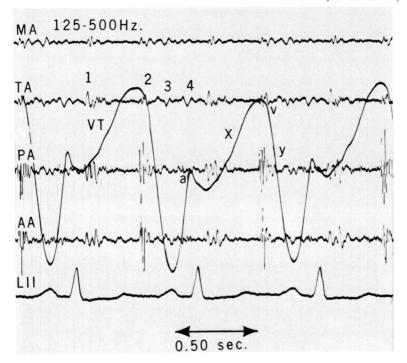

Figure 7.6. Simultaneously recorded phonocardiogram at the mitral (MA), tricuspid (TA), pulmonic (PA), and aortic areas (AA), jugular venous pulse tracing (VT), and lead II (LII) of the electrocardiogram in a 48-year-old patient with congestive heart failure and tricuspid insufficiency. The first heart sound is diminished. The second heart sound is single and accentuated. There are very prominent third and fourth heart sounds. The patient's rhythm is sinus. The jugular venous tracing shows a prominent A wave followed by a gradual upslope of the X descent, which is due to regurgitation of blood across the tricuspid valve transmitted to the superior vena cava and the jugular veins. The peak of the V wave is bigger than the A wave and is followed by a very rapid Y descent.

As soon as the tricuspid valve opens near the peak of the V wave, the Y descent begins. The Y descent is characteristically very rapid and terminates 0.08 to 0.16 sec after the peak of the V wave (Figs. 7.6 through 7.8). Following the Y descent, the tracing continues to rise, reaching a plateau during mid-diastole and terminating with a sharp H wave or with the A wave of the diastolic cycle. On the jugular and hepatic pulse tracings, these findings reflect the changes in pressure and flow in the right atrium, superior vena cava, and jugular vein. Great care must be exercised when interpreting the jugular venous pulse tracing in patients with atrial fibrillation. Most of the "characteristic" findings seen in patients with tricuspid insufficiency are nearly identical to tracings of patients with isolated atrial fibrillation without tricuspid insufficiency. Recording transcutaneous jugular vein velocity, using the Doppler flowmeter technique, is useful in differentiating between the two conditions because it records only the velocity of blood crossing the transducer (see Chap. 4).

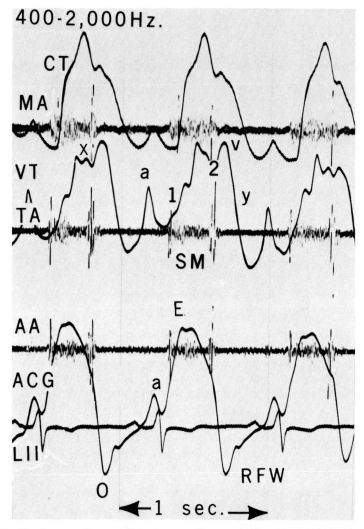

Figure 7.7. Simultaneously recorded phonocardiogram at the mitral (MA), tricuspid (TA), and aortic areas (AA), carotid pulse tracing (CT), jugular venous pulse tracing (VT), apexcardiogram (ACG), and lead II (LII) of the electrocardiogram in a 50-year-old patient with severe tricuspid insufficiency. Note the typical phonocardiographic features of the systolic murmur as described in the previous illustrations. The carotid pulse tracing has a normal contour. The jugular venous tracing shows a quite prominent A wave and a diminished X descent followed by a prominent V wave and a rapid Y descent. The apexcardiogram of the right ventricle shows a prominent A wave and a sustained systolic wave indicating right ventricular hypertrophy.

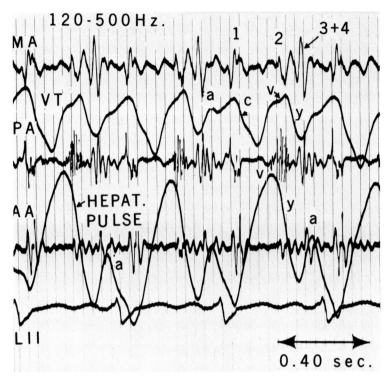

Figure 7.8. Simultaneously recorded phonocardiogram at the mitral (MA), pulmonic (PA), and aortic areas (AA), jugular venous pulse tracing (VT), hepatic pulse tracing (HEPAT. PULSE), and lead II (LII) of the electrocardiogram in a 32-year-old patient with severe tricuspid insufficiency. The rhythm is sinus tachycardia. The first and second heart sounds are normal. In mid-diastole, there is a very prominent vibration representing summation of the third and fourth heart sounds due to tachycardia. The jugular venous tracing shows an A wave that is followed by a C wave. The X descent is not particularly prominent in this recording. The V wave is prominent. The hepatic pulsations show a markedly prominent V wave and a rapid Y descent.

Apexcardiogram

The apexcardiogram of the left ventricle in patients with tricuspid insufficiency is normal and difficult to record because of enlargement of the right ventricle (Fig. 7.9). Most frequently, the technician records a right ventricular apexcardiogram. On a technically satisfactory right ventricular apexcardiogram, the abnormalities noted are: (1) The A wave will be slightly accentuated if the patient is in sinus rhythm; (2) the E point is not well recognized since it usually merges with a sustained, round systolic wave representing right ventricular hypertrophy or overloading; (3) the O point nearly coincides with the opening snap of the tricuspid valve; (4) the rapid filling wave is quite accentuated and its peak corresponds to the time of inscription of the right ventricular third heart sound; (5) the slow filling wave is normal.

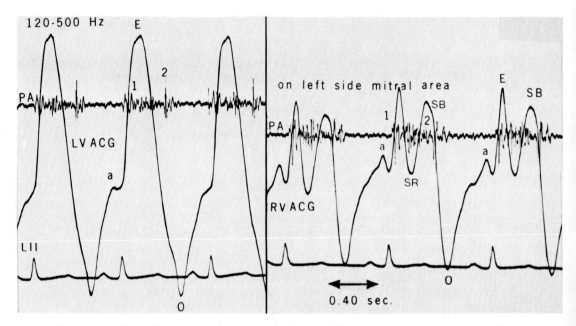

Figure 7.9. *Left:* Simultaneously recorded phonocardiogram at the pulmonic area (PA), left ventricular apexcardiogram (LV ACG), and lead II (LII) of the electrocardiogram in an 18-year-old patient with an atrial septal defect and tricuspid insufficiency. The first and second heart sounds are normal. There is a high frequency, high amplitude holosystolic murmur of the type seen in patients with tricuspid insufficiency. The left ventricular apexcardiogram is within the normal range. *Right:* Simultaneously recorded phonocardiogram at the pulmonic area (PA), right ventricular apexcardiogram (RV ACG), and lead II (LII) of the electrocardiogram. The apexcardiogram shows a conspicuous A wave. The normal E point is followed by a systolic retraction (SR) and a prominent late systolic bulge (SB). The rapid filling wave is prominent. For this recording the transducer was placed on the left side of the mitral area to record right ventricular motion, which is important in patients with a dilated right ventricle, commonly seen in patients with atrial septal defects.

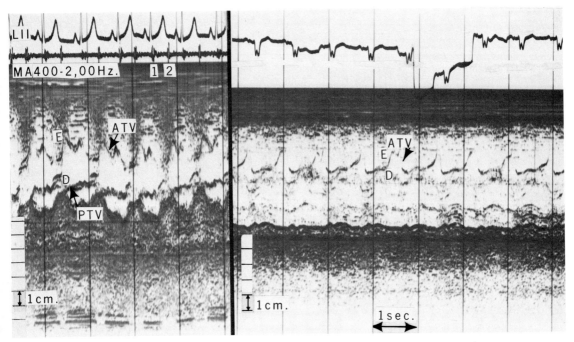

Figure 7.10. *Left:* Simultaneously recorded echocardiogram, mitral area (MA) phonocardiogram, and lead II (LII) of the electrocardiogram showing normal tricuspid motion. *Right:* Simultaneously recorded echocardiogram and lead II (LII) of the electrocardiogram in a 66-year-old patient with elevated initial right ventricular diastolic pressure. Note the premature closure of the tricuspid valve and prolongation of the A–C interval.

Systolic Time Intervals

The systolic time intervals are not altered significantly in patients with tricuspid insufficiency.

Vectorcardiogram

The vectorcardiogram is useful in this condition. It detects early signs of right ventricular hypertrophy that may not be present on the electrocardiogram. Patients with tricuspid insufficiency usually have large right ventricular and right atrial chambers and this can be recognized on the vectorcardiogram. Tricuspid insufficiency is most commonly seen in the late stage of diseases involving the mitral and aortic valve or primary involvement of the myocardium.

Echocardiogram

In tricuspid insufficiency, echocardiography is useful in measuring any increase of right ventricular size, which is quite frequently above the normal upper limit of 2.3 cm (Fig. 7.12). In addition, this technique is useful in detecting the presence of

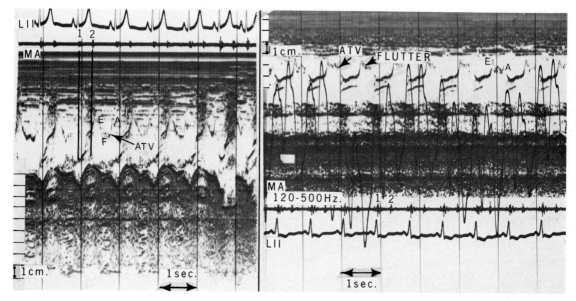

Figure 7.11. *Left:* Simultaneously recorded echocardiogram, mitral area (MA) phonocardiogram, and lead II (LII) of the electrocardiogram of a normal tricuspid valve. *Right:* Simultaneous recording of the pulmonic valve in a patient with tricuspid insufficiency and pulmonary hypertension. Note the fluttering motion of the tricuspid valve due to pulmonic insufficiency. This is similar to motion of the mitral valve in patients with aortic insufficiency.

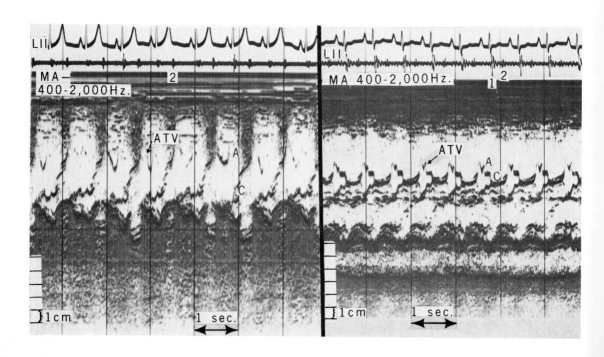

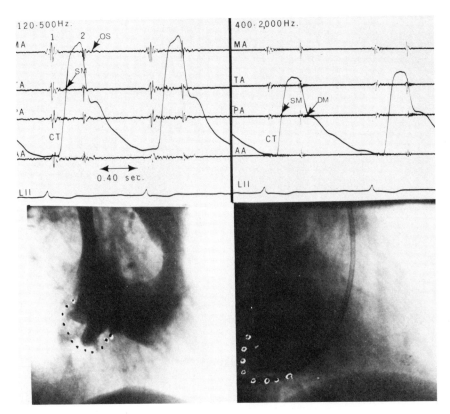

Figure 7.13. *Top Left:* Simultaneously recorded phonocardiogram at the mitral (MA), tricuspid (TA), pulmonic (PA), and aortic areas (AA), carotid pulse tracing (CT), and lead II (LII) of the electrocardiogram in a 58-year-old patient with valvular disease and tricuspid valve prolapse. The first and second heart sounds are normal. There is a midsystolic murmur (SM). An opening snap is best seen at the mitral area. The carotid pulse tracing is normal. *Top Right:* Simultaneously recorded phonocardiogram at the mitral (MA), tricuspid (TA), pulmonic (PA), and aortic areas (AA), carotid pulse tracing (CT), and lead II (LII) of the electrocardiogram. These tracings were recorded with the bandpass filter set at 400–2,000 Hz as compared with 120–500 Hz in the left panel, demonstrating the effect of filtering that eliminates high frequency components of the murmur. The murmur becomes small. There is also a faint diastolic murmur (DM) which, in this patient, was due to a small degree of aortic insufficiency. *Bottom:* Tricuspid valve angiograms showing the typical features of prolapsed tricuspid valve.

Figure 7.12. *Left:* Simultaneously recorded echocardiogram, mitral area (MA) phonocardiogram, and lead II (LII) of the electrocardiogram in a patient with a normal tricuspid valve. The A–C interval is normal. *Right:* Simultaneously recorded echocardiogram, mitral area phonocardiogram, and lead II of the electrocardiogram in a 30-year-old patient with tricuspid insufficiency, and pulmonary hypertension and elevated right ventricular end-diastolic pressure. Note the marked prolongation of the A–C interval, which is one of the important echocardiographic features of pulmonary hypertension.

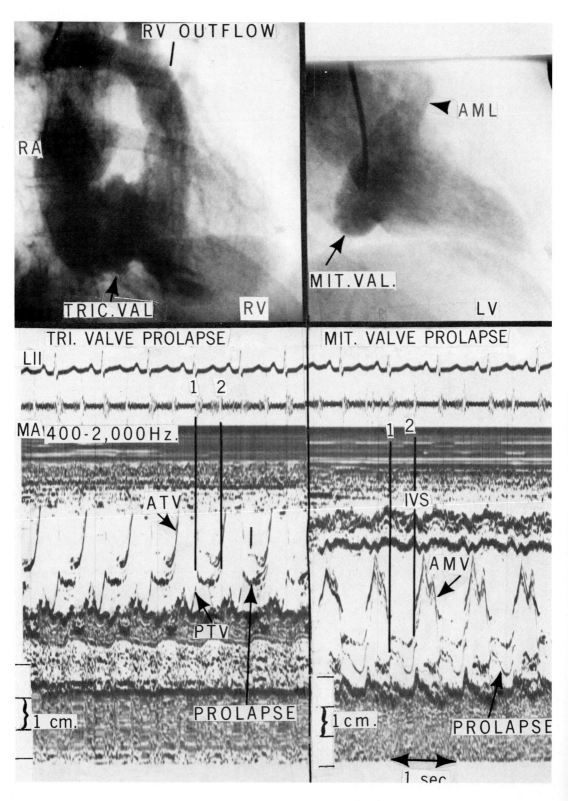

168

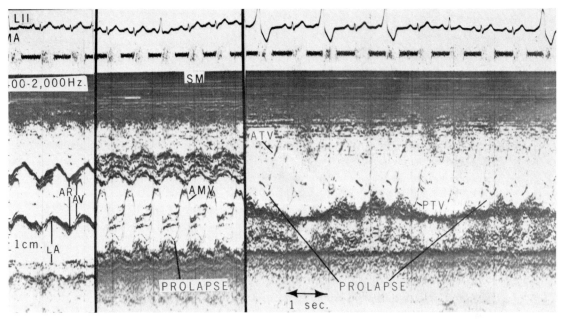

Figure 7.15. Simultaneously recorded echocardiogram, lead II (LII) of the electrocardiogram and mitral area (MA) phonocardiogram in a patient with Marfan's syndrome, mitral and tricuspid valve prolapse. *Left:* Echocardiogram of the aortic valve showing a normal aortic root (AR) and aortic valve (AV). LA = left atrium. *Middle:* Echocardiogram showing the typical features of prolapsed mitral valve including posterior displacement during systole. SM = systolic murmur, AMV = anterior mitral valve. *Right:* Echocardiogram showing tricuspid valve prolapse. The abnormalities of the valve during systole are the same as those seen in mitral valve prolapse. ATV = anterior tricuspid valve, PTV = posterior tricuspid valve.

pulmonary hypertension frequently seen in patients with tricuspid insufficiency (Figs. 7.10 through 7.12). The echocardiogram shows a diminished or absent A wave if pulmonary hypertension is present. In addition, the tricuspid valve may close prematurely in the presence of pulmonary hypertension.

Abnormalities of tricuspid valve motion are frequently noted with various cardiac arrhythmias. One such example is coarse fibrillation waves seen in patients with atrial fibrillation. Fine fibrillatory movements of the tricuspid valve in patients with pulmonic insufficiency are similar to the ones described for mitral valve motion in patients with aortic insufficiency (Fig. 7.11).

Figure 7.14. *Top Left:* Right side angiogram showing a prolapsed tricuspid valve, a normal right ventricle (RV), and pulmonary artery. *Top Right:* Left ventricular angiogram showing prolapse of the mitral valve (MIT. VAL.). *Bottom Left:* Echocardiogram of the tricuspid valve showing systolic posterior displacement of the valve. *Bottom Right:* Echocardiogram of the mitral valve on the same patient showing findings similar to those seen in tricuspid valve prolapse, i.e., the posterior motion of the valve during systole.

Points of Caution and Importance

1. Be sure you are recording the phonocardiogram and jugular venous tracing during inspiration and expiration. The murmur of tricuspid insufficiency increases with inspiration.

2. Be aware of the fact that the patient may have other associated valvular heart diseases.

3. Ask the physician what he is looking for.

4. On the echocardiogram, try hard to obtain a good recording of the tricuspid valve and of both the anterior and posterior leaflets. Be sure to obtain a good tricuspid valve recording so that measurements of various intervals can be made. They will be of value to the physician.

5. If the tricuspid valve cannot be recorded with the transducer in the standard location, try the subxyphoid approach. It is more difficult, but may provide additional useful diagnostic information.

6. Try to get a good echocardiographic recording so the right ventricular size can be measured.

7. Keep in mind that the physician may not be physically present during the recording of the echocardiogram and he has to rely on your recording technique.

8. In patients with chronic lung disease and secondary tricuspid valve disease, it may be very difficult to obtain a good tricuspid valve recording because the ultrasonic beam has to cross several structures including large masses of lung tissue.

TRICUSPID VALVE PROLAPSE

Tricuspid valve prolapse is rare as an isolated lesion. However, it has been recognized with increasing frequency in patients with associated mitral valve prolapse.

The auscultatory and phonocardiographic findings are essentially identical to the ones described in mitral valve prolapse, i.e., early, mid- or late systolic click followed by a late, high frequency systolic murmur. The first and second heart sounds are normal (Fig. 7.13).

The echocardiographic features of tricuspid valve prolapse are also identical to the ones described for mitral valve prolapse. The tricuspid leaflets move backward toward the right atrium during systole (Figs. 7.14, 7.15).

BIBLIOGRAPHY

Abinader, E.G.: Systolic venous reflux sounds. Am. Heart J. *85*:452, 1973.

Ainsworth, R.P., Hartman, A.F., Jr., Aker, U., and Schad, N: Tricuspid valve prolapse with late systolic tricuspid insufficiency. Radiology *107*:309, 1973.

Aravanis, C., and Michaelides, G.: Tricuspid insufficiency masquerading as mitral insufficiency in patients with severe mitral stenosis. Am. J. Cardiol. *20*:417, 1967.

Benchimol, A., Barreto, E.C., and Tio, S.:   Phasic right atrium and superior vena cava flow velocity in patients with tricuspid insufficiency. Am. Heart J. *79*:603, 1970.

Boicourt, O.W., Nagle, R.E., and Mounsey, J.P.:   The clinical significance of systolic retraction of the apical impulse. Br. Heart J. *27*:379, 1965.

Cairns, K.B., Kloster, F.E., Bristlow, J.D., Lees, M.H., and Griswold, H.E.:   Problems in the hemodynamic diagnosis of tricuspid insufficiency. Am. Heart J. *75*:173, 1968.

DeBrito, A.H.X., Sekeff, J.A.B., Toledo, A.N., Zaniol, W., Snitcowsky, R., DeLucena Costa, C.A., and DeCarvalho Azevedo, A.:   Early stage of tricuspid stenosis. Am. J. Cardiol. *18*:57, 1966.

Galvis, E.L., and Bouchard, F.:   Tricuspid insufficiency and congenital cardiopathies. Arch. Mal. Coeur *58*:100, 1965.

Gooch, A.S., Maranhao, V., Scampardonis, G., Cha, S.D., and Yang, S.S.:   Prolapse of both mitral and tricuspid leaflets in systolic murmur–click syndrome. N. Engl. J. Med. *287*:1218, 1972.

Gorinina, N.K., and Shcherba, S.G.:   Phonocardiography in the diagnosis of tricuspid stenosis. Kardiologia *4*:25, 1964.

Joyner, C.R., Jr., Hey, E.B., Jr., Johnson, J., and Reid, J.M.:   Reflected ultrasound in the diagnosis of tricuspid stenosis. Am. J. Cardiol. *19*:66, 1967.

Kavanagh-Gray, D., and Gerien, A.:   The preoperative assessment of multiple valve disease. Can. Med. Assoc. J. *91*:887, 1964.

Kawashima, U., Nakano, S., and Manabe, H.:   Tricuspid insufficiency; a study of hemodynamics. Am. J. Physiol. *74*:853, 1974.

Keefe, J.F., Wolk, M.J., and Levine, H.J.:   Isolated tricuspid valvular stenosis. Am. J. Cardiol. *25*:252, 1970.

Lisa, C.P., and Tavel, M.E.:   Tricuspid stenosis; graphic features which help in its diagnosis. Chest *61*:291, 1972.

Luisada, A.A.:   Internal and external phonocardiography; mitral stenosis, pulmonary hypertension, pulmonary and tricuspid insufficiency. Dis. Chest *54*:461, 1968.

Morgan, J.R., and Forker, A.D.:   Isolated tricuspid insufficiency. Circulation *43*:559, 1971.

Rios, J.C., Massumi, R.A., Breesmen, W.T., and Sarin, R.K.:   Auscultatory features of acute tricuspid regurgitation. Am. J. Cardiol. *23*:4, 1969.

Sanders, C.A., Harthorne, J.W., DeSanctis, R.W., and Austen, W.G.:   Tricuspid stenosis, a difficult diagnosis in the presence of atrial fibrillation. Circulation *33*:26, 1966.

Takabatake, Y., and Iizuka, M.:   Pathophysiology of tricuspid insufficiency—clinical and experimental study. Am. J. Physiol. *74*:843, 1974.

Toso, M., and Innocien, P.:   The Rivero–Carvallo maneuver in the diagnosis of tricuspid insufficiency; conventional and intracavitary phonocardiographic study. Cuore Circ. *50*:94, 1966.

Upshaw, C.B., Jr.:   Precordial honk due to tricuspid regurgitation. Am. J. Cardiol. *35*:85, 1975.

8
Prosthetic Cardiac Valves

Three basic types of prosthesis can be used to replace diseased cardiac valves: (1) caged ball, (2) caged disc, and (3) hetero- and homograft. Each of these implanted valves presents a variety of auscultatory, phonocardiographic, pulse wave, and echocardiographic findings. For this reason, it is important to know before the recording of these tracings which type of valve was implanted. Only the most commonly used valves will be described in this chapter. At the end of this chapter we have illustrated several types of prostheses that are commonly used.

The earliest models of caged ball type prostheses, used in patients with severe aortic insufficiency, were the Hufnagel, placed in the descending aorta, and the Harken, implanted in the subcoronary position. More recent types include the Starr–Edwards, and Cutter–Smeloff, which has a ball made of silicone placed in a double open cage structure; the Braunwald–Cutter, which has a silastic ball with an open cage; the DeBakey, a sutureless valve; and the Cooley–Liotta–Cromie, a titanium valve.

The most commonly used caged disc prostheses are the Kay–Shiley, a silastic caged disc protected with muscle guard; the Kay–Suzuki, a Teflon discoid valve with four small protusions within the orifice; the Cross–Jones caged lens, which has a titanium frame, a silicone lens shaped disc, and a woven Teflon fixation ring; the Wada–Cutter, which has a tilting disc and a titanium ring; the Beall disc valve; and the Björk–Shiley and Lillehei-Kaster valves with tilting discs.

Homografts, implanted in the mitral, tricuspid, or aortic positions, are valves preserved from human cadavers. Other types of homografts are made from stented fascia lata, pericardium or human dura mater. The most common type of heterograft is the stented Hancock-porcine valve, which can be implanted in the mitral, tricuspid, aortic, and pulmonary positions. Hancock-porcine conduits are used in the Rastelli and Fontan procedures for correction of some congenital heart diseases such as pulmonary and tricuspid atresia.

MITRAL VALVE PROSTHESES

Most of our experience has been in patients with a Starr–Edwards ball valve, Beall disc valve, and more recently, the Björk–Shiley tilting disc and Hancock-porcine valves.

172

Ball Valves—Clicks and Murmurs

Normally functioning ball valve prostheses usually produce sharp vibrations due to opening and closing of the valve (Fig. 8.1). The amplitude of these vibrations or clicks is approximately the same, but the opening click may be higher than the closing click in some recordings. The time interval from onset of the Q wave of the electrocardiogram to the onset of the valve closure is 40 msec or less in patients with sinus rhythm, 54 msec if the rhythm is atrial fibrillation (average the measurement of seven consecutive cardiac cycles). The interval from the aortic valve closure sound to the opening click ranges from 80–160 msec with a mean of 110 msec. In most patients this interval is fairly constant and quite independent of variation in cycle length, as seen in patients with atrial fibrillation. Amplitude of the closing click should be identical in several consecutive beats provided the patient is in sinus rhythm and has consistently regular R–R intervals. Minor variations in amplitude of the closing click may be seen in patients with a varying R–R interval such as in atrial fibrillation, atrial tachycardia with varying degree of AV block, etc., but this is not an indication of valve malfunction.

A prosthetic third heart sound can be heard in approximately 60% of patients. Multiple diastolic clicks are common and they are a normal feature in patients with this type of prosthesis, as shown in Figure 8.1.

A prosthetic fourth heart sound (Fig. 8.2), seen in 30–40% of patients in sinus rhythm, may have two components. The first component will have low amplitude,

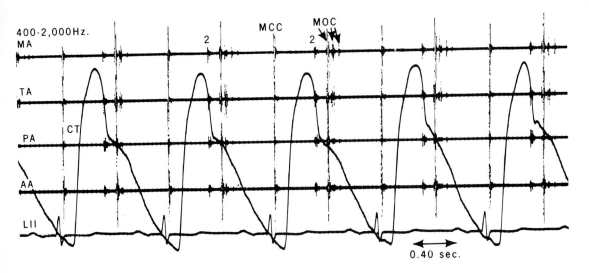

Figure 8.1. Simultaneously recorded phonocardiogram at the mitral (MA), tricuspid (TA), pulmonic (PA), and aortic areas (AA), carotid pulse tracing (CT), and lead II (LII) of the electrocardiogram in the 45-year-old patient with a Starr–Edwards mitral ball valve. Note the single mitral closing click (MCC) sound in systole. In diastole, there are several sounds. The first one, representing the opening click (MOC), is the most important one and the other two sounds are probably due to turbulent flow across the prosthesis. This is quite common in patients with a ball valve prosthesis, but is not necessarily an indication of valve malfunction. There are no murmurs. The carotid pulse tracing is normal.

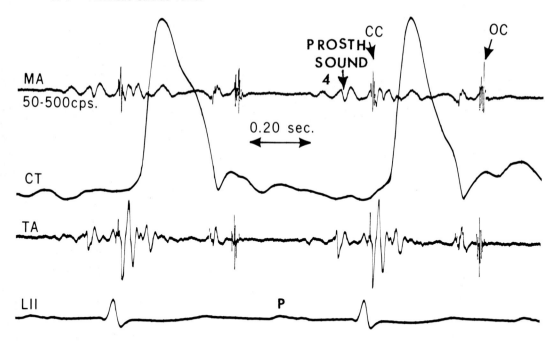

Figure 8.2. Simultaneously recorded phonocardiogram at the mitral (MA) and tricuspid areas (TA), carotid pulse tracing (CT), and lead II (LII) of the electrocardiogram in a 60-year-old patient with a prosthetic mitral Beall valve. Note the single closing (CC) and opening clicks (OC) of the prosthetic valve. There is also a prosthetic sound (PROSTH SOUND) after the atrial contraction. These are normal findings in patients with this type of prosthesis. The patient also has a fourth heart sound. There are no murmurs. The carotid pulse tracing is normal.

occurring 0.06–0.11 sec after the P wave of the electrocardiogram and the second most prominent component occurs 0.12–0.18 sec after the P wave.

All prosthetic valve sounds, which may be heard over the entire precordium, are most prominent at the mitral area and are well transmitted to the spine. They have a click-like characteristic and short duration, and are best recorded with the patient in a left lateral decubitus position.

Patients with normally functioning prosthetic mitral valves should not present with systolic murmurs. However, many patients with mitral valve disease who have been subjected to mitral valve replacement may have associated tricuspid insufficiency, in which case a systolic murmur may be recorded at the tricuspid area. If the diagnosis of tricuspid insufficiency can be excluded by other diagnostic techniques (see Chap. 7), the systolic murmur has important clinical implications because it may indicate prosthetic mitral valve malfunction. In this event, the physician should be informed promptly.

Disc Valves—Clicks and Murmurs

Disc valves, with the exception of the Björk–Shiley and Lillehei–Kaster, always present with the same auscultatory and phonocardiographic findings. The closing click is well recorded in most precordial areas (Fig. 8.3). The opening and closing click amplitude should be essentially identical. Amplitude of the closing click is inversely proportional to the preceding cycle length, i.e., the longer the preceding diastolic cycle, the smaller the amplitude of the opening click and vice versa (Fig. 8.4). This is a normal feature of most prosthetic disc valves in the mitral position. However, amplitude of the opening click should remain constant in a wide range of cycle lengths in patients with disc valve prostheses. Multiple clicks during mid-diastole or atrial contraction in patients with sinus rhythm are not part of the normal auscultatory and phonocardiographic findings in patients with prosthetic disc valves. The auscultatory and phonocardiographic features of the Björk–Shiley and the Lillehei–Kaster prostheses in the mitral position are illustrated in Figure 8.5.

Carotid Pulse Tracing—Ball and Disc Valves

The carotid pulse tracing should have a normal contour and ejection time should be normal provided the patient is not in heart failure (Figs. 8.1 through 8.3).

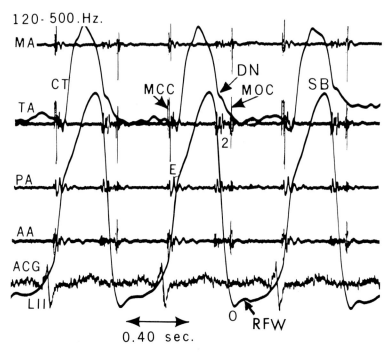

Figure 8.3. Simultaneously recorded phonocardiogram at the mitral (MA), tricuspid (TA), pulmonic (PA), and aortic areas (AA), carotid pulse tracing (CT), apexcardiogram (ACG), and lead II (LII) of the electrocardiogram in a 51-year-old patient with a prosthetic Beall mitral valve. Note the opening (MOC) and closing clicks (MCC) of the prosthetic valve without evidence of valve malfunction. There are no murmurs. The carotid pulse tracing is normal. The apexcardiogram shows a small rapid filling wave (RFW). There is a late systolic bulge (SB) and this is usually seen in patients with long-term left ventricular disease secondary to rheumatic heart disease.

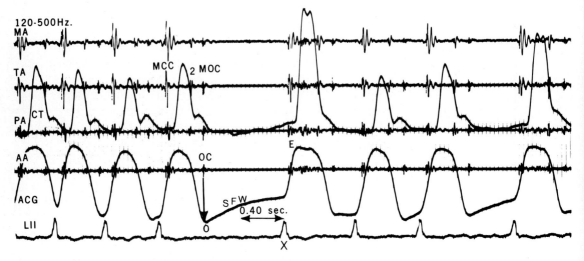

Figure 8.4. Simultaneously recorded phonocardiogram at the mitral (MA), tricuspid (TA), pulmonic (PA), and aortic areas (AA), carotid pulse tracing (CT), apexcardiogram (ACG) and lead II (LII) of the electrocardiogram in a 53-year-old patient with a prosthetic Beall mitral valve. The patient's rhythm is atrial fibrillation. Note the variations in amplitude of the carotid pulse in the beats that are preceded by a long cycle length as compared with those preceded by a short cycle length. There are no murmurs except in the beats followed by a long cycle length. The apexcardiogram is abnormal showing a sustained systolic wave that is probably secondary to left ventricular hypertrophy. The rapid filling wave is absent. This is not uncommon in patients with prosthetic mitral valves and simulates the tracings seen in mitral stenosis. MCC = mitral closing click, MOC = mitral opening click, OC = opening click, and SFW = slow filling wave.

Jugular Venous Pulse Tracing

The jugular venous pulse tracing cannot be utilized to determine normal or abnormal prosthetic valve function. It does help, at times, to determine the presence of tricuspid insufficiency in patients who present with systolic murmurs at the mitral and/or tricuspid areas. It is particularly valuable in patients with sinus rhythm, but is not a reliable indicator in patients with atrial fibrillation (see Chap. 7).

Apexcardiogram

The apexcardiogram usually exhibits a small rapid filling wave of short duration, or this wave may not be present, particularly in patients with mitral stenosis (Fig. 8.4). The systolic wave is normal provided the patient does not have left ventricular dyskinesis (abnormal contraction of the left ventricular walls). The apexcardiogram is valuable in determining the time of inscription of the first opening click in patients with prosthetic ball valves. The opening click should coincide with or shortly precede the O point of the apexcardiogram.

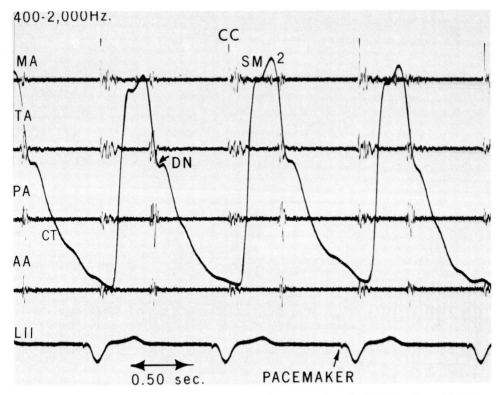

Figure 8.5. Simultaneously recorded phonocardiogram at the mitral (MA), tricuspid (TA), pulmonic (PA), and aortic areas (AA), carotid pulse tracing (CT), and lead II (LII) of the electrocardiogram in a 71-year-old patient with a Lillehei–Kaster mitral valve prosthesis and pacemaker rhythm. This type of valve usually does not cause an opening click. A closing click is inscribed near the first heart sound. There is a low amplitude, high frequency, systolic murmur probably due to a mild degree of periprosthetic insufficiency. There are no diastolic murmurs. The carotid pulse tracing is normal.

Homograft and Heterograft Valves—Mitral Position

The auscultatory and phonocardiographic features of these valves include the presence of two components of the first heart sound.

Third heart sounds that may be present in these patients are not indicative of heart failure. The interval from the aortic component of the second sound to the third heart sound is in the range of 0.12–0.18 sec. At times, mid-diastolic rumbles can be recorded in patients with Hancock-porcine prostheses and this finding does not necessarily indicate valve malfunction (Fig. 8.6).

Carotid and jugular venous pulse tracings, apexcardiogram, and systolic time intervals have not proven to be valuable in the early recognition of normal or abnormal function of homografts or heterografts (Fig. 8.7).

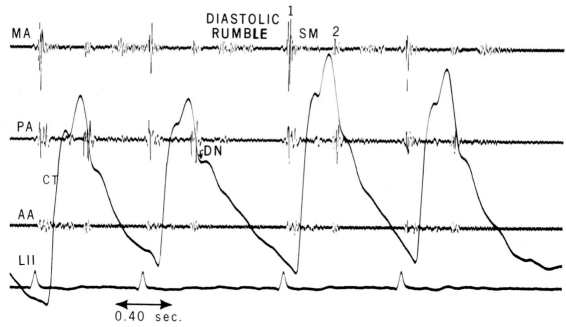

Figure 8.6. Simultaneously recorded phonocardiogram at the mitral (MA), pulmonic (PA) and aortic areas (AA), carotid pulse tracing (CT), and lead II (LII) of the electrocardiogram in a 41-year-old patient with a Hancock-porcine mitral valve prosthesis. The first heart sound is accentuated. The second heart sound is normal. There is an atrioventricular diastolic murmur. This type of murmur is sometimes seen in patients with a Hancock-porcine mitral valve and does not necessarily indicate the presence of valve malfunction. The patient also has a systolic high frequency murmur (SM), which could be due to either periprosthetic insufficiency or tricuspid insufficiency. The carotid pulse tracing is normal. DN = dicrotic notch.

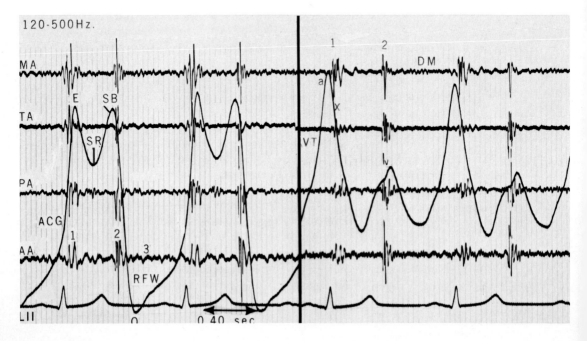

SUPRA STERNAL NOTCH

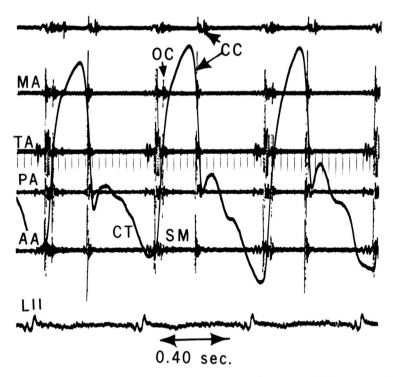

0.40 sec.

Figure 8.8. Simultaneously recorded phonocardiogram at the mitral (MA), tricuspid (TA), pulmonic (PA), and aortic areas (AA), carotid pulse tracing (CT), lead II (LII) of the electrocardiogram and another microphone placed near the suprasternal notch to show transmission of the click to that area. There are opening (OC) and closing clicks (CC) of the Starr–Edwards ball valve prosthesis, with a low amplitude, high frequency, systolic ejection murmur (SM) following the opening click. The carotid pulse tracing is normal. (From A. Benchimol: Non-Invasive Diagnostic Techniques in Cardiology. Copyright 1977 by The Williams & Wilkins Company, Baltimore. Used by permission.)

Figure 8.7. *Left:* Simultaneously recorded phonocardiogram at the mitral (MA), tricuspid (TA), pulmonic (PA) and aortic areas (AA), apexcardiogram (ACG), and lead II (LII) of the electrocardiogram in a 36-year-old patient with a #31 Hancock-porcine mitral valve prosthesis. This type of valve usually does not cause opening or closing clicks. The first and second heart sounds are normal. There are no murmurs. The apexcardiogram is abnormal showing a systolic retraction (SR) followed by a late systolic bulge (SB). This usually suggests left ventricular dyskinesis. The peak of the small rapid filling wave (RFW) coincides with the third heart sound on the phonocardiogram. *Right:* Simultaneously recorded phonocardiogram at the mitral, tricuspid, pulmonic and aortic areas, jugular venous tracing (VT), and lead II of the electrocardiogram. Note the slight increase in amplitude of the A wave (a) in relation to the V (v) wave. On this recording, the patient also had a low amplitude atrioventricular diastolic murmur (DM) best appreciated at the mitral area.

179

AORTIC VALVE PROSTHESES

Ball and Disc Valves—Clicks and Murmurs

Normally functioning aortic ball valve prostheses such as the Starr–Edwards result in high frequency, high amplitude opening and closing clicks that are transmitted to multiple precordial areas including the suprasternal notch area (Fig. 8.8). The opening click has higher amplitude than the closing click and the normal aortic-opening–aortic-closing click ratio ranges from 0.5–1.2, as seen in the logarithmic recording of the tricuspid area. This ratio is independent of variations in cycle length. It is not uncommon to observe multiple systolic clicks, particularly in early systole. They are probably the result of turbulent motion of the ball within the cage.

High frequency systolic ejection murmurs are uniformly present in patients with prosthetic aortic ball valves (Figs. 8.8, 8.9). The characteristics of the systolic ejection murmurs vary with the size of the prosthesis. Small ball valves usually produce a prominent systolic ejection murmur recorded over most precordial areas but most prominent at the mitral and aortic areas. This murmur is well transmitted to both carotid arteries and to the spine. The valves are available in various sizes, and the smaller the valve, the higher the amplitude of the systolic

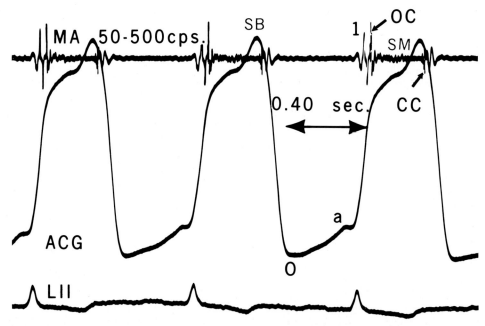

Figure 8.9. Simultaneously recorded phonocardiogram at the mitral area (MA), apexcardiogram (ACG), and lead II (LII) of the electrocardiogram in a 46-year-old patient with a Starr–Edwards aortic valve prosthesis. The opening (OC) and closing clicks (CC) are well recorded. The patient also has a low amplitude, high frequency, systolic murmur (SM) that is quite common in patients with prosthetic ball valves in the aortic position. The apexcardiogram is abnormal showing an inconspicuous E point and a late systolic bulge (SB) indicative of left ventricular hypertrophy.

ejection murmur. The larger the valve, the smaller the amplitude of the murmur. This is so because patients with small aortic ball valves have higher pressure gradients between the left ventricle and aorta, as opposed to smaller gradients in patients with large ball valves.

Diastolic murmurs resulting from prosthetic valve insufficiency are not uncommon in patients with a normally functioning Cutter–Smeloff ball valve prosthesis, but are rare in patients with a Starr–Edwards valve.

The disc valves most commonly used are the Björk–Shiley and Lillehei–Kaster prostheses. They usually produce very soft opening and closing sounds similar to the characteristics of normal heart sounds (Fig. 8.10). Systolic ejection clicks are rare (Fig. 8.11). Systolic ejection murmurs usually have low amplitude (Grade I–II/VI) and high frequency characteristics (Fig. 8.10) similar to those seen in patients with a mild degree of aortic valvular stenosis. These murmurs are recorded best at the aortic and mitral areas. Diastolic murmurs are rare in patients with aortic disc prostheses and, when present, suggest the possibility of prosthetic valve malfunction. Their presence must be correlated with the other clinical findings (Fig. 8.10).

Carotid Pulse Tracing

The carotid pulse tracing usually shows normal upstroke time, a prominent dicrotic notch, and a large dicrotic wave, which follows the second heart sound.

Jugular Venous Pulse Tracing

The jugular venous pulse tracing is only useful when the patient develops valve malfunction, congestive heart failure, or pulmonary hypertension, in which case it will show the characteristic findings seen in patients with pulmonary hypertension (see Chap. 10).

Apexcardiogram

The apexcardiogram is of some value in evaluating patients with prosthetic aortic ball and disc valves. Abnormalities usually present are of the type seen in patients with left ventricular hypertrophy, including a prominent A wave, inconspicuous E point, round and sustained systolic wave, and a small rapid filling wave (Fig. 8.12).

Systolic Time Intervals

Patients with aortic valvular disease have increased ejection time. Following aortic valve replacement systolic ejection time decreases considerably. The preejection period and left ventricular ejection time ratio tend to normalize following valve replacement.

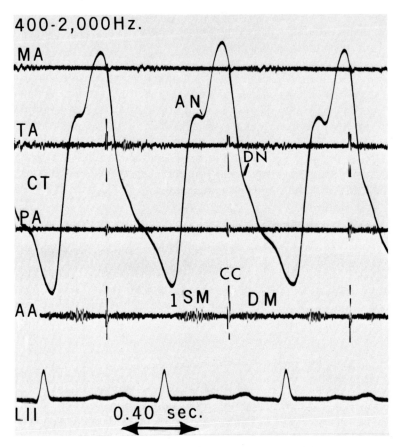

Figure 8.10. Simultaneously recorded phonocardiogram at the mitral (MA), tricuspid (TA), pulmonic (PA), and aortic areas (AA), carotid pulse tracing (CT), and lead II (LII) of the electrocardiogram in a 51-year-old patient with a Björk–Shiley aortic valve prosthesis. This prosthesis usually does not cause an opening click. One might record a closing click, which is present in this case at the second heart sound. The high frequency, medium amplitude, systolic ejection murmur (SM), best recorded at the aortic area, is not necessarily an indication of prosthetic valve malfunction. However, this patient may have some degree of prosthetic insufficiency, which in this case is represented by a diastolic murmur (DM) best recorded at the aortic area. The carotid pulse tracing shows a prominent anacrotic notch (AN) and an inconspicuous dicrotic notch (DN).

182

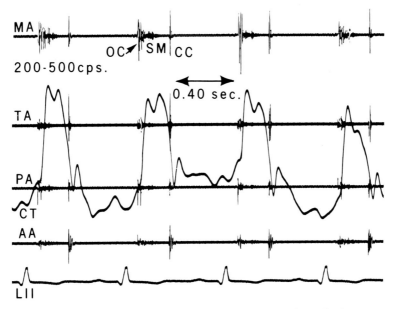

Figure 8.11. Simultaneously recorded phonocardiogram at the mitral (MA), tricuspid (TA), pulmonic (PA) and aortic areas (AA), carotid pulse tracing (CT), and lead II (LII) of the electrocardiogram in a 54-year-old patient with a Cutter aortic valve prosthesis, showing normal opening (OC) and closing clicks (CC). There is also a high frequency, low amplitude, early systolic ejection murmur (SM) recorded best at the mitral area. The carotid pulse tracing is normal.

HOMOGRAFT AND HETEROGRAFT VALVES— AORTIC POSITION

Homograft valves usually do not exhibit opening or closing clicks. However, low amplitude, high frequency systolic ejection murmurs are frequently noted due to turbulent blood flow across the prosthesis, or calcification of the valve, as shown in Figure 8.13. An ejection sound is usually present. The time interval from the Q or R wave of the electrocardiogram to the ejection sound with a range of 0.12–0.17 sec is probably due to motion of the valve and/or ring.

Arterial diastolic murmurs may be heard at varying times following valve replacement and are due to a mild degree of aortic valve insufficiency.

The auscultatory and phonocardiographic findings in patients with heterograft valves such as the Hancock-porcine have not been definitely established. In our experience with 40 cases, we have found that the majority of patients do not have any significant arterial diastolic murmurs but we have frequently observed systolic ejection murmurs (Fig. 8.14).

The carotid and jugular venous pulse tracings, apexcardiogram, and systolic time intervals have not proven to be of diagnostic value in determining valve malfunction (Fig. 8.15).

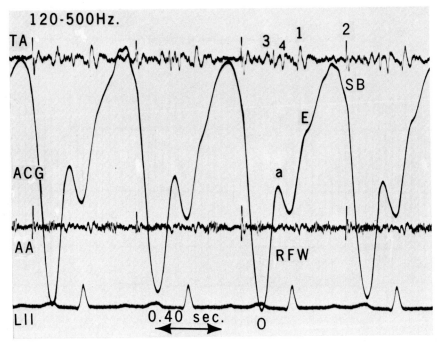

Figure 8.12. Simultaneously recorded phonocardiogram at the tricuspid (TA) and aortic areas (AA), apexcardiogram (ACG), and lead II (LII) of the electrocardiogram in a 51-year-old patient with a #23 aortic Björk–Shiley prosthetic valve. This patient was in heart failure when this tracing was taken. The opening and closing clicks are not well recorded. There are prominent third and fourth heart sounds on the phonocardiogram. The apexcardiogram is abnormal showing an inconspicuous A wave and a prominent late systolic bulge (SB) suggestive of left ventricular dyskinesis. There is also fusion of the rapid filling wave (RFW) with the A wave (a), both of which coincide with the third and fourth heart sounds recorded in the tricuspid area.

TRICUSPID VALVES

Tricuspid valve replacement is uncommon; therefore, the auscultatory and phonocardiographic findings are not well known. However, opening and closing clicks of the prosthetic ball or disc are usually similar to the ones seen when prostheses are implanted in the mitral position. An example of our findings in a patient with a Beall prosthesis in the tricuspid position is shown in Figure 8.16.

Our limited experience with the Hancock-porcine valve prosthesis in the tricuspid position indicates that the opening and closing clicks are not clearly identifiable.

Patients subjected to multiple valve replacement will exhibit the findings outlined for the types of prostheses implanted (Fig. 8.16).

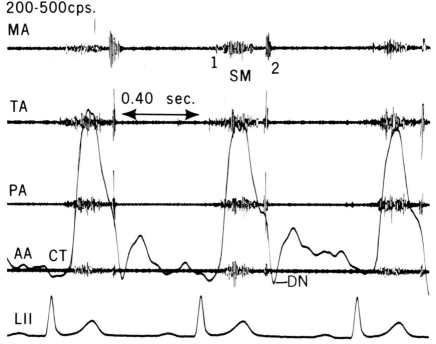

Figure 8.13. Simultaneously recorded phonocardiogram at the mitral (MA), tricuspid (TA), pulmonic (PA) and aortic areas (AA), carotid pulse tracing (CT), and lead II (LII) of the electrocardiogram in a 13-year-old patient with a homograft aortic valve. The first and second heart sounds are normal. The high frequency, high amplitude systolic ejection murmur (SM) recorded in all precordial areas was probably due to the patient's calcified aortic valve. The carotid pulse tracing is normal. (From A. Benchimol: Non-Invasive Diagnostic Techniques in Cardiology. Copyright 1977 by The Williams & Wilkins Company, Baltimore. Used by permission.)

PROSTHETIC MITRAL VALVE MALFUNCTION

Ball and Disc Valves

Valve variance is defined as valvular dysfunction secondary to physical and chemical alterations in the silastic disc or ball of the prosthesis or thrombus formation or detachment of the suture ring.

Delayed short, erratic, and absent opening clicks (Figs. 8.17 through 8.20) are the phonocardiographic criteria for mitral ball or disc variance. The relative amplitude of the opening and closing clicks is not always helpful.

Peri- and Intravalvular Insufficiency

A reduced A2–OC interval, diminished intensity of the opening click OC/CC < 0.35, a prominent systolic murmur at the mitral area, and reduced left ventricular ejection time are all very suggestive of perivalvular insufficiency. The systolic

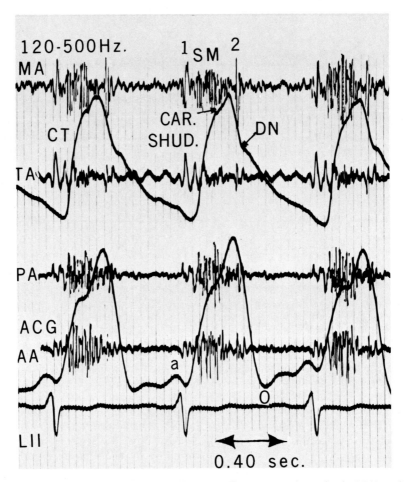

Figure 8.14. Simultaneously recorded phonocardiogram at the mitral (MA), tricuspid (TA), pulmonic (PA) and aortic areas (AA), carotid pulse tracing (CT), apexcardiogram (ACG), and lead II (LII) of the electrocardiogram in a 54-year-old patient with a #21 Hancock-porcine valve in the aortic position. The first and second heart sounds are normal. No diastolic murmurs are present. There is a high frequency, high amplitude, musical systolic ejection murmur (SM), recorded best at the mitral and aortic areas, that represents turbulent flow across the aortic prosthesis. Note the absence of a systolic ejection click. The carotid pulse shows a slight decrease in the upstroke with some high frequency components suggesting the presence of carotid shudder (CAR. SHUD.). The dicrotic notch (DN) is inconspicuous. The apexcardiogram is abnormal showing a small A wave. The E point is not well defined but is followed by a late systolic rise of the type seen in patients with left ventricular hypertrophy or dyskinesis. Systolic ejection murmurs are frequently seen in patients with this type of prosthesis but they do not necessarily indicate prosthetic valve malfunction.

186

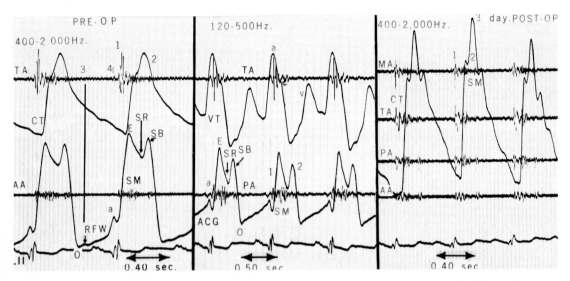

Figure 8.15. *Left*: Simultaneously recorded phonocardiogram at the tricuspid (TA) and aortic areas (AA), carotid pulse tracing (CT), apexcardiogram (ACG), and lead II (LII) of the electrocardiogram in a 60-year-old patient with aortic stenosis. The recording was taken prior to aortic valve replacement. The first heart sound is normal. The second heart sound is diminished. There is a high frequency, medium amplitude systolic ejection murmur (SM) best recorded at the aortic area. There are third and fourth heart sounds. The carotid pulse tracing is abnormal showing a high placed anacrotic notch and an inconspicuous dicrotic notch. The apexcardiogram is also abnormal showing a systolic retraction (SR) followed by a late systolic bulge (SB) usually suggestive of left ventricular hypertrophy or dyskinesis. *Middle*: Simultaneously recorded phonocardiogram at the tricuspid and pulmonic areas, jugular venous tracing (VT), apexcardiogram, and lead II of the electrocardiogram on the same patient prior to surgery. The jugular venous tracing is normal. The apexcardiogram shows the same features described in the left panel. *Right*: The tracing was recorded three days following valve replacement with an aortic Hancock-porcine prosthesis. Note the presence of a systolic murmur (SM), which can occur as early as three days following valve replacement. The first and second heart sounds are normal. There are no diastolic murmurs. The carotid pulse tracing is normal.

187

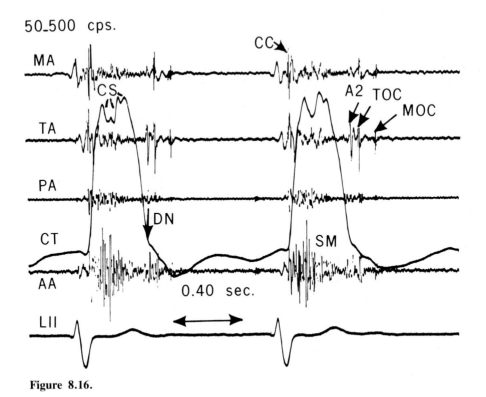

50–500 cps.

Figure 8.16.

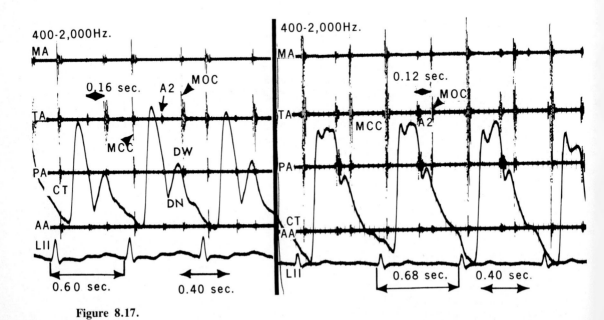

400-2,000Hz.

400-2,000Hz.

Figure 8.17.

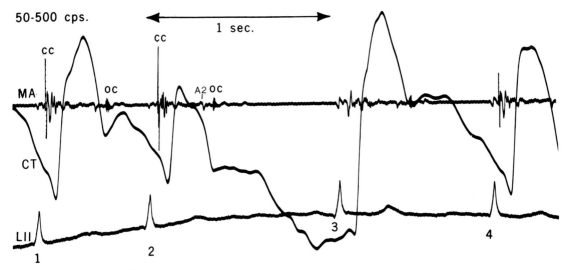

Figure 8.18. Simultaneously recorded phonocardiogram at the mitral area (MA), carotid pulse tracing (CT), and lead II (LII) of the electrocardiogram in a 47-year-old patient with a malfunctioning Beall mitral valve prosthesis. The closing click (CC) and the second heart sound are normal. However, the opening click (OC) has low amplitude and is inscribed very close to the second heart sound (A2). This is one of the signs of prosthetic valve malfunction. The carotid pulse tracing is normal. There are no murmurs.

Figure 8.16. Simultaneously recorded phonocardiogram at the mitral (MA), tricuspid (TA), pulmonic (PA) and aortic areas (AA), carotid pulse tracing (CT), and lead II (LII) of the electrocardiogram in a 53-year-old patient with mitral and tricuspid valve prostheses. Note the closing click (CC) of the mitral prosthesis. The closing click of the tricuspid prosthesis was not well recorded or may have been recorded simultaneously with the mitral closing click. Following the click, there is a high frequency, high amplitude systolic ejection murmur (SM) showing the typical features of the murmur of aortic stenosis. The aortic second sound (A2) is normal. Following aortic valve closure, the tricuspid opening click (TOC) is well recorded and is followed by the mitral opening (MOC) click. These clicks are normal. There are no diastolic murmurs. The carotid pulse tracing shows the features of aortic stenosis, i.e., carotid shudder (CS) and an inconspicuous dicrotic notch (DN).

Figure 8.17. *Left*: Simultaneously recorded phonocardiogram at the mitral (MA), tricuspid (TA), pulmonic (PA) and aortic areas (AA), carotid pulse tracing (CT), and lead II (LII) of the electrocardiogram in a 38-year-old patient who had a malfunctioning Beall mitral valve prosthesis. Note a decrease in the time interval from the second heart sound (A2) to the mitral opening click (MOC) (0.16 sec). *Right*: The patient was reoperated on 11/19/73. The second sound (A2) mitral opening click (MOC) interval was decreased to 0.12 sec. There is very little change in the cycle length between the two tracings. The contour of the carotid pulse tracing is within the normal limits, although the dicrotic wave (DW) following the dicrotic notch (DN) as compared with preoperative tracing is slightly prominent. MCC = mitral closing click.

189

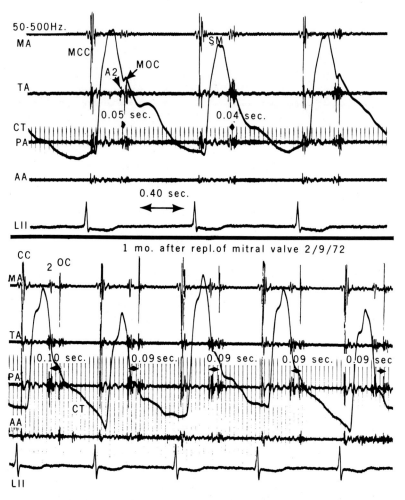

Figure 8.19. *Top*: Simultaneously recorded phonocardiogram at the mitral (MA), tricuspid (TA), pulmonic (PA) and aortic areas (AA), carotid pulse tracing (CT), and lead II (LII) of the electrocardiogram in a 42-year-old patient with Beall mitral valve prosthesis malfunction. The mitral closing click (MCC) and the second heart sound (A2) are normal. There is a high frequency, low amplitude systolic regurgitant murmur (SM) due to periprosthetic insufficiency. The mitral opening click (MOC) is recorded very close to the second heart sound and varies from beat to beat. The first beat is 0.05 sec and the second beat, 0.04 sec. *Bottom*: Phonocardiogram recorded one month after replacement with another Beall valve prosthesis. Now the opening click has normal amplitude, and despite the fact that the patient's rhythm is atrial fibrillation, the second sound–opening click interval remains fairly constant through several cardiac cycles. (From A. Benchimol: Non-Invasive Diagnostic Techniques in Cardiology. Copyright 1977 by The Williams & Wilkins Company, Baltimore. Used by permission.)

190

murmur is usually soft and of short duration in patients with a mild degree of insufficiency and holosystolic in moderate to severe mitral insufficiency (Fig. 8.20 through 8.22). A mid-diastolic murmur may infrequently be present. Dehiscence of mitral valve prostheses usually results in absence of the opening click and a very prominent systolic regurgitant murmur.

Mechanical obstruction may be due to thrombus formation or tissue ingrowth. Absence of the opening click, prolongation of the A2–OC interval (0.16–0.22 sec with a mean of 0.20), and less frequently, shortening of the A2–OC interval and a mid-diastolic murmur are indicative of mechanical obstruction.

Cocking of the disc may be defined as tilting of the disc in a fixed position. This usually occurs in the presence of severe aortic insufficiency. It results in absence of the opening and closing clicks and a loud systolic regurgitant murmur at the mitral area.

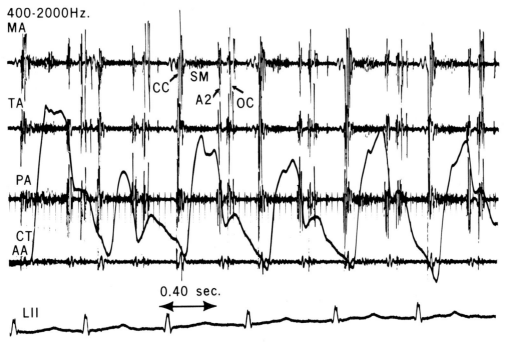

Figure 8.20. Simultaneously recorded phonocardiogram at the mitral (MA), tricuspid (TA), pulmonic (PA) and aortic areas (AA), carotid pulse tracing (CT), and lead II (LII) of the electrocardiogram in a 31-year-old patient with a malfunctioning Starr–Edwards mitral valve prosthesis. The closing click (CC) has normal amplitude. The second sound (A2)– opening click (OC) interval is short. There are several clicks in diastole. A high frequency, medium amplitude systolic regurgitant murmur (SM) recorded in all precordial areas is loudest at the mitral area indicating prosthetic insufficiency. The carotid pulse tracing is normal.

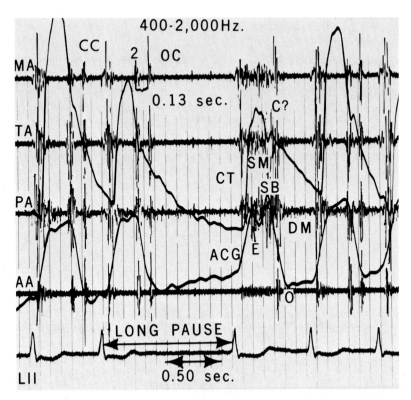

Figure 8.21. Simultaneously recorded phonocardiogram at the mitral (MA), tricuspid (TA), pulmonic (PA), and aortic areas (AA), carotid pulse tracing (CT), apexcardiogram (ACG), and lead II (LII) of the electrocardiogram in a patient with a malfunctioning Beall prosthetic valve. Note the opening (OC) and closing clicks (CC) of the prosthetic mitral valve. In most cycles the second sound–opening click interval averages approximately 0.13 sec. There is a very small systolic regurgitant murmur (SM) in the first two beats. The third beat is preceded by a long pause that causes diminution in amplitude of the closing click as seen at the mitral and pulmonic areas. This is followed by a high frequency, high amplitude systolic regurgitant murmur indicating prosthetic valve insufficiency. In the diastolic phase of the third beat, there is a diastolic murmur (DM) that probably indicates the presence of thrombus around the prosthesis creating some degree of stenosis. In addition, the opening click is no longer apparent. It is quite possible that what we are seeing as a second heart sound may represent the click plus the aortic closure sound. The carotid pulse tracing is normal. The apexcardiogram shows a sustained systolic wave. At surgery, this patient was found to have prosthetic insufficiency with clot formation around the prosthesis. SB = systolic bulge.

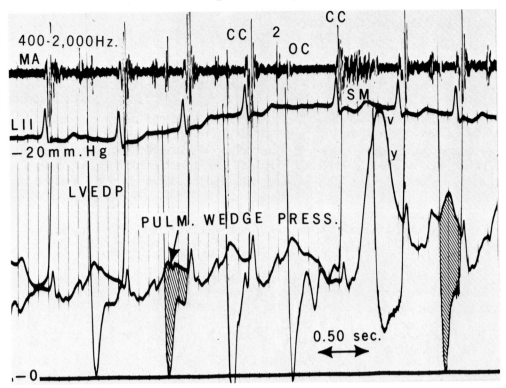

Figure 8.22. Simultaneously recorded phonocardiogram at the mitral area (MA), lead II (LII) of the electrocardiogram, left ventricular end-diastolic (LVEDP) and pulmonary "wedge" pressure recorded in the cardiac catheterization laboratory in a patient who had prosthetic Beall valve malfunction. Note the erratic opening click (OC), which at times is completely fused with the second heart sound or disappears. There is a prominent systolic murmur (SM). The V wave in the pulmonary "wedge" pressure tracing becomes prominent and the gradient is significant as compared with the small gradient in the shaded area. At the time of surgery, the patient had a moderate degree of periprosthetic insufficiency. CC = closing click.

HOMOGRAFT AND HETEROGRAFT MALFUNCTION—
MITRAL POSITION

Reported findings on the use of noninvasive techniques in patients with these prostheses are scarce. Investigators have found that these patients do not have opening clicks. The presence of prominent mitral systolic regurgitant or diastolic murmurs should be taken as possible evidence of mitral valve malfunction. However, this has not been proven.

A third heart sound is sometimes present and the time interval from aortic valve closure to the third heart sound (A2–S3) is 0.10–0.12 sec.

There have not been any definite reports on the value of carotid or jugular venous pulse tracings, the apexcardiogram, or systolic time intervals to determine normal or abnormal function of these prostheses.

AORTIC VALVE MALFUNCTION

Ball and Disc Valves

When malfunction is caused by lipid infiltration, cracking of the valve, ingrowth tissue formation, thrombus formation, or partial detachment of the valve, several findings can be detected by auscultation or phonocardiography. There is a progressive diminution in amplitude of the opening click up to the point where the click is intermittently or completely absent. The opening-to-closing click ratio decreases to less than 0.5 on a high frequency (250–500 Hz), logarithmic phonocardiogram recorded at the tricuspid area. In addition, there is prolongation of the time interval from the first, high frequency component of the first heart sound to the aortic opening click above 0.08 sec. The systolic ejection murmur may increase or decrease in amplitude and may vary from beat to beat. High frequency, high amplitude diastolic murmurs of aortic insufficiency suggest aortic valve malfunction due to periprosthetic insufficiency, particularly when they are associated with the above findings.

Pseudo ball variance has been described in patients with abnormal left ventricular function associated with low cardiac output, elevated left ventricular end-diastolic pressure.

Carotid Pulse Tracing

The carotid pulse tracing is useful only in the presence of thrombus formation around the cage. A significant left ventricular–aortic pressure gradient accompanies thrombus formation, causing an increase in ejection and upstroke times and an inconspicuous dicrotic notch. These findings are similar to what is seen in patients with aortic valvular stenosis (see Chap. 6). In patients with periprosthetic insufficiency, however, the carotid pulse tracing assumes the characteristics described for patients with aortic insufficiency, e.g., rapid upstroke time, pulsus bisferiens and a low placed and conspicuous dicrotic notch (Figs. 8.23, 8.24).

Jugular Venous Pulse Tracing

The jugular venous pulse tracing is useful to determine the presence of right heart failure and pulmonary hypertension. It will exhibit a quite prominent A wave and other abnormalities if the patient develops tricuspid insufficiency.

HOMOGRAFT AND HETEROGRAFT MALFUNCTION— AORTIC AND MITRAL POSITIONS

Very little has been described regarding the use of noninvasive techniques in detecting malfunction of these prostheses. On the phonocardiogram, patients with homografts (preserved cadaver valves) and heterografts (Hancock-porcine valves) present with high frequency, musical systolic murmurs with varying amplitude from beat to beat, unrelated to the preceding cycle length. This is due to the fact that these valves have a tendency to become calcified; therefore, the murmur will be similar to the one described for patients with calcific aortic valvular stenosis

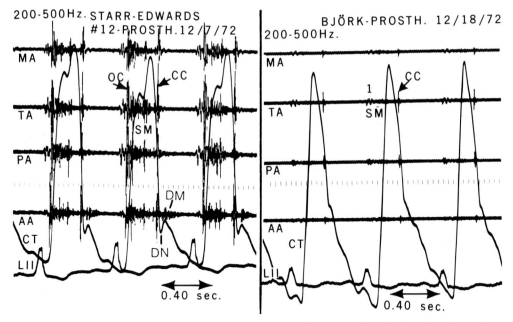

Figure 8.23. *Left*: Simultaneously recorded phonocardiogram at the mitral (MA), tricuspid (TA), pulmonic (PA) and aortic areas (AA), carotid pulse tracing (CT), and lead II (LII) of the electrocardiogram in a patient who had a #12 Starr–Edwards aortic valve prosthesis that was malfunctioning. The first heart sound, second heart sound, opening click (OC), and closing click (CC) are normal. A high frequency, high amplitude systolic ejection murmur (SM) is recorded in all precordial areas. A diastolic murmur (DM), well appreciated at the aortic area, is due to periprosthetic insufficiency. *Right*: Simultaneously recorded phonocardiogram at the mitral, tricuspid, pulmonic and aortic areas, carotid pulse tracing, and lead II of the electrocardiogram in the same patient after the valve was replaced with a Björk–Shiley prosthesis. With this prosthesis, the first heart sound is normal and there is no opening click. There is a closing click (CC), well recorded at the tricuspid area and a high frequency, low amplitude systolic ejection murmur recorded best at the tricuspid area. The carotid pulse tracing is normal.

(see Chap. 6). However, the presence of musical systolic murmurs is not always a definite indicator of valve malfunction, because they may also be recorded in patients with normally functioning homograft or heterograft valves.

High frequency, high amplitude (Grade III–IV/VI) arterial diastolic murmurs are usually significant and should make the examiner suspect the presence of prosthetic valve insufficiency. Murmurs similar to the Austin–Flint murmur have been described in these patients and probably represent a regurgitant jet of insufficiency against the mitral valve. Prominent third and fourth heart sounds are frequently noted.

Carotid Pulse Tracing

The carotid pulse tracing shows the abnormalities seen in patients with aortic insufficiency or aortic stenosis.

Jugular Venous Pulse Tracing

The jugular venous pulse tracing is useful in the diagnosis of homograft valve malfunction only when the patient presents with the clinical picture of right ventricular failure.

Apexcardiogram

The apexcardiogram usually exhibits prominent A and rapid filling waves, which coincide with the prominent fourth and third heart sounds.

Systolic Time Intervals

The systolic time intervals are essentially identical to the ones described for patients with aortic valvular disease and heart failure.

PROSTHETIC TRICUSPID VALVE MALFUNCTION

Ball and Disc Valves

Replacement of the tricuspid valve is uncommon and there are only a few reports of the normal and abnormal characteristics of tricuspid valve prostheses. These reports indicate that malfunction due to thrombus formation around the prosthesis results in findings similar to the ones seen in patients with tricuspid stenosis or insufficiency (see Chap. 7). On the phonocardiogram, these patients show a decrease in amplitude and wandering of the tricuspid opening click, and a low frequency, high amplitude atrioventricular diastolic murmur similar to what is seen in patients with tricuspid stenosis. When the valve does not close properly, the typical phonocardiographic features of tricuspid insufficiency are seen, such as a high frequency, high amplitude systolic regurgitant murmur, decrease in amplitude of the first heart sound, and a prominent third heart sound. Although the basic mechanism for this type of dysfunction has not been established, it has been suggested that it is the result of impingement of the valve cage or disc against the right ventricular myocardium or interventricular septum. In addition, there may be laceration of the myocardium or bacterial and fungal endocarditis. This is particularly common in patients with a prosthetic Cutter–Smeloff valve.

Carotid Pulse Tracing

The carotid pulse tracing shows decreased ejection time, probably secondary to diminished left ventricular stroke volume.

Jugular Venous Pulse Tracing

The jugular venous pulse tracing is valuable in determining the presence of tricuspid valve prosthesis malfunction. If the malfunction is primarily stenosis, it shows the typical features of tricuspid stenosis such as a very prominent A wave and a normal X descent, followed by a V wave and a very slow Y descent. If the malfunction results in insufficiency, the findings for tricuspid insufficiency will be evident (see Chap. 7).

Systolic Time Intervals

In patients with tricuspid valve prostheses the systolic time intervals are nonspecific and are only indicative of right and left ventricular failure.

ECHOCARDIOGRAPHY IN NORMAL AND ABNORMAL PROSTHETIC VALVE FUNCTION

It is important to obtain a baseline echocardiogram for each patient subjected to valve replacement prior to discharge from the hospital in order to determine normal values and the characteristics of the prosthesis implanted. This is very valuable because disc or ball excursions, diameters, and opening and closing velocities vary according to individual valve design and size. A technically satisfactory echocardiogram in the immediate postoperative period serves as each patient's control and any subsequent changes in the above parameters may be helpful in identifying valve malfunction. Transducer angulation and position for the baseline recording should be noted and subsequent tracings obtained utilizing the same technique. The transducer position varies from patient to patient in recording the same prosthetic valve. No definite position is considered best for recording any prosthesis.

Ball Valves—Mitral Position

Normal echocardiographic features of a Starr–Edwards mitral ball valve are shown in Figures 8.25 and 8.26. The findings usually include: (1) Opening and closing of the valves are related to approximate crossover pressure changes of the left atrium and left ventricle; (2) the ball moves to the open position (D–E slope) and to the closed position (B–C slope). The remainder of the echocardiographic recording is due to movement of the cage while the ball remains against the apex or the valve ring. The stenotic E–F slope of the prosthetic mitral ball valve resembles the E–F slope seen in patients with mitral stenosis, i.e., there is no significant rapid movement posteriorly during ventricular filling. The exact mechanism for this finding is not known.

Echocardiography has not been established as a tool in the definite diagnosis of prosthetic valve malfunction. However, a few reports have indicated that it is valuable in patients with normally functioning prosthetic mitral ball valves where the interventricular septum usually moves paradoxically. This finding can also be seen in patients with mild to moderate periprosthetic insufficiency, where the interventricular septum will show normal motion. The mechanism of paradoxical septal motion in patients with normally functioning prostheses is not well known. Caution should be exercised in interpreting this finding since many patients with normal functioning valves may have normal septal motion (Fig. 8.27). The usual echocardiographic features of patients with prosthetic valve malfunction include

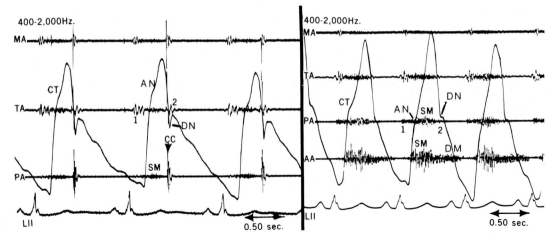

Figure 8.24. *Left*: Simultaneously recorded phonocardiogram at the mitral (MA), tricuspid (TA) and pulmonic areas (PA), carotid pulse tracing (CT), and lead II (LII) of the electrocardiogram in a patient who had a #25 Björk–Shiley aortic valve prosthesis. This tracing was recorded while the valve was functioning well. A systolic ejection murmur (SM) was recorded best at the pulmonic area. There is a normal closing click (CC). The carotid pulse tracing is normal. *Right*: Simultaneously recorded phonocardiogram at the mitral, tricuspid, pulmonic and aortic areas (AA), carotid pulse tracing, and lead II of the electrocardiogram when this patient developed prosthetic aortic valve dysfunction. A closing click is not present. Amplitude of the murmur has increased markedly. In addition, the patient developed an arterial diastolic murmur (DM) of aortic insufficiency. The carotid pulse tracing is abnormal, showing an anacrotic notch (AN), which is indicative of valvular obstruction. The dicrotic notch (DN) is inconspicuous as compared with the previous tracing.

multiple echoes derived from within the prosthesis, indicating the presence of thrombus formation. This causes obstruction of flow from the left atrium to left ventricle, resulting in an increase in left atrial pressure and in left atrial internal diameter. There may also be abnormal motion of the disc during systole or diastole (Fig. 8.28).

In the Cutter–Smeloff mitral ball prosthesis, delayed opening of the ball as well as delayed cage motion have been described in patients with valve malfunction. At operation, ingrowth of fibroid tissue or clot formation have been identified and these are most likely the causes that prevent proper ball excursion.

Ball Valves—Aortic Position

The following features have been described for normally functioning Starr–Edwards prostheses in the aortic position: (1) Motion of opening and closing of the ball valve and cage appear to be related to the appropriate crossover pressure changes between the aorta and left ventricle; (2) movement of the cage is much less evident in the aortic position as compared with the mitral. Rocking movement of the cage during diastole has been observed in patients with partial valve detachment.

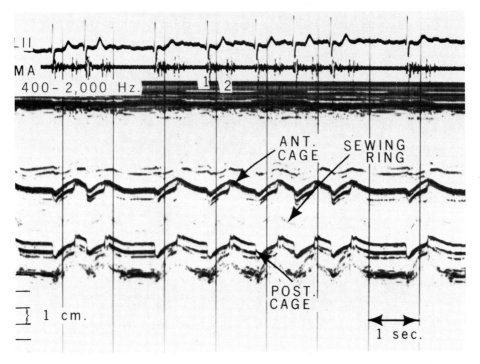

Figure 8.25. Echocardiogram recorded simultaneously with a mitral area (MA) phonocardiogram and lead II (LII) of the electrocardiogram showing normal opening and closing of a Starr–Edwards mitral valve prosthesis. The anterior and posterior cages and sewing ring are well recorded.

Beall Disc Valves—Mitral Position

Most disc valve prostheses present with nearly identical echocardiographic patterns. Our experience has been primarily in patients with a Beall prosthesis. The normal echocardiographic pattern of the Beall prosthesis in the mitral position is shown in Figure 8.26. The first echo arises from the anterior surface of one of the struts; the second echo from the anterior disc, which moves rapidly away from the anterior strut to the closed position. The third echo represents the suture ring. Another faint echo can be seen during systole and is located behind the anterior strut. During systole, all three echoes move synchronously and this represents movement of the mitral annulus.

Failure of the anterior echo of the disc to merge with the strut echo is usually indicative of incomplete disc opening and a 1 mm decrease in disc excursion is almost always an indicator of malfunction due to thrombus formation.

Dehiscence of the suture ring can be detected through echocardiography if the valve cage changes its motion pattern as compared with a previous echocardiogram, but disc motion may show a normal pattern in perivalvular insufficiency. A few reports have also indicated that significant perivalvular insufficiency may be recognized by a sudden or progressive increase in left atrial and left ventricular internal diameters.

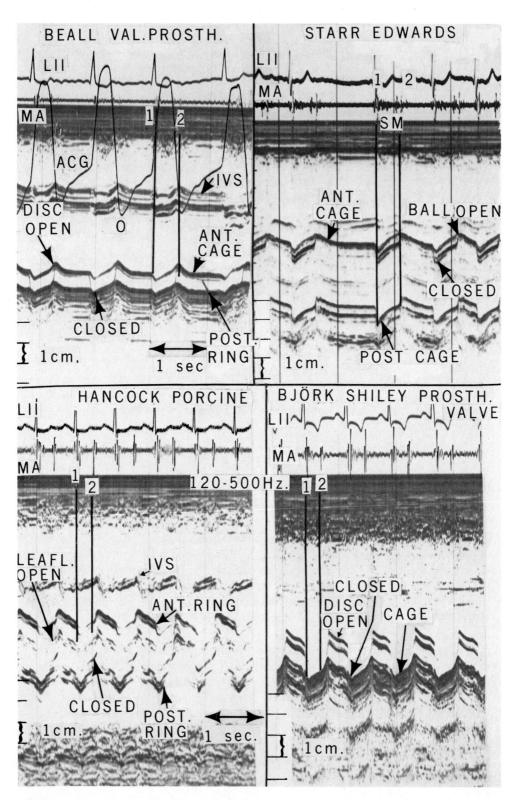

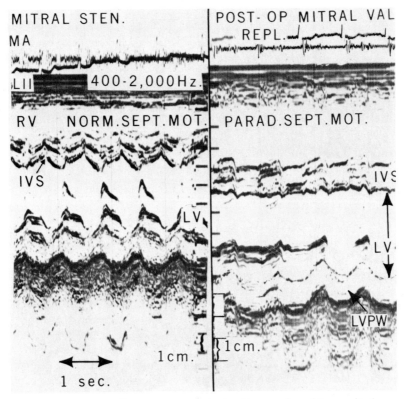

Figure 8.27. *Left:* Echocardiogram recorded simultaneously with a mitral area (MA) phonocardiogram and lead II (LII) of the electrocardiogram showing the typical findings seen in patients with mitral stenosis, including thickening of the anterior and posterior leaflets, anterior valve motion, and a decrease in the E–F slope. Prior to surgery, the patient had normal septal motion. *Right:* This tracing recorded following replacement of the valve shows paradoxical septal motion. This is not a sign of valve malfunction. It is seen in many patients with mitral valve prostheses. Left ventricular internal dimension is within normal limits. RV = right ventricle, IVS = interventricular septum, LVPW = left ventricular posterior wall, LV = left ventricle.

Figure 8.26. Echocardiogram recorded simultaneously with a mitral area (MA) phonocardiogram and lead II (LII) of the electrocardiogram in patients with various types of prostheses in the mitral position. *Top Left:* Example of a Beall valve disc prosthesis showing opening and closing of the disc. *Top Right:* Normal functioning Starr–Edwards prosthesis. Note that the valve remains in a closed position during systole and opens wide during diastole. *Bottom Left:* Hancock-porcine valve prosthesis. The configuration of the echocardiogram is quite different from the ones shown above. The motion of the valve is similar to a normally functioning mitral valve. *Bottom Right:* Tracing of a patient with a Björk–Shiley mitral valve prosthesis showing normal opening and closing of the disc. Echoes derived from the cage are also well seen.

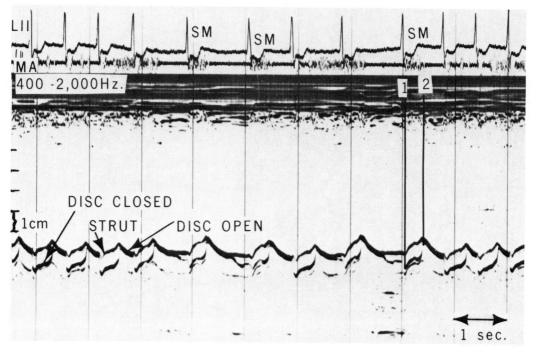

Figure 8.28. Simultaneously recorded echocardiogram, mitral area (MA) phonocardiogram, and lead II (LII) of the electrocardiogram in a 60-year-old patient with a malfunctioning Beall mitral valve prosthesis. The rhythm is atrial fibrillation. A systolic murmur that starts with the first heart sound and terminates with the second heart sound is due to insufficiency of the prosthesis. On the echocardiogram, the disc remains in an open position against the anterior strut of the valve shortly after the second heart sound. In some beats during systole, the valve appears to move anteriorly and open slightly, allowing insufficiency to occur. This is an indication of prosthetic valve malfunction.

Björk–Shiley Tilting Disc Valves— Mitral and Aortic Positions

The Björk–Shiley prosthetic disc valve can be implanted in the mitral (Fig. 8.29) or aortic (Fig. 8.30) positions. The valve is asymmetrical along the X (right–left), Y (superior–inferior) and Z axis (anterior–posterior) and the disc pivots about 60 degrees during ventricular ejection. During ventricular ejection, the larger segment of the disc exhibits greater excursion as compared with the lesser segment (Figs. 8.29 and 8.30). For aortic valves, a clear opening and closing point must be recorded because most aortic ball or disc prostheses look alike including Björk–Shiley valves, so no definite patterns are reliable. Usually, to record an aortic prosthesis with maximal disc excursion, the transducer is placed laterally near the apex and aimed up toward the aorta.

Optimal alignment of the transducer in relation to the valve for detecting maximal disc excursion, which occurs when the ultrasonic beam is perpendicular to the maximally opened disc, varies from patient to patient, e.g., 2 to 8 o'clock position in X–Z planes. It is usually possible to obtain satisfactory excursion of

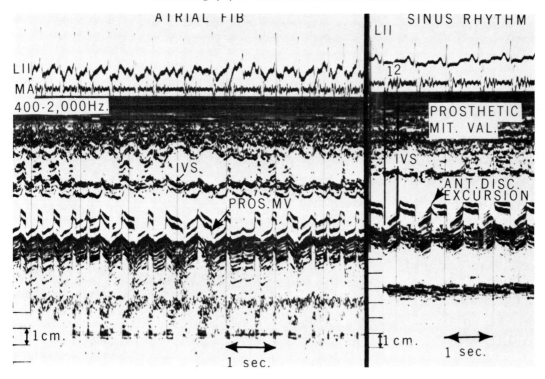

Figure 8.29. Echocardiogram, mitral area (MA) phonocardiogram, and lead II (LII) of the electrocardiogram recorded simultaneously in a patient with a #29 Björk–Shiley mitral valve prosthesis. *Left:* This tracing was recorded when the patient's rhythm was atrial fibrillation. There is normal motion of the valve. The configuration varies from beat to beat because of the atrial fibrillation. Disc motion is also normal. *Right:* Echocardiogram on the same patient after conversion to sinus rhythm. Note the normal excursion of the anterior disc, indicated by an arrow. IVS = interventricular septum.

the greater curvatures of the disc. The lesser opening portion of the disc is usually very difficult to record. It is best to record the valve at the transducer position where maximum anterior disc excursion is seen.

Definite criteria for detection of Björk–Shiley valve malfunction have not been established. However, the presence of strong and disorganized echoes within the valve structure may suggest clot formation.

Lillehei–Kaster Tilting Disc Valves— Mitral and Aortic Positions

Echocardiographic features of the Lillehei–Kaster valve have been described in a series of patients with normally functioning prostheses. Valve excursion and opening and closing velocities decrease with aging, and the valve velocity is not uniform. Considerable variation has been noted in patients who have apparently normal functioning prostheses. The average opening and closing velocities of Lillehei–Kaster valves exceed those of the Starr–Edwards and Beall valves.

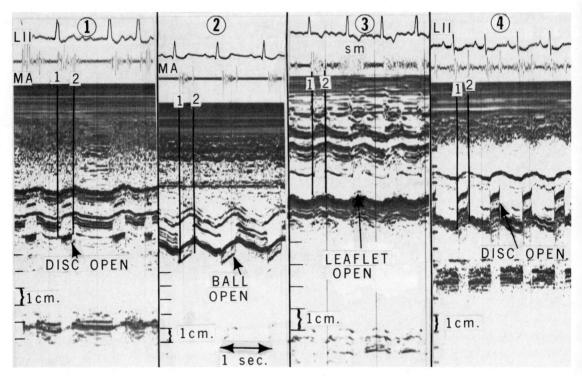

Figure 8.30. Echocardiogram, mitral area (MA) phonocardiogram, and lead II (LII) of the electrocardiogram in patients with different types of normally functioning valve prostheses. *Panel 1:* A Cutter valve. Note that the disc closes completely during ventricular diastole and opens wide during ventricular systole. *Panel 2:* A Starr–Edwards valve showing normal excursion of the prosthetic ball. *Panel 3:* A Hancock-porcine valve showing normal closing and opening of the leaflets. *Panel 4:* A #23 Björk–Shiley valve prosthesis. Note that the disc opens wide during systole and closes completely during diastole.

204

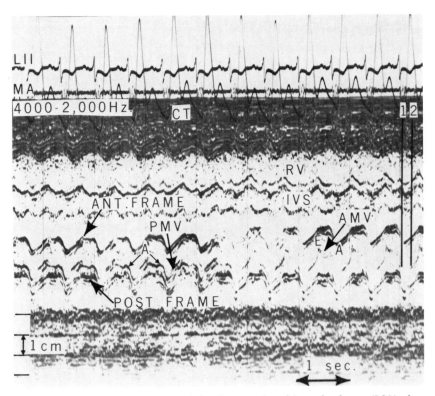

Figure 8.31. Echocardiogram recorded simultaneously with a mitral area (MA) phonocardiogram, carotid pulse tracing (CT), and lead II (LII) of the electrocardiogram in a 57-year-old patient with a Hancock-porcine mitral valve prosthesis. The anterior and posterior frame and anterior (AMV) and posterior (PMV) valve are well seen. Motion of the prosthesis resembles the motion of a normally functioning mitral valve. The interventricular septum (IVS) is recorded. RV = right ventricle.

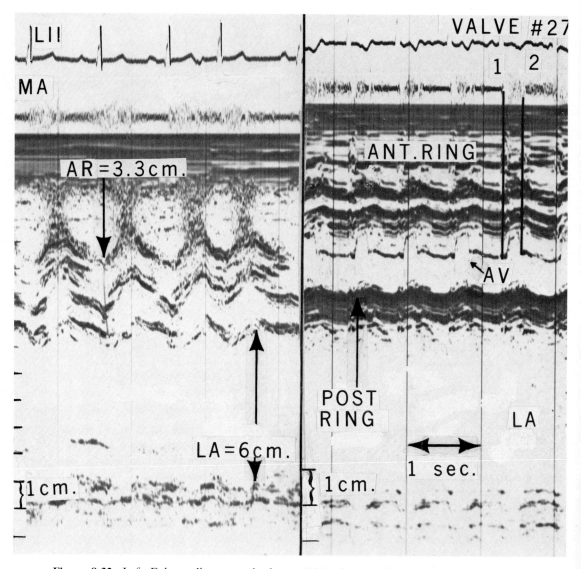

Figure 8.32. *Left:* Echocardiogram, mitral area (MA) phonocardiogram, and lead II (LII) of the electrocardiogram in a 43-year-old patient with aortic stenosis and insufficiency showing the typical echocardiographic features of aortic stenosis with narrowing of the aortic cusp excursion. Note that the left atrium (LA) is enlarged to 6 cm. *Right:* Echocardiogram recorded after aortic valve replacement with a #27 Hancock-porcine prosthesis. The prosthetic aortic valve looks very similar to a normal aortic valve with a box-like structure, open wide during systole and closing completely during diastole. AR = aortic root; AV = aortic valve.

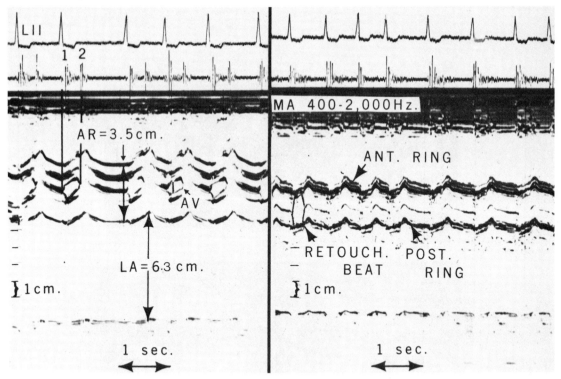

Figure 8.33. Echocardiogram recorded simultaneously with a phonocardiogram and lead II (LII) of the electrocardiogram in a 53-year-old patient with aortic stenosis who had an aortic valve replacement with a #25 Hancock-porcine prosthesis. *Left:* The echocardiogram prior to surgery shows a markedly stenotic aortic valve. The valve excursion is small and very heavy echoes around it indicate either fibrosis or calcification. The left atrium (LA) is enlarged to 6.3 cm. *Right:* Echocardiogram recorded after valve replacement. Note the normal box-like structure of the valve. It opens wide during systole and closes completely during diastole. The first beat on this recording has been retouched. AR = aortic root; AV = aortic valve.

Heterograft Valves

The most commonly used heterograft is the stented Hancock-porcine, a chemically preserved aortic valve of a pig, which can be implanted in the mitral (Fig. 8.31), tricuspid, or aortic positions (Figs. 8.30, 8.32, 8.33). There has not been a large series of reported echocardiographic findings for this prosthesis. In our experience, the valve exhibits the features seen in normally functioning human valves in the mitral, tricuspid, or aortic positions with the addition of a heavy band of echoes anterior and posterior to the leaflets representing the anterior and posterior ring. Definite patterns for recognition of malfunction have not been established. The Hancock-porcine valve is also used for the Rastelli and Fontan procedures for surgical correction of pulmonary and tricuspid atresia. The transducer position for recording these valves is basically the same as positions for recording normal valves.

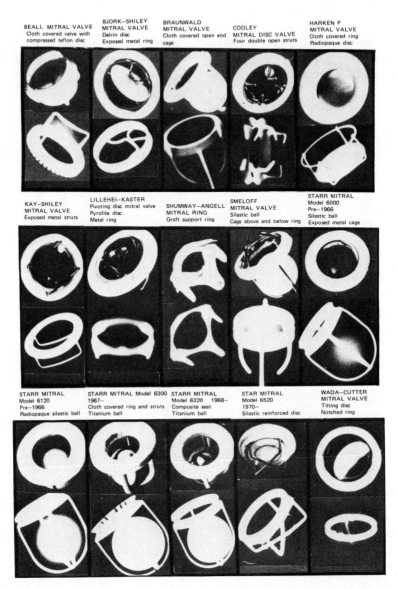

Figure 8.34. Illustration of several types of mitral valve prostheses. (Reproduced courtesy of Dryden Morse, M.D., Deborah Heart and Lung Center, Browns Mills, New Jersey.)

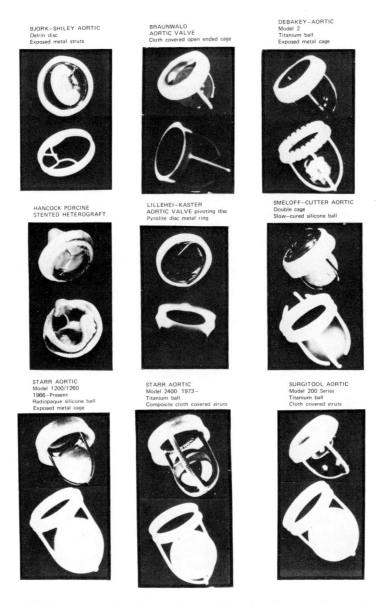

Figure 8.35. This is an example of several types of aortic valve prostheses. (Reproduced courtesy of Dryden Morse, M.D., Deborah Heart and Lung Center, Browns Mills, New Jersey.)

Homograft Valves

Echocardiograms of patients with stented fascia lata grafts in the mitral position have been reported. The diastolic closure rate (E–F slope) of the cusps revealed significant correlation with the effective valve area as calculated by standard formulas for valve area measurements using invasive techniques.

Autograft valves, made of human dura mater, have been used for mitral, aortic, and tricuspid valve replacement. The echocardiographic features are not well known, but the findings seem to be similar to the ones described for the heterograft Hancock-porcine valve.

Figures 8.34 and 8.35 illustrate several types of mitral and aortic valve prostheses.

BIBLIOGRAPHY

Angell, W.W., deLanerolle, P., and Shumway, N.E.:   Valve replacement; present status of homograft valves. Prog. Cardiovasc. Dis. *15*:589, 1973.

Aravanis, C., Toutouzas, P., and Stavrou, S.:   Disappearance of opening sound of Starr–Edwards mitral valve due to valvular detachment. Br. Heart J. *34*:1314, 1972.

Aston, S.J., and Mulder, D.G.:   Cardiac valve replacement: a seven-year follow up. J. Thorac. Cardiovasc. Surg. *61*:547, 1971.

Barratt-Boyes, B.G.:   Long-term follow-up of aortic valvular grafts. Br. Heart J. *33*:60, 1971 (Suppl.).

Beall, A.C. Jr., and Sheely, C.H. II: Current status of prosthetic valve replacement. Cardiovasc. Clin. *5*(2):319, 1973.

Behrendt, D.M., and Austen, W.G.:   Current status of prosthetics for heart valve replacement. Prog. Cardiovasc. Dis. *15*:369, 1973.

Belenkie, I.L., Carr, M., Schlant, R.C., Nutter, D.O., and Symbas, P.N.:   Malfunction of a Cutter–Smeloff mitral ball valve prosthesis: diagnosis by phonocardiography and echocardiography. Am. Heart J. *86*:399, 1973.

Björk, V.O.:   Aortic valve replacement with Björk–Shiley tilting disc valve prosthesis. Br. Heart J. *33*:42, 1971 (Suppl.).

Björk, V.O., and Henze, A.:   Encapsulation of the Björk–Shiley aortic disc valve prosthesis caused by the lack of anticoagulant treatment. Scand. J. Thorac. Cardiovasc. Surg. *7*:17, 1973.

Boicourt, O.W., Bristow, J.D., Starr, A., and Griswold, H.E.:   A phonocardiographic study of patients with multiple Starr–Edwards prosthetic valves. Br. Heart J. *28*:531, 1966.

Brown, D.F.:   Decreased intensity of closure sound in a normally functioning Starr–Edwards mitral valve prosthesis: observations on presystolic mitral valve closure. Am. J. Cardiol. *31*:93, 1973.

Cohen, A.I., Benchimol, A., and Brown, L.B.:   Clinical and phonocardiographic recognition of prosthetic aortic valve ball variance. Ariz. Med. *27*:90, 1970.

Dayem, M.K.A., and Raftery, E.B.:   Phonocardiogram of the ball-and-cage aortic valve prosthesis. Br. Heart J. *29*:446, 1967.

Delman, A.J.:   Aortic ball variance. Am. Heart J. *83*:291, 1972.

Douglas, J.E., and Williams, G.D.:   Echocardiographic evaluation of the Björk–Shiley prosthetic valve. Circulation *50*:52, 1974.

Fernandez, J., Morse, D., Maranhao, V., and Gooch, A.S.:   Results of use of the pyrolytic carbon tilting disc Björk–Shiley aortic prosthesis. Chest 65:640, 1974.

Fishman, N.H., Hutchinson, J.C., Massengale, M.M., and Roe, B.B.:   Follow-up evaluation of 100 consecutive mitral prosthesis implants. Arch. Surg. 97:691, 1968.

Fleming, J., Hamer, J., Hayward, G., Hill, I., and Tubbs, O.S.:   Long-term results of aortic valve replacement. Br. Heart J. 31:388, 1969.

Gibson, D.G., Broder, G., and Sowton, E.:   Phonocardiographic method of assessing changes in left ventricular function after Starr–Edwards replacement of aortic valve. Br. Heart J. 32:142, 1970.

Hamby, R.I., Aintablian, A., and Wisoff, B.G.:   Mechanism of closure of the mitral prosthetic valve and the role of atrial systole: phonocardiographic and cinefluorographic study. Am. J. Cardiol. 31:616, 1973.

Hildner, F.J.:   Detection of prosthetic valve dysfunction by bedside and laboratory evaluation. Cardiovasc. Clin. 5:289, 1973.

Hylen, J.C., Kloster, F.E., Starr, A., and Griswold, H.E.:   Aortic ball variance: diagnosis and treatment. Ann. Intern. Med. 72:1, 1970.

Isom, O.W., Williams, C.D., Falk, E.A., Glassman, E., and Spencer, F.C.:   Long-term evaluation of cloth-covered metallic ball prostheses. J. Thorac. Cardiovasc. Surg. 64:354, 1972.

Leachman, R.D., and Cokkinos, D.V.P.:   Absence of opening click in dehiscence of mitral valve prosthesis. New Engl. J. Med. 281:461, 1969.

Levy, M.J., Vidne, B., Salomon, J., and Eshkol, D.:   Long-term follow-up (one to four years) of heart valve prostheses (102) consecutive patients. Dis. Chest 56:440, 1969.

Mary, D.A.S., Pakrashi, B.C., Catchpole, R.W., and Ionescu, M.I.:   Echocardiographic studies of stented fascia lata grafts in the mitral position. Circulation 49:237, 1974.

Miller, H.C., Stephens, J., and Gibson, D.:   Echocardiographic features of mitral Starr–Edwards paraprosthetic regurgitation. Br. Heart J. 35:560, 1973.

Najmi, M., and Segal, B.L.:   Auscultatory and phonocardiographic findings in patients with prosthetic ball-valves. Am. J. Cardiol. 16:794, 1965.

Pileggi, F., Sosa, E.A., Bellotti, G., DelNero, E. Jr., Verginelli, G., Tranchesi, J., Puig, L.B. and Decourt, L.V.:   O fonomecanocardiograma da valva de dura-mater em posição mitral. Arq. Bras. Cardiol. 28(3):267, 1975.

Ross, D.N.:   Aortic valve replacements. Br. Heart J. 33:39, 1971 (Suppl.).

Stimmel, B., Stein, E., Katz, A.M., Litwak, R.S., and Donoso, E.:   Phonocardiographic manifestations of heterograft valve dysfunction in mitral area. Br. Heart J. 34:936, 1972.

Stross, J.K., Willis, P.W., and Kahn, D.R.:   Diagnostic features of malfunction of disc mitral valve prostheses. J.A.M.A. 217:305, 1971.

9
Coronary Artery Disease

Coronary artery disease is the most common cardiovascular abnormality in the western hemisphere. Techniques developed to delineate the anatomy of the coronary circulation include methods such as selective coronary arteriography and evaluation of cardiac functions through injection of contrast material into the left ventricle (left ventricular angiography). In addition, noninvasive methods such as vectorcardiography, electrocardiography, phonocardiography, echocardiography, holter monitoring, exercise stress testing, and perfusion studies utilizing isotopes have resulted in major improvements in diagnosis and determination of the degree of severity of the disease. The growing role of coronary artery surgery for treatment of symptomatic patients has helped us to improve our understanding of this pathologic condition.

Heart Sounds and Murmurs

The first heart sound is normal (Fig. 9.1). The second heart sound may be normal or show fixed or paradoxical (reverse) splitting. Paradoxical splitting of the second heart sound is characterized by a fixed A2–P2 interval during inspiration and expiration. The pulmonic component precedes the aortic component. This is particularly well seen during episodes of angina pectoris due to coronary insufficiency. The pulmonic component of the second heart sound may be abnormally accentuated if the patient is in heart failure and has elevated pulmonary artery pressures (normal range: 10/5 to 30/15 systolic and diastolic). Systolic ejection clicks, present in a small percentage ($\pm 3\%$) of patients with coronary artery disease, are probably due to dilatation of the ascending aorta. They are seen in patients with coronary artery disease and associated arterial hypertension. The presence of a fourth heart sound in patients with coronary artery disease has been related to abnormalities of left ventricular function at the time of atrial contraction (Fig. 9.2). The clinical importance of this sound has been questioned by several investigators since it may be present in a normal population without evidence of coronary artery disease. A simultaneously recorded phonocardiogram and apexcardiogram help to determine whether a fourth heart sound is of clinical importance. If the A wave of the apexcardiogram exceeds the normal upper value of 15% of total amplitude of the apexcardiogram (distance from the E to the O point), the fourth heart sound may have pathological significance (Figs. 9.2, 9.3). The

212

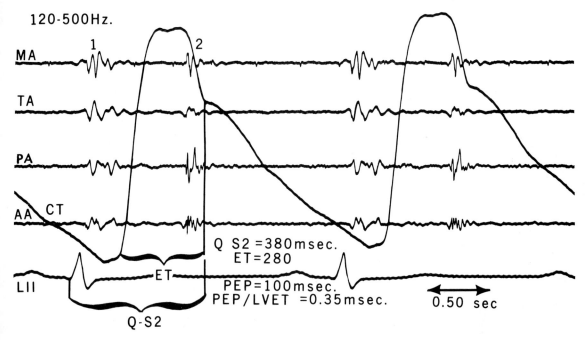

120-500Hz.

MA

TA

PA

AA   CT

Q S2 =380msec.
ET=280

LII

ET

PEP=100msec.
PEP/LVET =0.35msec.

0.50 sec

Q-S2

Figure 9.1. Simultaneously recorded phonocardiogram at the mitral (MA), tricuspid (TA), pulmonic (PA) and aortic areas (AA), carotid pulse tracing (CT), and lead II (LII) of the electrocardiogram in a 39-year-old patient with coronary artery disease. The first heart sound is split but is still within normal limits. The second heart sound is normal. The carotid tracing shows a normal ejection time and pre-ejection period. The pre-ejection period/left ventricular ejection time (PEP/LVET) ratio is normal.

presence of a third heart sound is almost always an abnormal finding in patients with coronary artery disease (Fig. 9.3). It usually indicates the presence of left ventricular dyskinesis and/or ventricular aneurysm with elevated left ventricular end-diastolic pressure, decreased cardiac output, stroke volume, and ejection fraction (Figs. 9.2, 9.3).

Characteristic murmurs have not been described in patients with chronic coronary artery disease. However, some patients have mitral insufficiency due to abnormal motion of the mitral leaflets secondary to a lack of sustained tension of the papillary muscle, which allows insufficiency to occur late in systole. In addition, these patients may present with a systolic murmur that starts after the first heart sound, has a late systolic accentuation, and terminates with the second heart sound. The systolic regurgitant murmur of anterior papillary muscle dysfunction (Fig. 9.4) tends to radiate to the axillary line, and the murmur of posterior papillary muscle dysfunction radiates toward the sternum. It is a high frequency murmur, usually Grade II–III/VI, heard best when the patient is placed in a left lateral decubitus position.

The systolic ejection murmurs in these patients are transmitted to all precordial areas (Fig. 9.5), and are probably due to turbulent flow across a slightly sclerotic, thickened or calcified aortic valve. At cardiac catheterization, most patients do not have a significant gradient across the aortic valve.

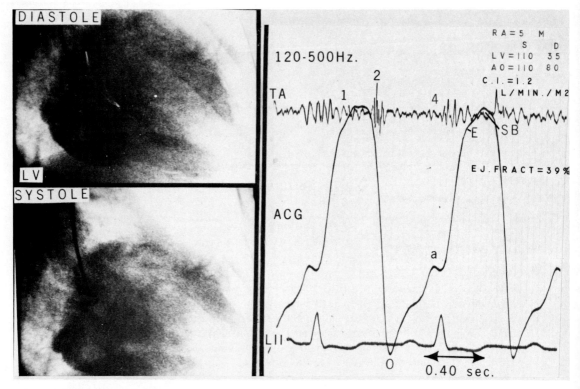

Figure 9.2. *Left:* Left ventricular angiogram in a patient with coronary artery disease. During systole and diastole significant abnormalities on this angiogram were documented in the right anterior oblique projection. There is very little change in the size of the left ventricle during systole and diastole, indicating poor left ventricular function. *Right:* Simultaneously recorded phonocardiogram at the tricuspid area (TA), apexcardiogram (ACG), and lead II (LII) of the electrocardiogram. There are normal first and second heart sounds, and a fourth heart sound that coincides with a prominent A wave on the apexcardiogram. The measurements obtained during cardiac catheterization showed normal right atrial pressure (RA 5). The systolic left ventricular pressure is 110, the diastolic is 35, which is markedly elevated. The upper limit of normal for left ventricular end-diastolic pressure is 12. The aortic pressure is normal. The cardiac index is diminished to 1.2 L/Min/M2. The normal cardiac index is 2.2:4.

214

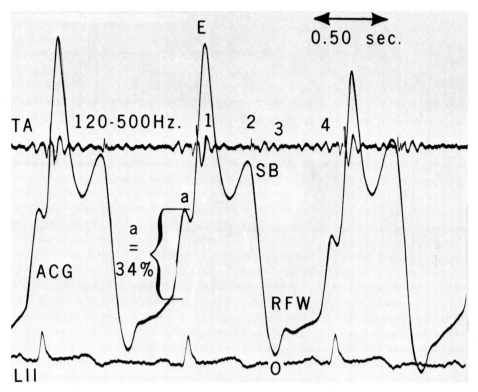

Figure 9.3. Simultaneously recorded phonocardiogram at the tricuspid area (TA), apexcardiogram (ACG), and lead II (LII) of the electrocardiogram in a 59-year-old patient with coronary artery disease. The first and second heart sounds are normal. A prominent third heart sound, which is definitely an abnormal finding in patients with coronary artery disease for this age group, coincides with the peak of the rapid filling wave (RFW) on the apexcardiogram. There is also a prominent fourth heart sound that coincides with the peak of the A wave on the apexcardiogram. The apexcardiogram is abnormal showing a prominent A wave and a systolic retraction followed by a late systolic bulge (SB).

215

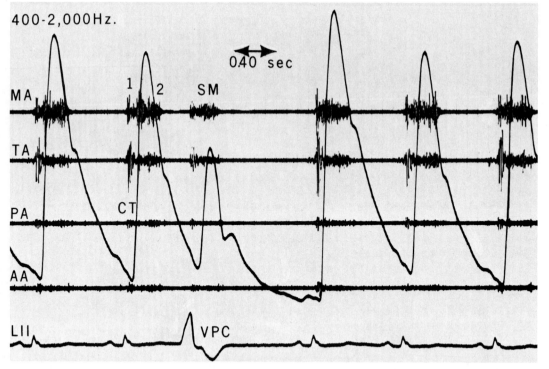

Figure 9.4. Simultaneously recorded phonocardiogram at the mitral (MA), tricuspid (TA), pulmonic (PA) and aortic areas (AA), carotid pulse tracing (CT), and lead II (LII) of the electrocardiogram in a 71-year-old patient with coronary artery disease and papillary muscle dysfunction due to mitral insufficiency. The first heart sound is slightly diminished. The second heart sound is single and normal. There is a high frequency, high amplitude systolic regurgitant murmur (SM). During the recording the patient had a ventricular premature contraction (VPC), which causes a decrease in amplitude of the systolic murmur. The carotid pulse tracing is normal.

The murmur of a ruptured papillary muscle or of the chordae tendineae that attach the mitral valve to the papillary muscle may occur during myocardial infarction particularly in patients with anterior wall involvement of the left ventricle. It resembles the murmur of mitral insufficiency due to rheumatic heart disease. The murmur is usually musical, has high amplitude, and radiates to all precordial areas. It may be preceded by an ejection or midsystolic click in approximately 20 to 30% of cases. The rupture of chordae tendineae is usually a catastrophic event during the acute stage of myocardial infarction and should be recognized immediately through auscultation or other noninvasive techniques because it requires immediate aggressive medical or surgical therapy.

If rupture of the interventricular septum occurs during acute myocardial infarction, a prominent pansystolic murmur will be present. It is identical to the one seen in patients with congenital ventricular septal defects. Low frequency, mid-diastolic rumbling murmurs may be present and usually indicate the presence of a large left-to-right shunt through the acquired septal defect (Fig. 9.6).

400-2,000Hz.

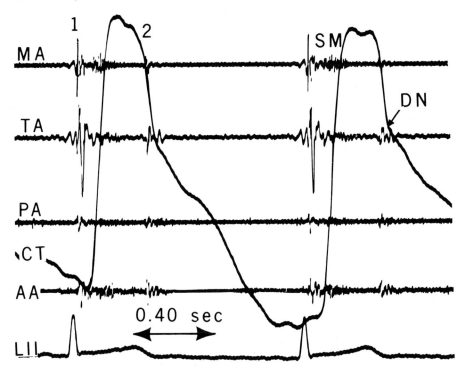

Figure 9.5. Simultaneously recorded phonocardiogram at the mitral (MA), tricuspid (TA), pulmonic (PA) and aortic areas (AA), carotid pulse tracing (CT), and lead II (LII) of the electrocardiogram in a 55-year-old patient with aortic sclerosis. The first and second heart sounds are normal. There is a high frequency, medium amplitude systolic ejection murmur (SM) that starts shortly after the first heart sound, reaches a peak in early to midsystole and terminates prior to the second heart sound. The carotid pulse tracing shows a slight delay in upstroke time. The dicrotic notch is inconspicuous. This is not an unusual finding for patients in this age group.

Carotid Pulse Tracing

The carotid pulse tracing is usually normal (Figs. 9.1, 9.4, 9.5). However, it may show a slow or notched upstroke time (Fig. 9.1) and an inconspicuous dicrotic notch probably related to decreased distensibility of the carotid artery with or without associated aortic or carotid artery sclerosis. Ejection time may be decreased during periods of angina pectoris. Pulsus alternans, which is characterized by high amplitude beats followed by low amplitude beats, may be seen in the terminal stages of this disease and is indicative of left heart failure (Fig. 9.7).

Jugular Venous Pulse Tracing

The jugular venous pulse tracing is normal unless the patient has congestive heart failure, pulmonary hypertension, or tricuspid insufficiency. Pulsus alternans seen

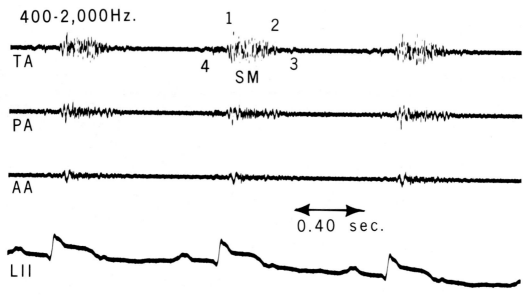

Figure 9.6. Simultaneously recorded phonocardiogram at the tricuspid (TA), pulmonic (PA) and aortic areas (AA), and lead II (LII) of the electrocardiogram in a 77-year-old patient with acute myocardial infarction and rupture of the interventricular septum causing a left-to-right shunt of 1.7:1. The first heart sound is normal. The second heart sound is diminished. A high frequency, high amplitude systolic regurgitant murmur (SM) is recorded best at the tricuspid area. There are prominent third and fourth heart sounds. Note the marked elevation of the ST-segments on the electrocardiogram indicative of a current of injury. An autopsy documented a rupture of the interventricular septum due to massive anterior wall myocardial infarction.

on the jugular venous pulse tracing can be observed in the late stages of this disease and indicates right heart failure.

Apexcardiogram

In 1962, we observed that an increase in amplitude of the A wave of the apexcardiogram was seen during spontaneous episodes of chest pain due to coronary insufficiency. As angina pectoris subsided, there was a progressive diminution in size of the A wave to the preanginal level. Amplitude of the A wave, at rest, measured from its beginning rise to the peak, should not exceed 15% of the total amplitude of the apexcardiogram as measured from the E (maximal excursion of the tracing) to the O points (lowest deflection), as shown in Figure 9.3.

Since then, abnormalities of the A wave on the apexcardiogram have become a useful tool for diagnosis of coronary artery disease, even though this is not seen exclusively in these patients. The abnormal A wave seen on the apexcardiogram is a reflection of abnormal left ventricular contraction commonly seen in patients with coronary artery disease (Figs. 9.2, 9.8). Subsequent studies have shown that in addition to abnormalities of the A wave, the systolic component and rapid filling wave are important in this disease state (Figs. 9.8 through 9.12). Various combina-

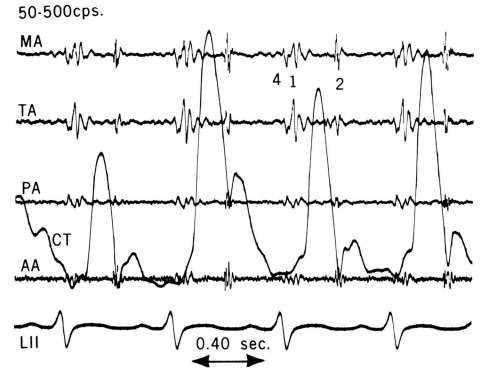

50-500cps.

MA

TA

PA

CT

AA

LII   0.40 sec.

4 1   2

Figure 9.7. Simultaneously recorded phonocardiogram at the mitral (MA), tricuspid (TA), pulmonic (PA) and aortic areas (AA), carotid pulse tracing (CT), and lead II (LII) of the electrocardiogram in a 53-year-old patient with ischemic cardiomyopathy due to coronary artery disease and pulsus alternans. Amplitude of the first beat is low, in the next beat it is higher, and then there is another beat with low amplitude. This type of tracing is seen in patients in the terminal stage of congestive heart failure due to coronary artery disease or in patients with primary myocardial disease.

tions of abnormalities of the A, systolic, and rapid filling waves are shown in Figure 9.12. They usually reflect the hemodynamic state of the left ventricle. If abnormalities are not present in the resting tracing, they may be induced by exercise stress testing, smoking, Valsalva maneuver, or in the beats following a premature atrial or ventricular contraction (Figs. 9.8, 9.10). These changes may be reversed by administration of nitroglycerin or other coronary vasodilators, or changes in cycle length.

The apexcardiogram is also a useful technique in studying patients prior to and after coronary bypass surgery. If there is significant improvement in left ventricular function following myocardial revascularization, amplitude of the A wave diminishes and there is a decrease in the size of the late systolic bulge. However, ventricular function may be unaltered or actually deteriorate if the patient develops intra- or postoperative myocardial infarction and the apexcardiogram may detect these changes.

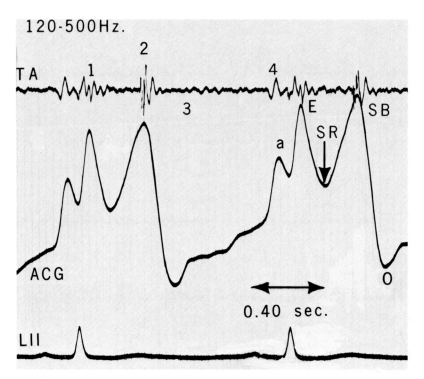

Figure 9.8.

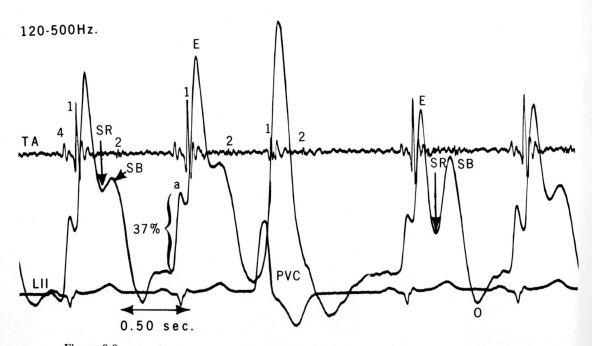

Figure 9.9.

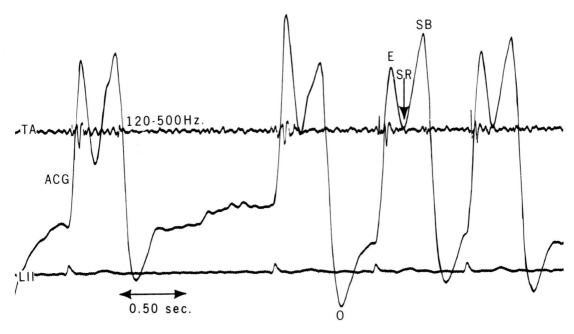

Figure 9.10. Simultaneously recorded tricuspid area (TA) phonocardiogram, apexcardiogram (ACG), and lead II (LII) of the electrocardiogram in a patient with coronary artery disease and atrial fibrillation. Note the variations in cycle length due to atrial fibrillation and the artifacts in the baseline during diastole. The first and second heart sounds are normal. The second beat, preceded by a long cycle length, is very prominent and shows a tall E point followed by a downward deflection or systolic retraction (SR) and a late systolic bulge (SB). In the beats preceded by a short cycle length, there is an exaggeration of the systolic bulge as compared with those preceded by a long cycle length. This points out the importance of recording tracings during cardiac arrhythmias.

Figure 9.8. Simultaneously recorded phonocardiogram at the tricuspid area (TA), apexcardiogram (ACG), and lead II (LII) of the electrocardiogram in a patient with coronary artery disease and severe left ventricular dyskinesis. The first and second heart sounds are normal. A small third heart sound coincides with the rapid filling wave on the apexcardiogram. The A wave is quite prominent. The E point is followed by a downward deflection called systolic retraction (SR). After the systolic retraction, there is a prominent systolic bulge (SB) that reaches a peak near the second heart sound. This is one of the abnormalities seen on the apexcardiogram in patients with severe coronary artery disease.

Figure 9.9. Simultaneously recorded phonocardiogram at the tricuspid area (TA), apexcardiogram (ACG), and lead II (LII) of the electrocardiogram in a 46-year-old patient with coronary artery disease. The first and second heart sounds are normal. A prominent fourth heart sound coincides with the A wave of the apexcardiogram. Amplitude of the A wave is increased to 37% of the total amplitude of the tracing as measured from the E to the O point. Following the ventricular premature contraction, note that the A wave still has increased amplitude, but now there is a major systolic retraction (SR) followed by a late systolic bulge (SB), which was not as prominent in the beat before the ventricular premature contraction. This tracing indicates the importance of recording the phonocardiogram and pulse waves during cardiac arrhythmias because they can precipitate changes that may not be seen during regular sinus beats.

221

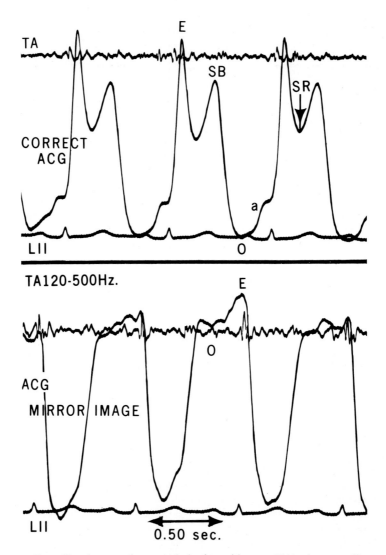

Figure 9.11. *Top:* Simultaneously recorded tricuspid area (TA) phonocardiogram, apexcardiogram (ACG), and lead II (LII) of the electrocardiogram in a 67-year-old patient with coronary artery disease. The apexcardiogram is abnormal. There is a large A wave and a midsystolic retraction (SR) followed by a late systolic bulge (SB). *Bottom:* A mirror image of the apexcardiogram as seen on the top tracing. This illustration indicates the importance of locating the transducer exactly in the center of the apex beat rather than in the periphery where you record a paradoxical motion of the apex.

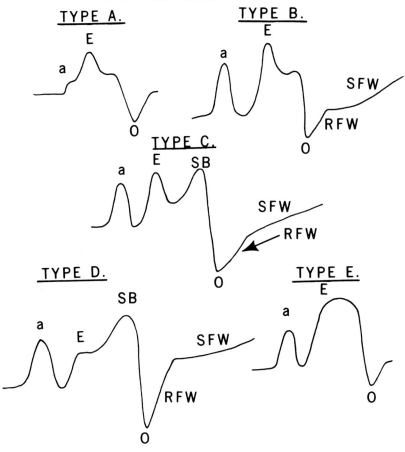

Figure 9.12. Diagrammatic representation of various abnormalities on the apexcardiogram. Type A is a normal apexcardiogram. Type B is seen in patients with elevated left ventricular end-diastolic pressure without significant left ventricular dyskinesis. Types C and D are seen in patients with elevated left ventricular end-diastolic pressure and a moderate to severe degree of left ventricular dyskinesis. Type E is seen in patients with coronary artery disease, elevated left ventricular end-diastolic pressure, and left ventricular hypertrophy.

Systolic Time Intervals

Measurements of systolic time intervals are useful in evaluating left ventricular function. Measurements of the pre-ejection period and corrected ejection time, or pre-ejection period/left ventricular ejection time ratio in patients with coronary artery disease without coronary insufficiency are usually normal (Fig. 9.1). The time interval between the Q wave of the electrocardiogram and the aortic component of the second heart sound (Q–S2 interval) is shortened slightly in patients with chronic coronary artery disease, but this has not proven to be of clinical value in our large series of patients. Shortening of ejection time and prolongation of the pre-ejection period may be seen in patients with coronary artery disease and significant impairment of ventricular function. Following myocardial revascularization using an aortocoronary saphenous vein bypass graft or a left-internal-mammary–left-anterior-descending-artery anastomosis (Green procedure) with resultant improvement in left ventricular performance, the pre-ejection period/ejection time ratio moves toward normal.

Maneuvers, Pharmacologic Agents, Cycle Length

Exercise stress testing is useful in the diagnosis of patients with coronary artery disease. Through increased use of treadmill exercise testing, correlations have been made between abnormalities of the ST segments and T waves on the electrocardiogram and the apexcardiogram and systolic time intervals. Earlier studies demonstrated that exercise testing resulted in a significant increase in the amplitude of the A and rapid filling waves on the apexcardiogram. Cigarette smoking also causes an increase in the amplitude of the A wave on the apexcardiogram. These changes are probably a reflection of diminished left ventricular compliance with elevated left ventricular end-diastolic pressure. Many patients subjected to some form of coronary artery surgery develop myocardial infarction and some of these abnormalities may become even more prominent. Administration of vasopressor agents, which increase the afterload, make these changes more prominent on the apexcardiogram and in the systolic time intervals. Administration of vasodilators such as nitroglycerin and amyl nitrite causes a reduction in amplitude of the A wave on the apexcardiogram, shortening of the pre-ejection period and prolongation of the other time intervals. The influence of cycle length on the murmur of papillary muscle dysfunction is shown in Figure 9.10. With atrial fibrillation at a rapid ventricular rate, the systolic regurgitant murmur of papillary muscle dysfunction is almost inaudible and not recordable. However, in beats preceded by a long diastolic pause, there is a significant increase in amplitude of the systolic murmur as well as an increase in amplitude of the carotid pulse tracing.

Vectorcardiogram

The vectorcardiogram has a great application in evaluating patients with coronary artery disease with or without associated myocardial infarction. This is a superior technique as compared with the electrocardiogram in the diagnosis of this condition, as shown in Tables 9.1 through 9.6. This is a very sensitive technique

Table 9.1. Area of Left Ventricular Contraction Abnormality and Nutrient Coronary Artery Occlusion

Area of Contraction Abnormality	Expected Coronary Lesion
Anterior	LAD
Lateral	LAD or LCx
Posterior	RCA or LCx (if dominant left coronary system)
Inferior	RCA or LCx (if dominant left coronary system)

LAD = left anterior descending coronary artery.
LCx = left circumflex coronary artery.
RCA = right coronary artery.

Table 9.2. Sensitivity of ECG and VCG for Detecting Appropriate Area of Left Ventricular Contraction Abnormality

Area of Contraction Abnormality	No. of Cases (N)	Record Diagnostic of Infarction	
		ECG N(%)	VCG N(%)
Inferior	80	50(63%)	71(89%)
Posterior	38	6(16%)	21(55%)
Anterior	32	17(53%)	20(63%)
Lateral	6	4(67%)	6(100%)
Total	156	77(49%)	118(76%)

Table 9.3. Sensitivity of ECG and VCG for Detecting Appropriate Areas of Left Ventricular Contraction Abnormality in the Presence of Two Occluded Coronary Arteries

Areas of Contraction Abnormality	No. of Cases (N)	Record Diagnostic of Infarctions	
		ECG N(%)	VCG N(%)
Anterior–Inferior	19	7(37%)	12(63%)
Posterior–Inferior	14	2(14%)	8(57%)
Anterior–Posterior	3	0(0%)	2(67%)
Inferior–Lateral	2	1(50%)	2(100%)
Anterior–Lateral	13	9(69%)	12(92%)
Total	51	19(37%)	36(71%)

Table 9.4. Sensitivity of ECG and VCG for Detecting Appropriate Area of Left Ventricular Contraction Abnormality When Degree of Coronary Obstruction Ranged Between 70 and 95%

Coronary Artery Involved	No. of Vessels (N)	Record Diagnostic of Infarction	
		ECG N(%)	VCG N(%)
Left Anterior Descending	60	34(57%)	40(67%)
Left Circumflex	21	12(57%)	19(90%)
Right	103	52(50%)	76(74%)
Total	184	98(53%)	135(73%)

Table 9.5. Sensitivity of ECG and VCG for Detecting Two Appropriate Areas of Left Ventricular Contraction Abnormality in Presence of Double Vessel Disease (70 to 95% Obstruction)

Coronary Arteries Involved	No. of Cases (N)	Record Diagnostic of Infarction	
		ECG N(%)	VCG N(%)
LAD + RCA	37	10(27%)	18(49%)
LAD + LCx	18	10(56%)	14(78%)
LCx + RCA	26	3(12%)	11(42%)
Total	81	23(28%)	43(53%)

Table 9.6. Incidence of Positive ECG or VCG Diagnoses of Infarction When Angiography Demonstrated No Significant Coronary Artery Disease and Absence of Myocardial Contraction Abnormality

	ECG	VCG
Anterior	4	2
Inferior	1	1
Posterior	0	2
Lateral	0	1
Total	5	6

particularly for the diagnosis of inferior or posterior wall myocardial infarction (Figs. 9.13 through 9.15). A great deal of care should be exercised in making this diagnosis since approximately 10% of normal subjects can exhibit findings identical to the ones seen in patients with posterior wall myocardial infarction. The most important plane for diagnosing this condition is the horizontal, which shows an increase in the anterior forces (Fig. 9.15). The vectorcardiogram is also quite helpful in patients with infarction involving the anterior or lateral wall of the left ventricle (Figs. 9.16 through 9.18). In patients with inferior wall (diaphragmatic) myocardial infarction, the vectorcardiogram is superior to the electrocardiogram. For recognition of an inferior wall myocardial infarction, measure the 25 and 30 msec vectors in the frontal plane (Figs. 9.13, 9.14). If these vectors are located above the O point, it is highly suggestive of an inferior wall myocardial infarction.

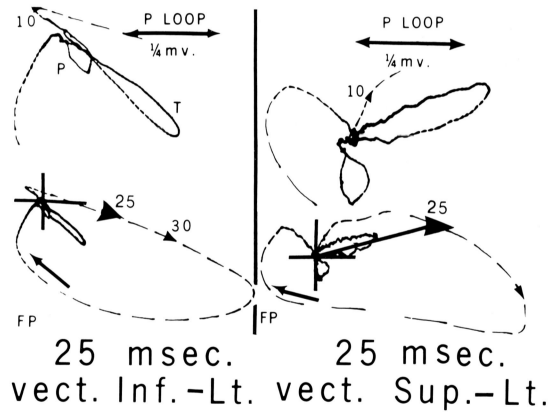

Figure 9.13. *Left:* Frontal plane (FP) vectorcardiogram in a normal subject with clockwise rotation of the QRS loop. The 25 and 30 msec QRS vectors are located inferiorly and to the left. *Right:* Frontal plane vectorcardiogram showing abnormal superior displacement of the 25 msec QRS vector. It is located above the O point, which is at the center of the axis indicator. Abnormal superior location of the 25 msec vector in this quadrant is one of the diagnostic features of an inferior wall myocardial infarction. Rotation of the entire QRS loop is clockwise. On the magnified portion of this vectorcardiogram at the top of the picture, note that the T loop is located superior to the O point in keeping with the diagnosis of myocardial ischemia.

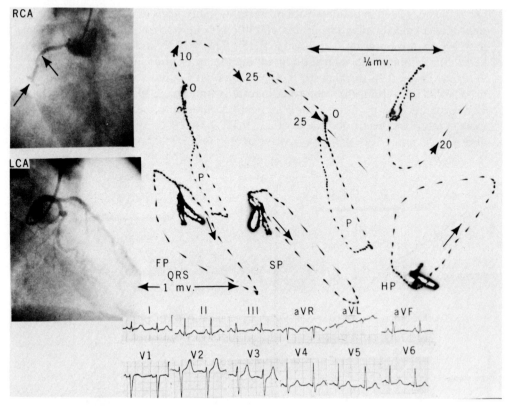

Figure 9.14. Coronary arteriogram, vectorcardiogram, and electrocardiogram in a 51-year-old patient with an inferior wall myocardial infarction. The electrocardiogram shows sinus rhythm. There is no evidence of inferior wall myocardial infarction. The frontal plane (FP) vectorcardiogram shows superior orientation of the 25 msec vector in the left sagittal plane (SP) indicating the presence of an inferior wall myocardial infarction. The coronary arteriogram shows total occlusion of the proximal right coronary artery. This patient had a clinical history of myocardial infarction in the past.

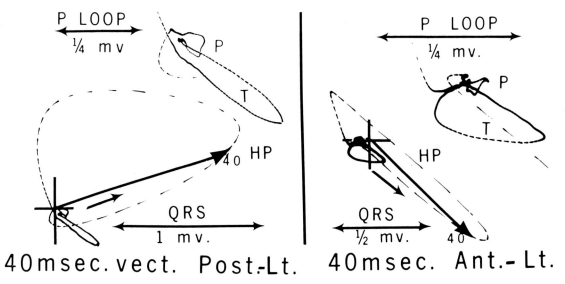

Figure 9.15. *Left:* Normal vectorcardiogram. Note the orientation of the 40 msec vector, which is located posteriorly and to the left, indicated by an arrow. *Right:* Horizontal plane (HP) vectorcardiogram showing the typical findings seen in patients with posterior or dorsal myocardial infarction. The 40 msec vector is located anteriorly and to the left as indicated by the arrow. The rotation is counterclockwise. Another feature of this recording diagnostic for posterior wall myocardial infarction is the fact that more than 50% of the area within the QRS loop is located anteriorly. This type of tracing can be seen in patients with right ventricular hypertrophy. One of the findings that can help differentiate posterior wall myocardial infarction from right ventricular hypertrophy is that in patients with right ventricular hypertrophy, the P loop should show signs of right ventricular strain, and right atrial hypertrophy, and the T loop is usually located posteriorly and to the left. In this case the P loop is normal and the T loop is oriented in the same direction as the QRS loop, which is also normal.

Vectorcardiography is also useful to detect the presence of fibrosis involving the left ventricle. It can be detected in an unfiltered tracing in all three planes. Be sure to obtain a good recording of the QRS loop in all three planes without filtering, because most of the high frequency components are in the range of 400–1000 Hz. If the filter is used, you will eliminate the high frequency components of the QRS loop, which indicate the presence of myocardial disease. If it is difficult to obtain a recording without artifacts because of 60 cycle interference or somatic tremor, you should still record a tracing without filtering and then a second one with filtering. Large numbers of patients with coronary artery disease demonstrate mild to moderate abnormalities of myocardial contractility, which can only be appreciated by recording the high fidelity "bite" (Fig. 9.18). Unfortunately, because of poor frequency response on the electrocardiogram, many of these high frequency components cannot be obtained on a standard electrocardiograph. In addition, be sure to obtain a good recording with a high degree of magnification of the P loop. Many patients with coronary artery disease have abnormal left ventricular contractions, thus requiring a forceful contraction to accomplish good

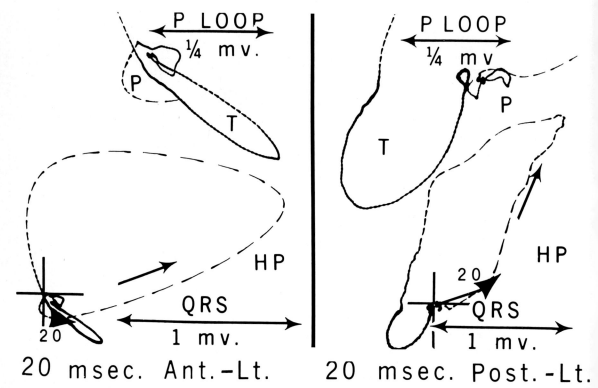

Figure 9.16. *Left:* Horizontal plane (HP) vectorcardiogram showing normal direction and location of the 20 msec vector anteriorly and to the left. The loop rotates counterclockwise. *Right:* Vectorcardiogram in the horizontal plane (HP) of a patient with an anteroseptal myocardial infarction. The 20 msec vector is located posteriorly and to the left as indicated by an arrow. The entire QRS loop rotates counterclockwise. In the magnified portion at the top of the illustration, note that the loop is open, i.e., the terminal QRS loop does not come near the beginning of the loop. This represents an abnormal ST vector, in keeping with the diagnosis of myocardial ischemia. The T loop is quite large and is located anteriorly and to the left. Compare the QRS and T loops with the normal ones in the left panel.

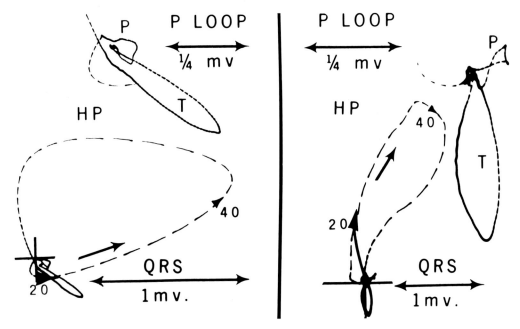

20msec.vect. Ant.-Lt.   20msec. Post.- Rt.

Figure 9.17. *Left:* Vectorcardiogram in the horizontal plane (HP) showing normal orientation of the 20 msec vector, which is located anteriorly and to the left, and counterclockwise rotation of the QRS loop. *Right:* Horizontal plane (HP) vectorcardiogram showing abnormal direction of the 20 msec vector posteriorly and to the right, as well as abnormal clockwise rotation of the QRS loop. This recording is characteristic for patients with anterolateral myocardial infarction, which is usually associated with medium to large lesions in the myocardium. An anterolateral infarction has much more severe clinical implications than an anteroseptal myocardial infarction. Compare the abnormal orientation of the T loop with the normal tracing. In the right panel it is located anteriorly indicating the presence of myocardial ischemia. The P loop is normal.

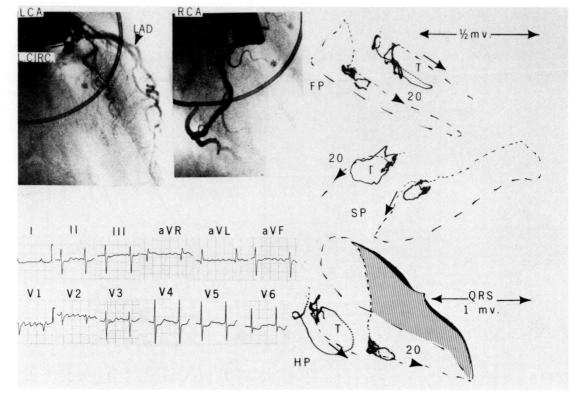

Figure 9.18. Vectorcardiogram and electrocardiogram in a 74-year-old patient with coronary artery disease. The electrocardiogram shows atrial fibrillation, slight left axis deviation, and abnormal T waves and ST segments suggesting digitalis effect or myocardial ischemia. The vectorcardiogram in the frontal plane (FP) shows normal initial forces. However, there are some late superior and rightward forces that are abnormal. The sagittal plane (SP) shows a counterclockwise rotation with superior displacement of the terminal forces. On this vectorcardiogram the horizontal plane (HP) is important. The initial portion of the QRS loop begins to rotate counterclockwise and suddenly changes direction and rotates clockwise. Coronary arteriograms show severe segmental disease of the left anterior descending artery.

filling in the late phase of diastole. This can be manifested in the vectorcardiogram by an increase in size of the P loop, which is particularly well seen in the horizontal plane.

Echocardiogram

Echocardiography has become more valuable in the diagnosis of coronary artery disease. The findings are not specific for this disease state; however, it is useful under certain circumstances, particularly in evaluating left ventricular function, abnormal patterns of interventricular septal and posterior wall motion, and measurement of intracavitary diameters, and elevated early or late left ventricular diastolic pressure.

Patients with coronary artery disease may exhibit abnormalities of the interventricular septum with flat (Fig. 9.19) or paradoxical (Fig. 9.20) motion during systole. Decreased (Fig. 9.21) excursion of the posterior wall of the left ventricle may also be seen (Fig. 9.22). Abnormal increased motion of the anterior leaflet of the mitral valve at the time of atrial contraction may be seen in patients with elevated left ventricular initial diastolic pressure above 15–20 mmHg (normal 1–12 mmHg). In these recordings, amplitude of the A wave must be higher than the E point (Fig. 9.23). Measurement of the P–R interval on the electrocardiogram minus the A–C interval on the echocardiogram will be shorter than normal (normal 60 mm/sec or greater) in patients with elevated left ventricular end-diastolic pressure.

Echocardiographic studies obtained in patients with acute myocardial infarction have shown abnormalities of the interventricular septal (Fig. 9.24) and posterior wall motion and an increase in left ventricular internal diameter. Detection and quantitation of left ventricular aneurysm is difficult to appreciate on the echocardiogram in most patients. This diagnosis can be suspected if there is abnormal systolic anterior motion (SAM) of the mitral valve during systole associated with increased motion of the posterior wall of the left ventricle and diminished or paradoxical motion of the interventricular septum (Fig. 9.25). In addition, a good scan from the aorta to the apex of the left ventricle may show an increase in the left ventricular internal dimension or apical dilatation, which is highly suggestive of left ventricular aneurysm (Figs. 9.26, 9.27). Also, a good recording of the tricuspid and pulmonic valves is very important in evaluating right ventricular function because many of these patients may have heart failure and pulmonary hypertension. In this instance, the right ventricular size will be increased and motion of the tricuspid and pulmonic valves will be abnormal.

Points of Importance and Caution

A good recording of both leaflets of the mitral valve must be recorded to demonstrate the opening and closing points. This is helpful to determine elevated left ventricular pressures.

A technically good recording of the septum and posterior wall of the left ventricle, below the mitral valve level where the mitral chordae echoes are seen, is essential.

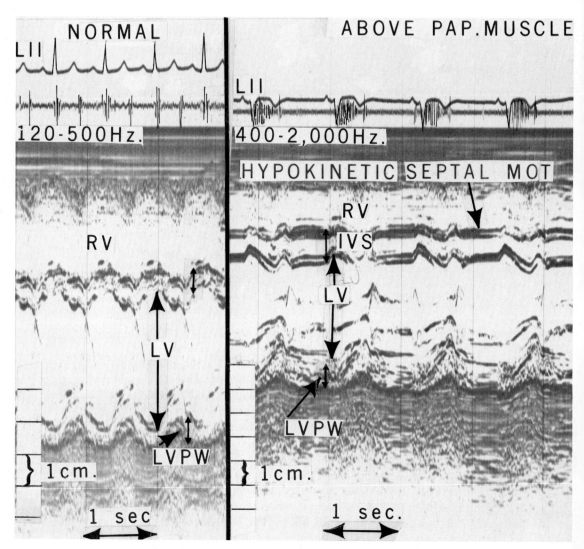

Figure 9.19. *Left:* Echocardiogram recorded simultaneously with the phonocardiogram and lead II of the electrocardiogram in a subject with normal left ventricular internal dimension and normal motion of the interventricular septum. *Right:* Echocardiogram in a patient with coronary artery disease showing where the septum should be measured, i.e., above the papillary muscle, but below the mitral valve. This shows a hypokinetic interventricular septum.

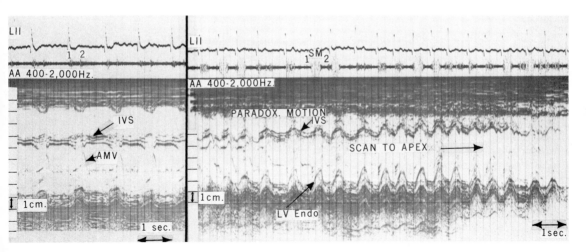

Figure 9.20. *Left:* Echocardiogram of the mitral valve (AMV) in a 63-year-old patient prior to surgery, demonstrating a hypokinetic interventricular septum (IVS). *Right:* Following aortocoronary bypass surgery, there is paradoxical motion of the interventricular septum, indicating further deterioration of left ventricular contraction.

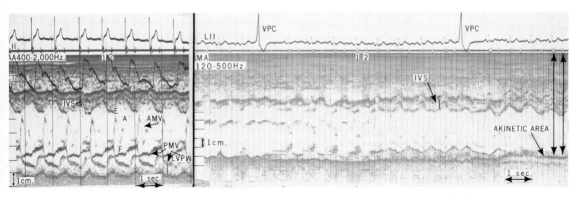

Figure 9.21. *Left:* Echocardiogram showing normal motion of the interventricular septum and the posterior wall of the left ventricle. The tracing was recorded simultaneously with the carotid pulse tracing (CT), lead II (LII) of the electrocardiogram, and a phonocardiogram at the mitral area (MA). *Right:* Echocardiogram recorded simultaneously with the phonocardiogram and lead II of the electrocardiogram in a patient with coronary artery disease. The scan from the aorta to the apex shows a progressive decrease in motion of the posterior wall of the left ventricle to an area of akinesis which is indicated by an arrow. Two ventricular premature contractions (VPC) are recorded on the electrocardiogram.

235

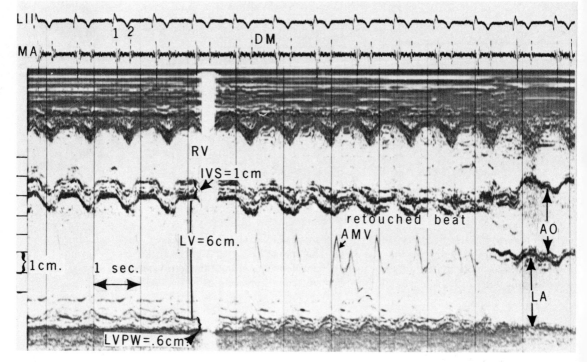

Figure 9.22.

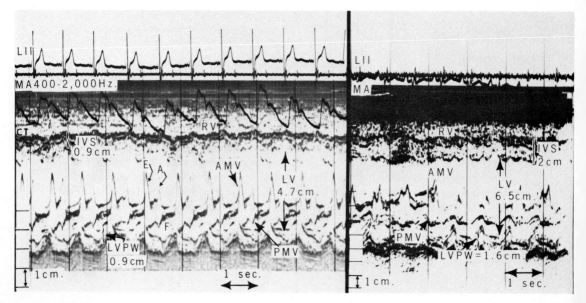

Figure 9.23.

236

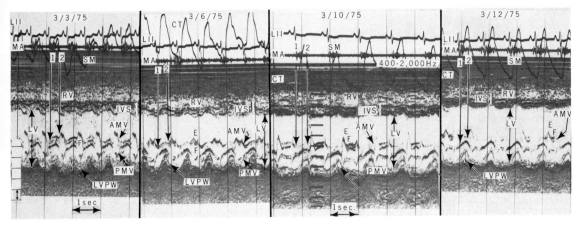

Figure 9.24. This is a series of echocardiograms recorded simultaneously with a mitral area (MA) phonocardiogram, carotid pulse tracing (CT), and lead II (LII) of the electrocardiogram in a 66-year-old patient who sustained an acute anteroseptal myocardial infarction and developed mitral insufficiency secondary to papillary muscle dysfunction. The initial tracing shows a fairly good excursion of the interventricular septum (IVS). In the subsequent tracings on 3/6, 3/10, and 3/12/75, there is a further decrease in motion of the interventricular septum. RV = right ventricle, AMV = anterior mitral valve, PMV = posterior mitral valve, LVPW = left ventricular posterior wall, SM = systolic murmur, LV = left ventricle.

Figure 9.22. Echocardiogram recorded simultaneously with a mitral area (MA) phonocardiogram and lead II (LII) of the electrocardiogram in a 48-year-old patient with inferior and posterior wall myocardial infarctions. Observe the reduced motion of the posterior wall of the left ventricle (LVPW) and the increase in left ventricular (LV) internal dimension to 6 cm. RV = right ventricle, IVS = interventricular septum, AMV = anterior mitral valve, AO = aorta, LA = left atrium, and DM = diastolic murmur.

Figure 9.23. *Left:* Echocardiogram showing normal motion of the mitral valve (AMV/PMV), interventricular septum (IVS), left ventricular posterior wall (LVPW), and normal left ventricular (LV) internal dimension recorded simultaneously with a mitral area (MA) phonocardiogram, carotid pulse tracing (CT) and lead II (LII) of the electrocardiogram. *Right:* Echocardiogram in a patient with coronary artery disease and elevated initial left ventricular end-diastolic pressure. Note the abnormal motion of the mitral valve with a tall A wave and an increase in dimensions of the left ventricle (6.5 cm) and left ventricular posterior wall (1.6 cm). The septum has flat motion and an increased dimension of 2 cm. RV = right ventricle.

237

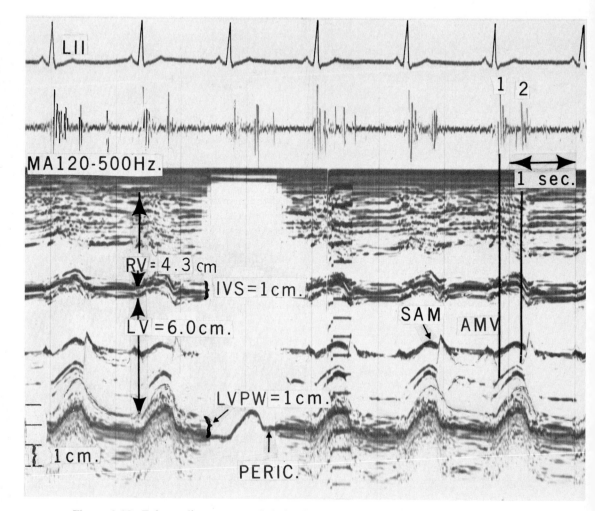

Figure 9.25. Echocardiogram recorded simultaneously with a mitral area (MA) phonocardiogram and lead II (LII) of the electrocardiogram in a patient with a left ventricular aneurysm secondary to coronary artery disease. Note the paradoxical septal motion, abnormal systolic anterior motion (SAM) of the mitral valve, and increased left ventricular (LV) internal dimension, 6 cm. RV = right ventricle, LVPW = left ventricular posterior wall, AMV = anterior mitral valve, Peric = pericardium.

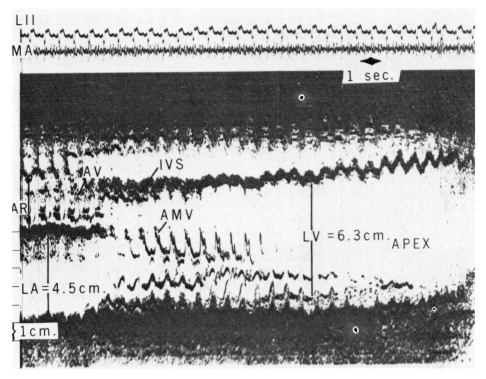

Figure 9.26. Echocardiographic scan from the aorta to the apex showing the presence of an apical aneurysm. There is a progressive enlargement of the left ventricle. This structure measures 6.3 cm at the apex. LA = left atrium, AR = aortic root, AV = aortic valve, IVS = interventricular septum, AMV = anterior mitral valve, LV = left ventricle.

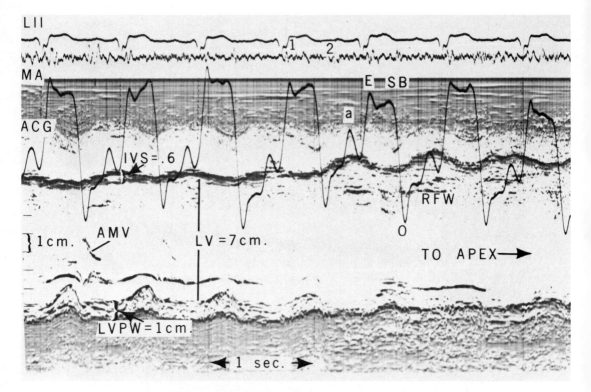

Figure 9.27. Echocardiogram recorded simultaneously with a mitral area (MA) phonocardiogram, apexcardiogram (ACG), and lead II (LII) of the electrocardiogram in a 65-year-old patient with an apical aneurysm. On the scan from the mitral valve toward the apex there is progressive enlargement of the left ventricle (LV); in some areas it measures 7 cm. At the point of the apex the aneurysm is clearly seen. There is reduced motion of the posterior wall of the left ventricle (LVPW). The apexcardiogram shows prominent A and rapid filling waves (RFW). SB = systolic bulge, AMV = anterior mitral valve, IVS = interventricular septum.

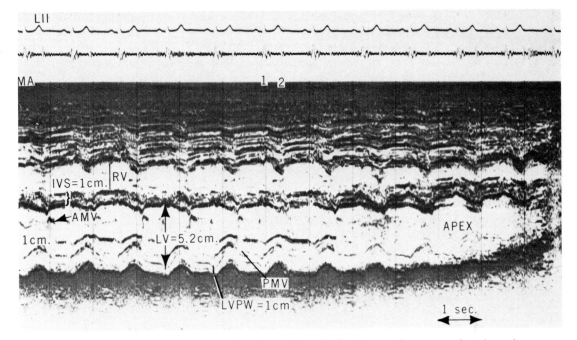

Figure 9.28. Echocardiographic scan from the mitral valve to the apex using the subxyphoid approach recorded simultaneously with a mitral area (MA) phonocardiogram and lead II (LII) of the electrocardiogram. Note the decreased excursion of the interventricular septum (IVS). The left ventricular (LV) internal dimension measures 5.2 cm. The left ventricular posterior wall (LVPW) measures 1 cm. AMV = anterior mitral valve, PMV = posterior mitral valve.

The subxyphoid approach is often helpful to examine the heart from another view (Fig. 9.28). This approach can be helpful in patients with ventricular aneurysms.

Scanning to the apex is important for exhibiting a dilated apex. This approach is valuable when technical difficulties are encountered when using the sternal approach.

BIBLIOGRAPHY

Abbasi, A.S., Eber, L.M., MacAlpin, R.N., and Kattus, A.A.: Paradoxical motion of interventricular septum in left bundle branch block. Circulation *49*:423, 1974.

Abrams, H.L.: Aortocoronary saphenous bypass. New Engl. J. Med. *282*:456, 1970.

Agress, C.M., Wegner, S., Forrester, J.S., Chatterjee, K., Parmley, W.W., and Swan, H.J.C.: An indirect method for evaluation of left ventricular function in acute myocardial infarction. Circulation *46*:291, 1972.

Anderson, J.W.: Ischemic electrocardiographic changes with reversion after removal of diseased gallbladders. Minn. Med. *55*:211, 1972.

Aronow, W.S., Bowyer, A.F., and Kaplan, M.A.: External isovolumic contraction times and left ventricular ejection time/external isovolumic contraction time ratios at rest and after exercise in coronary artery disease. Circulation 43:59, 1971.

Balcon, R., Bennett, E.D., and Sowton, G.E.: Comparison of pulmonary artery diastolic and left ventricular end-diastolic pressures in patients with ischaemic heart disease. Brit. Heart J. 33:615, 1971.

Bamrah, V.S., Bahler, R.C., and Rakita, L.: Hemodynamic response to supine exercise in patients with chest pain and normal coronary arteriograms. Amer. Heart J. 87:147, 1974.

Beilin, L., and Mounsey, P.: The left ventricular impulse in hypertensive heart disease. Brit. Heart J. 24:409, 1962.

Benchimol, A., Asendorf, A., and Dimond, E.G.: The apex cardiogram in coronary artery disease. Heart Bulletin 19:69, 1970.

Benchimol, A., Buxbaum, A., Maroko, P.R., Pedraza, A., and Brener, L.: Chest pain with or without abnormal electrocardiograms in patients with normal coronary arteriograms. Ariz. Med. 26:341, 1969.

Benchimol, A., Desser, K.B., and Harris, C.L.: Coronary artery spasm—a case report. Ariz. Med. 31:356, 1974.

Benchimol, A., and Dimond, E.G.: The apex cardiogram in ischemic heart disease. Brit. Heart J. 24:581, 1962.

Benchimol, A., and Dimond, E.G.: The apex cardiogram in "normal older" subjects and in patients with arteriosclerotic heart disease. Effect of exercise on the "a" wave. Amer. Heart J. 65:789, 1963.

Benchimol, A., and Maroko, P.: The apex cardiogram. The value of the apex cardiogram in coronary artery disease. Dis. Chest 54:378, 1968.

Benchimol, A., Matsuo, S., Desser, K.B., Wang, T.F., and Gartlan, J.L. Jr.: Coronary artery blood flow velocity during ventricular tachycardia in man. Amer. J. Med. Sci. 264:277, 1972.

Benchimol, A., and Tippit, H.C.: The clinical value of the jugular and hepatic pulses. In: Friedberg, C.K. (ed.): Physical diagnosis in cardiovascular diseases. New York: Grune and Stratton, 1969.

Bennet, E.D., Smithen, C.R., and Sowton, E.: Significance of atrial sound in acute myocardial infarction. Brit. Heart J. 34:202, 1972.

Bristow, J.D., Van Soparate Zee, B.E., and Judkins, M.P.: Systolic and diastolic abnormalities of the left ventricle in coronary artery disease. Studies in patients with little or no enlargement of ventricular volume. Circulation 42:219, 1970.

Burch, G.E., Giles, T.D., and Colcolough, H.L.: Ischemic cardiomyopathy. Amer. Heart J. 79:291, 1970.

Burch, G.E., Giles, T.D., and Martinez, E.: Echocardiographic detection of abnormal motion of the interventricular septum in ischemic cardiomyopathy. Amer. J. Med. 57:293, 1974.

Buyukozturk, K., Kimbiris, D., and Segal, B.L.: Systolic time intervals; relation to severity of coronary artery disease, intercoronary collateralization and left ventricular dyskinesia. Amer. J. Cardiol. 28:183, 1971.

Carlsten, A., Forsberg, S.A., Paulin, S., Varnauskas, E., and Werko, L.: Coronary angiography in the clinical analysis of suspected coronary disease. Amer. J. Cardiol. 19:509, 1967.

Caulfield, W.H., Jr., Smith, R.H., and Franklin, R.B.: The second heart sound in coronary artery disease. A phonocardiographic assessment. Amer. Heart J. 77:187, 1969.

Cheng, T.O.:   Incidence of ventricular aneurysm in coronary artery disease. An angiographic appraisal. Amer. J. Med. *50*:340, 1971.

Cheng, T.O.:   Murmurs in coronary-artery disease. New. Engl. J. Med. *283*:1054, 1970.

Cohn, P.F., Gorlin, R., Cohn, L.H., and Collins, J.J., Jr.:   Left ventricular ejection fraction as a prognostic guide in surgical treatment of coronary and valvular heart disease. Amer. J. Cardiol. *34*:136, 1974.

Cohn, P.F., Levine, J.A., Bergeron, G.A., and Gorlin, R.:   Reproducibility of the angiographic left ventricular ejection fraction in patients with coronary artery disease. Amer. Heart J. *88*:713, 1974.

Collins, M., Obeid, A., Ryan, G.F., Smulyan, H., and Eich, R.H.:   Hemodynamic effects of increasing the heart rate in patients with arteriosclerotic heart disease. Amer. Heart J. *77*:466, 1969.

Corya, B.C., Feigenbaum, H., Rasmussen, S., and Black, M.J.:   Anterior left Ventricular wall echoes in coronary artery disease. Linear scanning with a single element transducer. Amer. J. Cardiol. *34*:652, 1974.

Diamant, B., and Killip, T.:   Indirect assessment of left ventricular performance in acute myocardial infarction. Circulation *42*:579, 1970.

Dimond, E.G., and Benchimol, A.:   Correlation of intracardiac pressure and precordial movement in ischaemic heart disease. Brit. Heart J. *25*:389, 1963.

Dimond, E.G., and Benchimol, A.:   The exercise apex cardiogram in angina pectoris; its possible usefulness in diagnosis and therapy. Dis. Chest *43*:92, 1963.

Dimond, E.G., Duenas, A., and Benchimol, A.:   Apex cardiography; a review. Amer. Heart J. *72*:124, 1966.

Dimond, E.G., Li, Y., and Benchimol, A.:   Tourniquets and abdominal binders in ischemic heart disease. Effects on the apex cardiogram. J.A.M.A. *187*:981, 1964.

Dowling, J.T., Sloman, G., and Urquhart, C.:   Systolic time interval fluctuations produced by acute myocardial infarction. Brit. Heart J. *33*:765, 1971 (Suppl.).

Eddleman, E.E., Jr.:   Kinetocardiographic changes in ischemic heart disease. Circulation *32*:650, 1965.

Ellestad, M.H., Allen, W., Wan, M.C., and Kemp, G.L.:   Maximal treadmill stress testing for cardiovascular evaluation. Circulation *39*:517, 1969.

Fabian, J., Epstein, E.J., Coulshed, N., and McKendrick, C.S.:   Duration of phases of left ventricular systole using indirect methods. II. Acute myocardial infarction. Brit. Heart J. *34*:882, 1972.

Gahl, K., Caspari, P., Pearson, M., Sutton, R., and McDonald, L.:   Apical systolic murmurs related to mitral regurgitation at angiography in ischaemic heart disease. Brit. Heart J. *34*:965, 1972.

Garrard, C.L., Jr., Weissler, A.M., and Dodge, H.T.:   The relationship of alterations in systolic time intervals to ejection fraction in patients with cardiac disease. Circulation *42*:455, 1970.

Greenwald, J., Yap, J.F., Franklin, M., and Lichtman, A.M.:   Echocardiographic mitral systolic motion in left ventricular aneurysm. Brit. Heart J. *37*:684, 1975.

Hamosh, P., Cohn, J.N., Engelman, K., Broder, M.I., and Freis, E.D.:   Systolic time intervals and left ventricular function in acute myocardial infarction. Circulation *45*:375, 1972.

Harrison, T.R.:   Some clinical and physiologic aspects of angina pectoris. Bull. Johns Hopkins Hosp. *104*:275, 1959.

Harrison, T.R., and Hughes, L.:   Precordial systolic bulges during anginal attacks. Trans. Assoc. Am. Physicians *71*:174, 1958.

Heikkila, J., Luomanmaki, K., and Pyorala, K.:   Serial observations on left ventricular dysfunction in acute myocardial infarction. II. Systolic time intervals in power failure. Circulation *44*:343, 1971.

Hellerstein, H.K., Prozan, G.B., Liebow, I.M., Doan, A.E., and Henderson, J.A.:   Two step exercise test as a test of cardiac function in chronic rheumatic heart disease and in arteriosclerotic heart disease with old myocardial infarction. Amer. J. Cardiol. *7*:234, 1961.

Hill, J.C., O'Rourke, R.A., Lewis, R.P., and McGranahan, G.M.:   The diagnostic value of the atrial gallop in acute myocardial infarction. Amer. Heart J. *78*:194, 1969.

Hodges, M., Halpern, B.L., Friesinger, G.C., and Dagenais, G.R.:   Left ventricular preejection period and ejection time in patients with acute myocardial infarction. Circulation *45*:933, 1972.

Hornsten, T.R., and Bruce, R.A.:   Computed ST forces of Frank and bipolar exercise electrocardiograms. Amer. Heart J. *78*:346, 1969.

Hutchinson, R.G.:   The apexcardiogram in the diagnosis of coronary artery disease; a review. Angiology *25*:381, 1974.

Inoue, K., Smulyan, H., Mookherjee, S., and Eich, R.H.:   Ultrasonic measurement of left ventricular wall motion in acute myocardial infarction. Circulation *43*:778, 1971.

Inoue, K., Young, G.M., Grierson, A.L., Smulyan, H., and Eich, R.H.:   Isometric contraction period of the left ventricle in acute myocardial infarction. Circulation *42*:79, 1970.

Jain, S.R., and Lindahl, J.:   Apex cardiogram and systolic time intervals in acute myocardial infarction. Brit. Heart J. *33*:578, 1971.

Jeresaty, R.M., and Liss, J.P.:   Midsystolic clicks and coronary artery disease. Chest *63*:297, 1973.

Kattus, A.A., Jr., Hanafee, W.N., Longmire, W.P., Jr., MacAlpin, R.N., and Rivin, A.U.:   Diagnosis, medical and surgical management of coronary insufficiency. Ann. Intern. Med. *69*:114, 1968.

Kazamias, T.M., Gander, M.P., Ross, J. Jr., and Braunwald, E.:   Detection of left-ventricular-wall motion disorders in coronary-artery disease by radarkymography. New. Engl. J. Med. *285*:63, 1971.

Khaja, F., Parker, J.O., Ledwich, R.J., West, R.O., and Armstrong, P.W.:   Assessment of ventricular function in coronary artery disease by means of atrial pacing and exercise. Amer. J. Cardiol. *26*:107, 1970.

Legler, J.F., and Benchimol, A.:   The significance of extrasystoles in coronary artery disease. Geriatrics *19*:468, 1964.

Lewis, R.P., Boudoulas, H., Forester, W.F., and Weissler, A.M.:   Shortening of electromechanical systole as a manifestation of excessive adrenergic stimulation in acute myocardial infarction. Circulation *46*:856, 1972.

Likoff, W.:   Myocardial revascularization. A critique. New York J. Med. *70*:1983, 1970.

Likoff, W., Kasparian, H., Segal, B.L., Forman, H., and Novack, P.:   Coronary arteriography; correlation with electrocardiographic response to measured exercise. Amer. J. Cardiol. *18*:160, 1966.

Lipp, H., Gambetta, M., Schwartz, J., Domingo de la Fuente, D., and Resnekov, L.:   Intermittent pansystolic murmur and presumed mitral regurgitation after acute myocardial infarction. Amer. J. Cardiol. *30*:690, 1972.

Ludbrook, P., Karliner, J.S., London, A., Peterson, K.L., Leopold, G.R., and O'Rourke, R.A.:   Posterior wall velocity; an unreliable index of total left ventricular performance in patients with coronary artery disease. Amer. J. Cardiol. *33*:475, 1974.

Luisada, A.A., and Magri, G.:   The low frequency tracings of the precordium and epigastrium in normal subjects and cardiac patients. Amer. Heart J. *44*:545, 1952.

Lynn, T.N., and Wolf, S.:   The prognostic significance of the ballistocardiogram in ischemic heart disease. Amer. Heart J. *88*:277, 1974.

McCallister, B.D., Richmond, D.R., Saltups, A., Hallermann, F.J., Wallace, R.B., and Frye, R.L.:   Left ventricular hemodynamics before and 1 year after internal mammary artery implantation in patients with coronary artery disease and angina pectoris. Circulation *42*:471, 1970.

McConahay, D.R., Martin, C.M., and Cheitlin, M.D.:   Resting and exercise systolic time intervals. Correlations with ventricular performance in patients with coronary artery disease. Circulation *45*:592, 1972.

McKusic, V.A.:   Cardiovascular sound in health and disease. Baltimore: William & Wilkins, 1958.

Margolis, C.:   Significance of ejection period/tension period as a factor in the assessment of cardiac function and as a possible diagnostic tool for the uncovering of silent coronary heart disease. A study of 111 cases. Dis. Chest *46*:706, 1964.

Martinez-Rios, M.A., Da Costa, B.C., Cecena-Seldner, F.A., and Gensini, G.G.:   Normal electrocardiogram in the presence of severe coronary artery disease. Amer. J. Cardiol. *25*:320, 1970.

Mounsey, P.:   Praecordial pulsations in relation to cardiac movement and sounds. Brit. Heart J. *21*:457, 1959.

Muller, O., and Rorvik, K.:   Haemodynamic consequences of coronary heart disease; with observations during anginal pain and on the effect of nitroglycerine. Brit. Heart J. *20*:302, 1958.

Nixon, P.G.F., and Bethell, H.J.N.:   Atrial gallop in diagnosis of early coronary heart disease. Brit. Heart J. *34*:202, 1972.

Pasternac, A., Gorlin, R., Sonnenblick, E.H., Haft, J.I., and Kemp, H.G.:   Abnormalities of ventricular motion induced by atrial pacing in coronary artery disease. Circulation *45*:1195, 1972.

Piessens, J., Van Mieghem, W., Kesteloot, H., and De Geest, H.:   Diagnostic value of clinical history, exercise testing and atrial pacing in patients with chest pain. Amer. J. Cardiol. *33*:351, 1974.

Pouget, J.M., Harris, W.S., Mayron, B.R., and Naughton, J.P.:   Abnormal responses of the systolic time intervals to exercise in patients with angina pectoris. Circulation *43*:289, 1971.

Ratshin, R.A., Rackley, C.E., and Russell, R.O.:   Serial evaluation of left ventricular volumes and posterior wall movement in the acute phase of myocardial infarction using diagnostic ultrasound. Amer. J. Cardiol. *29*:286, 1972.

Rosa, L.M., and Nevzat, K.:   Precordial pulsatory mechanism in coronary heart disease. Circulation *22*:801, 1960.

Ross, R.S., and Friesinger, G.C.:   Coronary arteriography. Amer. Heart J. *72*:437, 1966.

Rushmer, R.F.:   Initial ventricular impulse: A potential key to cardiac evaluation. Circulation *29*:268, 1964.

Samson, R.:   Changes in systolic time intervals in acute myocardial infarction. Brit. Heart J. *32*:839, 1970.

Sangster, J.F., and Oakley, C.M.:   Diastolic murmur of coronary artery stenosis. Brit. Heart J. *35*:840, 1973.

Sawayama, T., Marumoto, S., Niki, I., and Matsuura, T.:   The clinical usefulness of the amyl nitrite inhalation test in the assessment of the third and atrial heart sounds in ischemic heart disease. Amer. Heart J. *76*:746, 1968.

Shelburne, J.C., Rubinstein, D., and Gorlin, R.:   A reappraisal of papillary muscle dysfunction; correlative clinical and angiographic study. Amer. J. Med. *46*:862, 1969.

Sonnenblick, E.H.:   Non-invasive evaluation of regional ventricular dysfunction. New Engl. J. Med. *285*:114, 1971.

Spodick, D.H.:   Coronary bypass operations. New Engl. J. Med. *285*:55, 1971.

Spodick, D.H.:   Coronary surgery. Amer. Heart J. *79*:579, 1970.

Tippit, H.C., and Benchimol, A.:   The apex cardiogram. J.A.M.A. *201*:24, 1967.

Toutouzas, P., Gupta, D., Samson, R., and Shillingford, J.:   Q-second sound interval in acute myocardial infarction. Brit. Heart J. *31*:462, 1969.

Turner, P.P., and Hunter, J.:   The atrial sound in ischaemic heart disease. Brit. Heart J. *35*:657, 1973.

Weissler, A.M., and Garrard, C.L. Jr.:   Systolic time intervals in cardiac disease. (II) Mod. Concepts Cardiovasc. Dis. *40*:5, 1971.

Weissler, A.M., Peeler, R.G., and Roehill, W.H.:   Relationships between left ventricular ejection time and patients with cardiovascular disease. Amer. Heart J. *62*:367, 1961.

Wood, P.:   Diseases of the heart and circulation. Philadelphia: J.B. Lippincott, 1956.

Yurchak, P.M., and Gorlin, R.:   Paradoxical splitting of the second heart sound in coronary disease. New Engl. J. Med. *269*:741, 1963.

10
Congenital
Heart Disease

There are two types of atrial septal defects, ostium secundum and ostium primum. In both conditions, patients have a left-to-right shunt at the atrial level causing diastolic volume overloading of the left ventricle. The ostium primum type is also called endocardial cushion defect. In these patients, associated congenital malformations of either the mitral and/or tricuspid valve are present, causing insufficiency of the valve.

ATRIAL SEPTAL DEFECTS—OSTIUM SECUNDUM

Heart Sounds and Murmurs

The first heart sound is split; therefore, two major components should be clearly identified on the logarithmic recording. The tricuspid component is accentuated and best analyzed from the tricuspid area phonocardiogram. In about 25% of cases, a systolic ejection click due to dilatation of the pulmonary artery or abnormal pulmonary valve motion is present. This sound occurs 0.02 to 0.04 sec after the first high frequency vibration of the first heart sound. The incidence of ejection clicks increases in patients with elevated pulmonary artery pressure and may be inscribed very early in systole (0.01–0.03 sec) after the initial vibration of the first heart sound. In many patients, it is impossible to identify an ejection click because it is inscribed too close to, or at the same time as, the first heart sound. The second heart sound is widely split and fixed in most patients. The A2–P2 interval ranges from 0.04 to 0.08 sec (Fig. 10.1). The aortic component is normal. The pulmonic component of the second heart sound has normal intensity in the absence of pulmonary hypertension and it is usually transmitted well to the mitral area. The fixed splitting of the second sound means that the A2–P2 interval does not change significantly during the respiratory cycle.

A tricuspid opening snap is rare in this condition and is seen only in patients with large left-to-right shunts. The best anatomical area for its recording is at the third intercostal space using a high frequency filter. Prominent third heart sounds are frequently heard and recorded best at the tricuspid area. Fourth heart sounds in patients below age 30 are rare, but are frequently heard in patients with elevated pulmonary artery pressure.

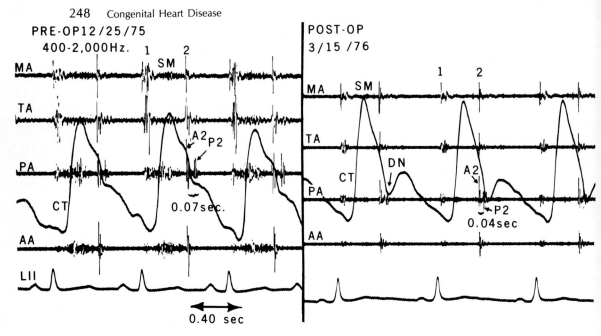

Figure 10.1. *Left:* Simultaneously recorded phonocardiogram at the mitral (MA), tricuspid (TA), pulmonic (PA) and aortic areas (AA), carotid pulse tracing (CT), and lead II (LII) of the electrocardiogram in a patient with atrial septal defect, secundum type. The first (1) heart sound is normal. The second (2) heart sound shows a fixed splitting. The A2–P2 interval is 0.07 sec. There is a high frequency, medium amplitude systolic ejection murmur (SM) recorded in all precordial areas. There are no diastolic murmurs. The carotid pulse tracing is normal. *Right:* Simultaneously recorded phonocardiogram at the mitral, tricuspid, pulmonic and aortic areas, carotid pulse tracing, and lead II of the electrocardiogram on the same patient following closure of the atrial septal defect. Note that the systolic murmur is practically absent. The A2–P2 interval has decreased to 0.04 sec. The carotid pulse tracing continues to be normal.

A systolic ejection murmur heard in patients with secundum type atrial septal defects is the result of increased blood flow across the outflow tract of the right ventricle causing a large amount of blood flow across a normal pulmonic valve. This murmur varies in intensity but it is recorded best at the pulmonic and tricuspid areas (Figs. 10.1 through 10.4). Diastolic murmurs may be present in mid-diastole or during atrial systole. They can be recorded in patients with large left-to-right shunts and are due to increased blood flow through a normal tricuspid valve. In patients with pulmonary hypertension, there is progressive disappearance of the right ventricular third heart sound and diastolic murmur because of decreased magnitude of the left-to-right shunt. In addition, amplitude of the systolic ejection murmur decreases and the A2–P2 interval becomes very short. However, another diastolic murmur due to pulmonic insufficiency is seen in patients with marked dilatation of the pulmonary artery or in those with severe pulmonary hypertension. It differs from the diastolic murmur described above because this murmur starts with the second heart sound. A systolic regurgitant murmur representing tricuspid insufficiency is usually indicative of a large left-to-

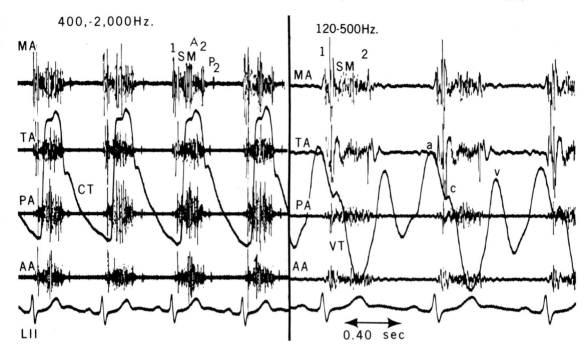

Figure 10.2. *Left:* Simultaneously recorded phonocardiogram at the mitral (MA), tricuspid (TA), pulmonic (PA) and aortic areas (AA), carotid pulse tracing (CT), and lead II (LII) of the electrocardiogram at a filter setting of 400–2,000 Hz in a 26-year-old patient with an atrial septal defect, secundum type. The first (1) heart sound is normal. The second (2) heart sound is widely split and the pulmonic component is transmitted to all precordial areas. There is a high frequency, high amplitude systolic ejection murmur (SM) recorded in all precordial areas. The carotid pulse tracing is normal. *Right:* Recording of the same patient using a filter setting of 120–500 Hz with a jugular venous pulse tracing (VT). The jugular venous pulse has essentially normal contour since the pulmonary artery pressure in this patient was within normal range.

right shunt or severe pulmonary hypertension. This type of murmur is seen in patients with marked dilatation of the right ventricle. The postoperative phonocardiogram after closure of an atrial septal defect shows a decrease in amplitude or disappearance of the systolic murmur (Fig. 10.4), or a decrease in the A2–P2 interval (Fig. 10.1) and disappearance of the atrioventricular diastolic murmur. It is very important to obtain a postoperative tracing because it can be used as a control record for subsequent follow-up.

Carotid Pulse Tracing

The carotid pulse tracing is of no diagnostic value in secundum type atrial septal defects except for timing and identification of the components of the second heart sound (Figs. 10.1, 10.2).

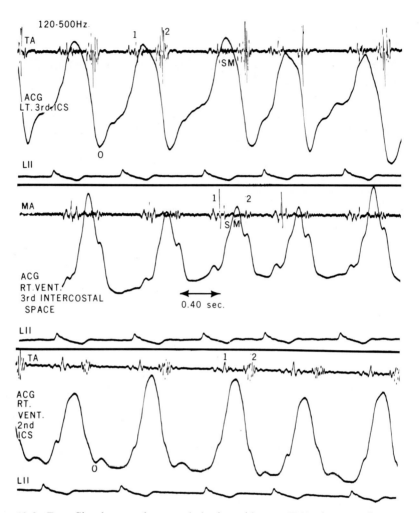

Figure 10.3. *Top:* Simultaneously recorded tricuspid area (TA) phonocardiogram, apex-cardiogram (ACG) with the transducer placed at the left third intercostal space (Lt 3rd ICS) and lead II (LII) of the electrocardiogram. With the transducer at this location, the apexcardiogram has a round systolic wave and a distinct O point. The phonocardiogram shows normal first (1) and second (2) heart sounds, and a systolic ejection murmur (SM). *Middle:* In this recording the transducer was moved closer to the right sternal border. In this area, one begins to record a right ventricular apexcardiogram where the systolic wave is not as round. The phonocardiogram shows the same features as described above. *Bottom:* Recording of the precordial pulsations with the transducer placed at the second right intercostal space. This most likely represents a recording of the outflow tract of the right ventricle. Note the sustained systolic wave, which is suggestive of right ventricular hypertrophy. The phonocardiographic findings are identical to the ones described above.

250

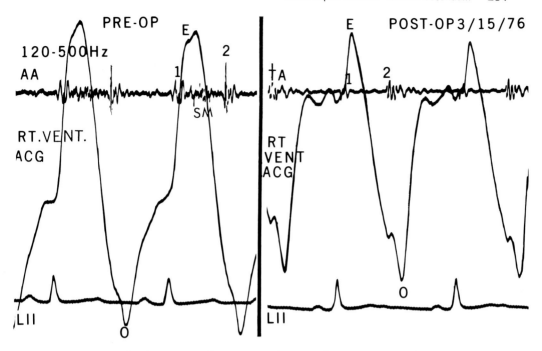

Figure 10.4. *Left:* Simultaneously recorded phonocardiogram at the aortic area (AA), right ventricular apexcardiogram (RT. VENT ACG), and lead II (LII) of the electrocardiogram in a 14-year-old patient with an atrial septal defect. The first (1) and second (2) heart sounds are normal. There is a high frequency, low amplitude systolic ejection murmur (SM). On the apexcardiogram the E point and downward deflection are normal. The O point is distinctly recorded after the second heart sound. *Right Panel:* This tracing was recorded after closure of the atrial septal defect. The right ventricular apexcardiogram shows a rapid systolic retraction following the E point, and the O point moves closer to the second heart sound. This type of apexcardiogram closely resembles a normal right ventricular apexcardiogram. On the phonocardiogram recorded at the tricuspid area (TA), the systolic murmur is not seen.

Jugular Venous Pulse Tracing

The jugular venous pulse tracing is frequently abnormal, showing prominent A and V waves (Fig. 10.2). A relative increase is recognized by measuring the amplitude of these waves in relation to the C wave. These A and V waves reflect the amplitude of the left-to-right shunt occurring during atrial contraction and early ventricular diastole. When pulmonary artery pressure begins to rise, the V wave becomes progressively smaller and the A wave larger. Tricuspid insufficiency occurs late in the natural history of this disease. Abnormalities of the venous pulse are the same as those described for tricuspid insufficiency (see Chap. 7), except that the A wave components are quite large, and the A wave becomes the predominant wave of the tracing, provided the patient is in sinus rhythm.

Apexcardiogram

An apexcardiogram of the left ventricle has no value in the diagnosis of secundum type atrial septal defects and is very difficult to record. However, right ventricular precordial motion can be recorded with a transducer placed over the tricuspid or subxyphoid area or over the third or fourth intercostal space near the sternum (Figs. 10.3, 10.4). When a good recording is obtained, it shows a prominent systolic retraction followed by a late systolic bulge and a conspicuous rapid filling wave. In patients with severe right ventricular hypertrophy with or without pulmonary hypertension, the systolic wave has a round shape and the A wave is quite prominent.

Systolic Time Intervals

Systolic time intervals are of no value in the diagnosis of atrial septal defects. However, when patients develop severe pulmonary hypertension, the left ventricular ejection time decreases.

Vectorcardiogram

The vectorcardiogram is quite helpful for noninvasive evaluation of patients with congenital heart disease because of its sensitivity in detecting signs of chamber enlargement. This is particularly true in patients with mild to moderate pulmonary stenosis in whom the vectorcardiogram shows an increase in size of the P loop with most of the forces in the horizontal plane located in front of the O point, and signs of right ventricular hypertrophy (Fig. 10.5). This technique is, of course, not specific for any type of congenital heart disease and simply indicates the type of chamber enlargement that may be present in a given case.

Echocardiogram

Echocardiography is a useful noninvasive technique in the diagnosis of secundum type atrial septal defects. The most common findings include: (1) Increase in right ventricular internal diameter due to increased diastolic volume loading, usually indicative of a large left-to-right shunt (Figs. 10.6, 10.7, 10.8); (2) abnormal motion of the interventricular septum. Two types of septal motion may be seen in patients with right ventricular volume loading. In Type A (paradoxical), the septum moves anteriorly in systole and posteriorly in diastole (Figs. 10.6, 10.8). Type B septal motion is flat throughout systole with a brief posterior deflection in early diastole. Caution should be exercised in the interpretation of these findings because normal septal motion has been seen in patients with atrial septal defects, but when present, it might be a clue that the left-to-right shunt is small. It is important to obtain a good recording of the mitral valve. A decrease in the D–E slope of the anterior and posterior mitral leaflets and systolic anterior motion (SAM) have been observed in patients with atrial septal defect. These abnormalities of mitral valve motion simulate the ones seen in patients with idiopathic hypertrophic subaortic stenosis. Systolic anterior motion is present in approximately 35–40% of

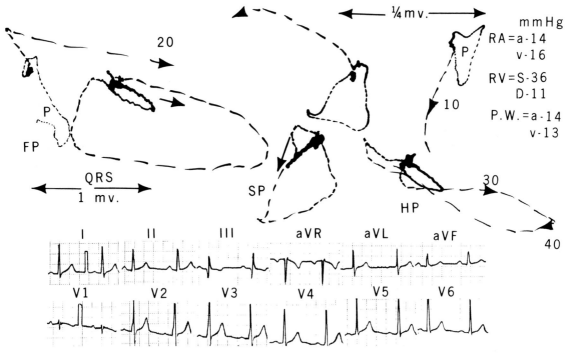

Figure 10.5. Vectorcardiogram and electrocardiogram in a 45-year-old patient with an atrial septal defect. The vectorcardiogram shows signs of right ventricular hypertrophy, primarily seen in the horizontal plane (HP) with most of the forces located in front of the O point. The P loop is located anteriorly indicating right atrial hypertrophy. The right atrial, right ventricular, and pulmonary "wedge" pressures are indicated. The electrocardiogram shows sinus rhythm and possible signs of right ventricular hypertrophy.

patients with this disease. Patients with atrial septal defects may also show some of the echocardiographic features seen in patients with prolapse of the mitral valve. The tricuspid valve may have an increased opening excursion (Fig. 10.7) or may flutter in diastole from the shunting blood hitting the leaflets.

ATRIAL SEPTAL DEFECTS—OSTIUM PRIMUM OR ENDOCARDIAL CUSHION DEFECTS

Endocardial cushion defects are also called ostium primum septal defects. The most severe form is an atrioventricular canal, but defects also include a variety of cardiac lesions that should be considered in generic terms. Most of these lesions are due to a lack of fusion of the anatomical endocardial cushion that eventually forms the interventricular septum. Therefore, a variety of combined malformations may be seen. Most patients will have a blood shunt from the left ventricle to the right atrium. Due to the variety and combination of anatomical defects seen in these patients, the auscultatory, phonocardiographic, pulse wave and echocardiographic abnormalities may not be identical.

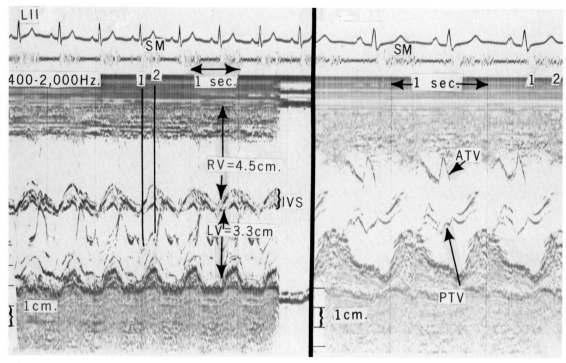

Figure 10.6. *Left:* Echocardiogram of a patient with an atrial septal defect recorded simultaneously with a phonocardiogram and lead II (LII) of the electrocardiogram. Note the increase in right ventricular (RV) internal dimension to 4.5 cm and the paradoxical motion of the interventricular septum. *Right:* Echocardiogram at the tricuspid valve of the same patient showing a large excursion of the tricuspid valve, which is one of the important echocardiographic features of patients with atrial septal defect. There is a large flow of blood due to a left-to-right shunt. SM = systolic murmur, LV = left ventricle, IVS = interventricular septum, ATV = anterior tricuspid valve, PTV = posterior tricuspid valve.

Heart Sounds and Murmurs

The first heart sound is normal in patients with endocardial cushion defects. If the patient has significant mitral insufficiency, the first heart sound is diminished and the second heart sound is usually widely split and fixed (Fig. 10.9). A third heart sound, frequently recorded at the mitral and tricuspid areas, is secondary to increased early diastolic right ventricular filling. Fourth heart sounds and systolic ejection clicks are not generally heard unless there is associated pulmonary hypertension.

Typical murmurs associated with ostium primum defects are mitral and/or tricuspid insufficiency due to congenital anatomical deformities of these valves, usually caused by lack of tissue fusion. The systolic murmur of mitral or tricuspid insufficiency starts with the first heart sound, reaches a plateau during early or midsystole, and terminates with the aortic or pulmonic valve closure sound (Fig. 10.9). Systolic ejection murmurs are frequently present due to increased flow across the pulmonary valve. A diastolic murmur is frequently recorded in mid-

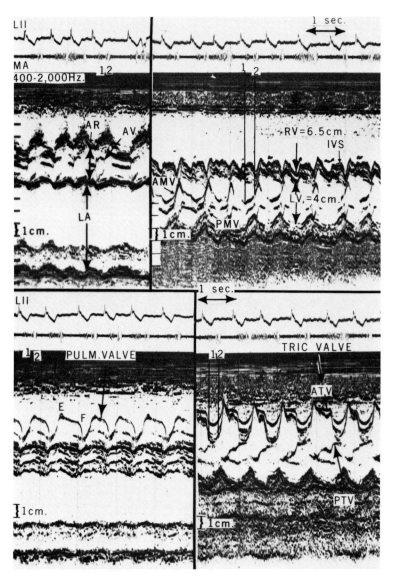

Figure 10.7. *Top Left:* Echocardiogram of the aortic valve (AV) and left atrium (LA) showing a normal aortic valve. The left atrium is enlarged. *Top Right:* This recording shows a marked increase in right ventricular (RV) internal dimension to 6.5 cm. The left ventricular (LV) internal dimension is normal. *Bottom Left:* Echocardiogram of the pulmonic valve on the same patient showing a reduced e–f slope, which is usually seen in patients with pulmonary hypertension. *Bottom Right:* Echocardiogram of the tricuspid valve showing tricuspid valve prolapse which is one of the features seen in patients with atrial septal defect. ATV = anterior tricuspid valve; PTV = posterior tricuspid valve.

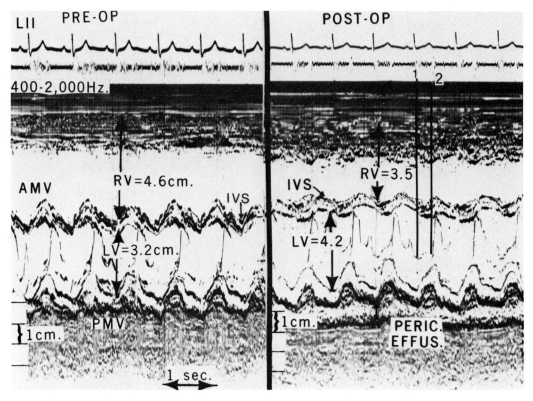

Figure 10.8. *Left:* Echocardiogram recorded prior to closure of a secundum type atrial septal defect in a 37-year-old patient showing an increase in right ventricular (RV) internal dimension to 4.6 cm and paradoxical motion of the interventricular septum (IVS). The left ventricular (LV) internal dimension of 3.2 cm is below normal. *Right:* After closure of the atrial septal defect, the right ventricular internal dimension decreased to 3.5 cm. Left ventricular internal dimension increased to 4.2 cm, which is normal. The interventricular septum now has normal motion. PMV = posterior mitral valve; AMV = anterior mitral valve.

diastole and indicates increased flow across the mitral or tricuspid valves. This murmur is usually preceded by a prominent third heart sound and terminates prior to atrial contraction. Diastolic murmurs of pulmonary insufficiency are associated with a very large left-to-right shunt and/or severe pulmonary hypertension.

Carotid Pulse Tracing

The carotid pulse tracing does not have any diagnostic value in patients with ostium primum atrial septal defects.

Jugular Venous Pulse Tracing

The jugular venous pulse tracing usually shows an abnormal contour similar to the findings described for secundum type atrial septal defects, including prominent A and V waves.

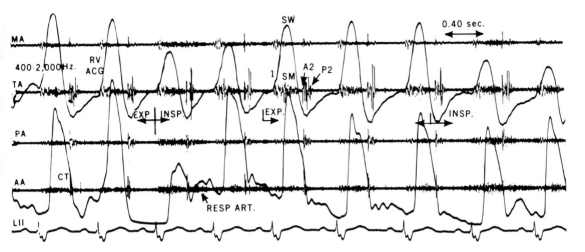

Figure 10.9. Simultaneously recorded phonocardiogram at the mitral (MA), tricuspid (TA), pulmonic (PA) and aortic areas (AA), right ventricular apexcardiogram (RV ACG), carotid pulse tracing (CT), and lead II (LII) of the electrocardiogram in a 12-year-old patient with an endocardial cushion defect and a large left-to-right shunt. A high frequency high amplitude systolic regurgitant murmur (SM) seen best at the mitral and tricuspid areas is due to mitral insufficiency. Amplitude of the first (1) heart sound is slightly diminished. The second (2) heart sound is widely split and fixed (approximately 0.07 sec). Duration of the split does not change significantly during inspiration (INSP) and expiration (EXP). The right ventricular apexcardiogram shows a sustained systolic wave (SW) of the type seen in patients with right ventricular hypertrophy. The carotid pulse tracing is normal. (From A. Benchimol: Non-Invasive Diagnostic Techniques in Cardiology. Copyright 1977 by The Williams & Wilkins Company, Baltimore. Used by permission.)

Systolic Time Intervals

Systolic time intervals are of no diagnostic value in patients with endocardial cushion defects; however, in the presence of mitral insufficiency with a large left-to-right shunt, left ventricular ejection time decreases secondary to diminished left ventricular forward stroke volume.

Vectorcardiogram

The vectorcardiogram in these patients shows forces oriented superiorly only in the frontal plane and conduction defects in the right bundle called complete or incomplete right bundle branch block.

Echocardiogram

The echocardiogram in patients with endocardial cushion defects varies depending upon the types of lesions associated with the disease. The most common type of ostium primum septal defect is usually associated with right ventricular volume overloading. In these patients, the echocardiogram may show multiple mitral valve echoes during systole and diastole with normal posterior left atrial wall motion, exaggeration of the anterior mitral valve opening excursion that comes close to the interventricular septum, and decreased excursion of the tricuspid leaflet. The outflow tract of the left ventricle is narrow in almost all cases (Fig. 10.10).

Paradoxical (type A) septal motion (Fig. 10.10) is frequently seen and right ventricular internal diameter may be increased. The various anatomical landmarks for mitral valve motion, such as recording of the E–F slope, are difficult to identify. The D–E slope can usually be recorded and is abnormal. In advanced forms of endocardial cushion defects such as atrial ventricular canal, patients will exhibit an unusual atrial–ventricular valve motion pattern. In these instances, the mitral and tricuspid leaflets seem to join together at the level of the aortic root during the systolic phase of the cardiac cycle. During diastole, the mitral valve moves posteriorly and the tricuspid valve moves anteriorly. The interventricular septum is absent in patients with common atrial–ventricular canal (Fig. 10.11).

TOTAL ANOMALOUS PULMONARY VENOUS RETURN

Anomalous pulmonary venous return can be partial or total. Most frequently in this type of congenital heart disease, the pulmonary veins will drain into the right atrium, superior vena cava or coronary sinus, and rarely into the inferior vena cava.

The phonocardiographic and pulse wave abnormalities are quite similar to the ones described in patients with secundum type atrial septal defects. A high amplitude, high frequency atrioventricular diastolic murmur may be present representing markedly increased flow across the tricuspid valve.

Echocardiogram

No definite echocardiographic pattern has been established in patients with total anomalous pulmonary venous return. Some reports have indicated a decrease in left atrial internal diameter. Paradoxical septal motion has been described in a few isolated cases, but this has not been demonstrated by all investigators. The right ventricular dimension is increased (Fig. 10.12).

VENTRICULAR SEPTAL DEFECT

Noninvasive techniques are valuable in evaluating patients with ventricular septal defects.

Heart Sounds and Murmurs

The first heart sound is normal. The second heart sound is single or shows a narrow split (0.04 sec or less). Splitting of the second heart sound in this condition is not wide as it is in patients with atrial septal defects or pulmonary valvular stenosis, and there is little variation, if any, during the two phases of the respiratory cycle. A progressive increase in pulmonary artery pressure and decrease in

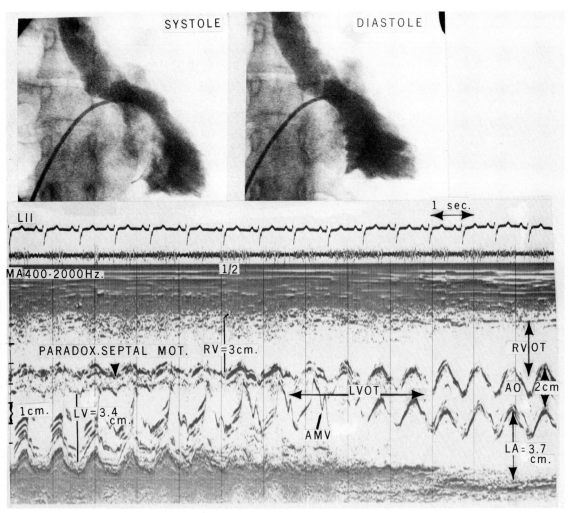

Figure 10.10. *Top:* Left ventricular angiogram with the patient in a right anterior oblique projection during systole and diastole showing narrowing of the outflow tract of the left ventricle, which is one of the features seen in patients with ostium primum type endocardial cushion defect. *Bottom:* Echocardiogram of the same patient recorded simultaneously with a mitral area (MA) phonocardiogram and lead II (LII) of the electrocardiogram showing paradoxical septal motion and an increase in left ventricular (LV) internal dimension to 3.4 cm. When the mitral valve opens, it touches the septum in the left ventricular outflow tract. RV = right ventricle, LVOT = left ventricular outflow tract, RVOT = right ventricular outflow tract, AO = aorta, LA = left atrium, AMV = anterior mitral valve.

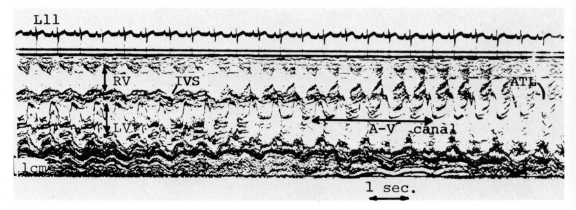

Figure 10.11. Echocardiogram of a patient with complete A–V canal. Note that the mitral and tricuspid valve leaflets (ATL) tend to join together and appear to be the same valve. This phenomenon is especially well seen during the systolic phase of the cardiac cycle. RV = right ventricle, IVS = interventricular septum, LV = left ventricle, LII = lead II of the electrocardiogram.

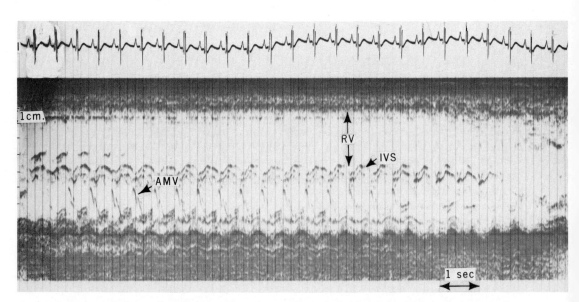

Figure 10.12. Echocardiogram of a patient with total anomalous pulmonary venous return showing a marked increase in right ventricular (RV) internal dimension. IVS = interventricular septum, LII = lead II of the electrocardiogram.

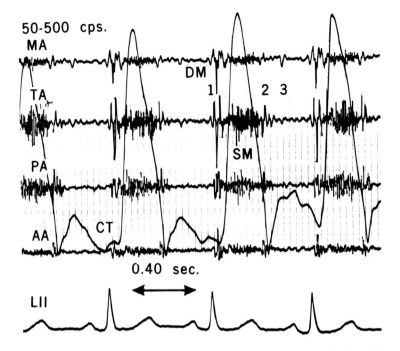

Figure 10.13. Simultaneously recorded phonocardiogram at the mitral (MA), tricuspid (TA), pulmonic (PA) and aortic areas (AA), carotid pulse tracing (CT), and lead II (LII) of the electrocardiogram in a 12-year-old patient with a ventricular septal defect and a left-to-right shunt without evidence of pulmonary hypertension. The first (1) heart sound is normal. The second (2) heart sound is single and normal. There is a third (3) heart sound. A high frequency, high amplitude systolic murmur (SM) reaches a maximal peak in midsystole and terminates prior to the aortic component of the second heart sound. In mid-diastole, there are some low frequency vibrations following the third heart sound, which probably represent increased turbulent flow across the mitral valve due to large recirculating volume of blood through the valve. The carotid pulse tracing is normal. DM = diastolic murmur. (From A. Benchimol: Non-Invasive Diagnostic Techniques in Cardiology. Copyright 1977 by The Williams & Wilkins Company, Baltimore. Used by permission.)

magnitude of the left-to-right shunt results in early pulmonary valve closure and the second heart sound becomes single and accentuated.

Prominent third heart sounds, frequently present in patients with large ventricular septal defects, are best recorded at the mitral and tricuspid areas.

Fourth heart sounds and systolic ejection clicks are rare in patients below age 20 provided they do not have pulmonary hypertension.

A systolic murmur is the most striking finding in patients with ventricular septal defects. It has the combined characteristics of a systolic regurgitant and ejection murmur (Fig. 10.13). The regurgitant feature is due to the fact that the murmur starts with the first heart sound, during the period of isovolumic contraction, when the left-to-right shunt is already present. The ejection feature is due to turbulent blood flow across a relatively small orifice, specifically, the ventricular septal defect, resulting in a diamond-shaped murmur that has a maximal peak during midsystole (Fig. 10.13). This murmur terminates with the aortic component of the second heart sound. It is recorded best at the tricuspid area with a log filter setting and is transmitted well to most precordial areas. As pulmonary hypertension develops and magnitude of the left-to-right shunt decreases, there is a progressive diminution of intensity and duration of the systolic murmur because less blood flows through the septal defect (Fig. 10.14). In cases with severe pulmonary hypertension, right ventricular systolic pressure equals the left ventricular systolic pressure and the systolic murmur may not be present, because the amount of blood crossing the septal defect is quite small or there may be no blood flow at all.

A low amplitude, low frequency diastolic murmur is recorded only in patients with large left-to-right shunts. The explanation for this murmur is that a large amount of blood flows through the pulmonary circulation and has to return to the left heart. As a result, this high volume of blood will cross the mitral valve, thus creating turbulent flow during diastole, resulting in a diastolic murmur. As pulmonary artery pressure increases, the diastolic murmur decreases because there is a smaller shunt, sometimes to the point where the murmur is no longer present. Murmurs of pulmonic insufficiency, present in approximately 20–30% of patients with severe pulmonary hypertension, are usually due to dilatation of the pulmonary valve.

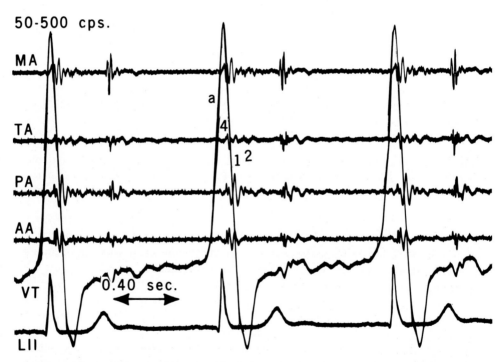

Figure 10.14. Simultaneously recorded phonocardiogram at the mitral (MA), tricuspid (TA), pulmonic (PA) and aortic areas (AA), jugular venous tracing (VT), and lead II (LII) of the electrocardiogram in a 38-year-old patient with a ventricular septal defect and severe pulmonary hypertension. Note that the systolic murmur is practically absent. The first (1) and second (2) heart sounds are single and normal. There is a fourth (4) heart sound. The jugular venous tracing shows a prominent A wave due to right ventricular hypertension.

Carotid Pulse Tracing

The carotid pulse tracing has a normal contour in ventricular septal defects.

Jugular Venous Pulse Tracing

The jugular venous pulse tracing is useful in identifying the degree of elevation of pulmonary artery pressure. If pulmonary artery pressure is normal, the jugular venous tracing is normal. With an increase in pulmonary pressure and resistance, the A wave becomes progressively larger (Fig. 10.14). Giant A waves, seen only when the mean pulmonary artery pressure exceeds 80 to 100 mm Hg, are due to abnormal, late right ventricular end-diastolic compliance requiring a forceful atrial contraction.

Apexcardiogram

The apexcardiogram of the left ventricle may show slight exaggeration of the rapid filling wave with the peak coinciding with the third heart sound. This may be a normal finding, however, in young subjects with small left-to-right shunts (Roger's type ventricular septal defect), representing a normal physiological third heart sound. The right ventricular apexcardiogram, recorded at the tricuspid area, third left intercostal space, or subxyphoid area is valuable. It may show exaggeration of the A wave, a sustained systolic wave, and a diminished rapid filling wave if the left-to-right shunt is large and the patient has right ventricular hypertrophy.

Systolic Time Intervals

Systolic time intervals are not useful in evaluating uncomplicated ventricular septal defects because no definite abnormalities have been described for the pre-ejection period (PEP) or pre-ejection period/left ventricular ejection time (PEP/LVET) ratio in these patients.

Vectorcardiogram

The vectorcardiogram usually shows signs of left ventricular hypertrophy in patients with moderate left-to-right shunts. However, if pulmonary hypertension develops, signs of right ventricular hypertrophy will be seen, i.e., the QRS forces are oriented anteriorly, inferiorly and to the right (Fig. 10.15).

Echocardiogram

Echocardiography has not been completely established as a diagnostic tool in evaluating patients with ventricular septal defects. In patients with normal pulmonary artery pressures and small left-to-right shunts, pulmonic valve motion is normal and the "a" dip has normal amplitude in the range of 2–8 mm. In patients with moderate-to-severe pulmonary hypertension, the pulmonic valve exhibits abnormal motion with a progressive decrease in amplitude of the "a" dip (Fig. 10.16), or it may be absent. Abnormal systolic notching of the pulmonic valve and

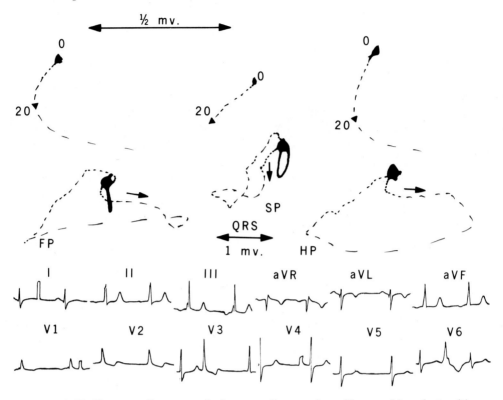

Figure 10.15. Vectorcardiogram and electrocardiogram in a 23-year-old patient with a ventricular septal defect and severe pulmonary hypertension. On the vectorcardiogram, all of the forces are located in front of the O point, indicative of right ventricular hypertrophy. The electrocardiogram also shows signs of right ventricular hypertrophy with tall R waves in V1 and V2.

a flat e–f diastolic slope are also commonly seen. If a good recording of the tricuspid valve is obtained, one may detect a prolonged a–c interval. This technique is also useful in demonstrating an increase in left atrial and left ventricular internal diameters, particularly in patients with large left-to-right shunts. Left and right ventricular wall thickness, and interventricular septal motion are usually normal.

PRIMARY OR IDIOPATHIC PULMONARY HYPERTENSION

In primary or idiopathic pulmonary hypertension, there is a marked increase in pulmonary artery pressure and resistance with associated dilatation of the main pulmonary artery. The etiology of this condition is unknown. The phonocardiographic (Fig. 10.17), auscultatory, pulse wave, and echocardiographic features in this condition are quite similar to the ones described in patients with ventricular septal defects and severe pulmonary hypertension (see ventricular septal defects).

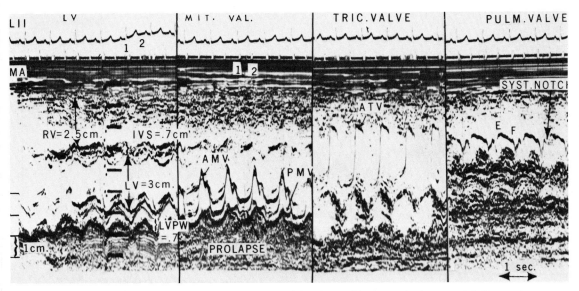

Figure 10.16. Echocardiogram in a 15-year-old patient with a ventricular septal defect and pulmonary hypertension recorded simultaneously with a mitral area (MA) phonocardiogram and lead II (LII) of the electrocardiogram. On the left is an echocardiogram of the left ventricular (LV) cavity showing normal left ventricular internal dimension, 3 cm. The right ventricular (RV) internal dimension is 2.5 cm. The echocardiogram of the mitral valve shows a prolapse of this valve, which is one of the features seen in patients with ventricular septal defect. The tricuspid valve echocardiogram also shows prolapse of the valve. The echocardiogram of the pulmonic valve shows a decrease in the e–f slope and systolic notching of the valve demonstrating pulmonary hypertension. LVPW = left ventricular posterior wall, IVS = interventricular septum, AMV/PMV = anterior and posterior mitral valve, ATV = anterior tricuspid valve.

Vectorcardiogram

The vectorcardiogram usually shows signs of right atrial and right ventricular hypertrophy, which are best appreciated in the horizontal plane. The P and QRS loops are oriented anterior to the O point. In the frontal plane, the QRS forces are directed inferiorly and to the right.

PATENT DUCTUS ARTERIOSUS

The first and second heart sounds are normal. If the second heart sound is split and there is associated pulmonary hypertension, the pulmonic component is accentuated and transmits well to the aortic and mitral areas. Multiple high frequency systolic sounds are recorded in mid- and/or late systole representing turbulent flow across the ductus arteriosus. This has been attributed to eddies through the ductus. A third heart sound is present at the mitral area in patients with large left-to-right shunts. Fourth heart sounds are rarely recorded. Systolic ejection clicks are present only in patients with severe pulmonary hypertension

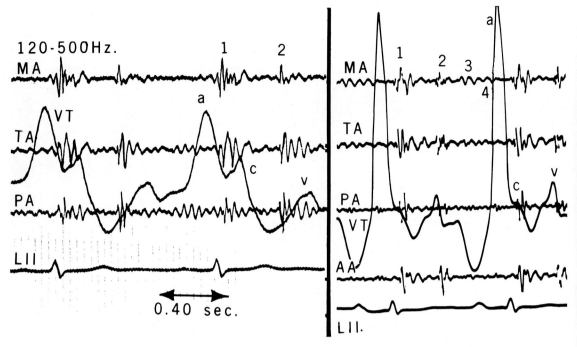

Figure 10.17. *Left:* Simultaneously recorded phonocardiogram at the mitral (MA), tricuspid (TA) and pulmonic areas (PA), jugular venous tracing (VT) and lead II (LII) of the electrocardiogram in a normal subject. The first (1) and second (2) heart sounds are normal and there are no murmurs. The jugular venous tracing is normal. *Right:* Recordings of a patient with a ventricular septal defect and severe pulmonary hypertension showing a quite prominent A wave that coincides with the fourth (4) heart sound. There is a third heart sound. The first (1) and second (2) heart sounds are not remarkable. The jugular venous tracing shows a giant A wave, as compared with the left panel.

and these patients usually have marked dilatation of the pulmonary arteries. A continuous machinery murmur throughout systole and diastole is commonly recorded. It is called a machinery murmur because it simulates the sound of a moving train. This high frequency murmur starts immediately after the first heart sound, reaches maximal intensity at the time of the second heart sound, continues throughout diastole and terminates prior to atrial contraction (Fig. 10.18). It is recorded best at the pulmonic or left infraclavicular area and is well transmitted to the spine. It is difficult to differentiate this murmur from arteriovenous fistula (abnormal communication between an artery and vein) and aortic–pulmonary window (consummated communication between the ascending aorta and the pulmonary artery), because they may also be continuous murmurs. In patients with patent ductus arteriosus and large left-to-right shunts, a low frequency mid-diastolic rumbling murmur is recorded at the mitral area corresponding to increased flow across the mitral valve. The murmur is usually preceded by a prominent third heart sound. In patients with pulmonary hypertension, the systolic and diastolic components of the machinery murmur disappear. This condition is called "silent" patent ductus arteriosus. The Graham–Steel murmur of

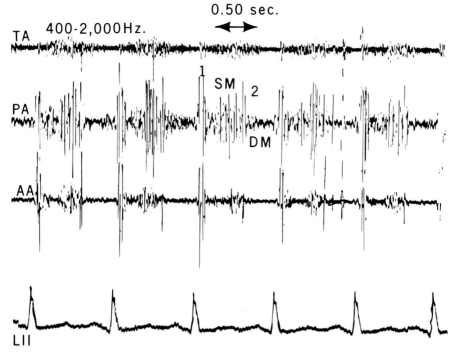

Figure 10.18. Simultaneously recorded phonocardiogram at the tricuspid (TA), pulmonic (PA) and aortic areas (AA), and lead II (LII) of the electrocardiogram in an 8-month-old patient with patent ductus arteriosus. Note the typical features of the so-called machinery murmur of patent ductus including a systolic murmur (SM) with a maximal peak at the end of the second (2) heart sound, continuing throughout diastole and terminating with the P wave of the electrocardiogram. This is best seen at the pulmonic area. DM = diastolic murmur.

pulmonic insufficiency, seen in only a few cases in the late stage of the natural history of this disease, is due to dilatation of the pulmonary valve secondary to pulmonary hypertension.

Carotid Pulse Tracing

The carotid pulse tracing may show the same features described in patients with aortic insufficiency, including a rapid systolic rise, and mid-systolic retraction followed by a late systolic bulge. The dicrotic notch is sharp and followed by a large early diastolic wave.

Jugular Venous Pulse Tracing

The jugular venous pulse tracing is normal in patients with normal pulmonary artery pressures. With elevated pulmonary and right ventricular pressures, the A wave becomes quite prominent.

Apexcardiogram

The apexcardiogram of the left ventricle shows a normal E point and systolic wave. In the presence of left ventricular hypertrophy, seen in patients with large left-to-right shunts, the systolic wave is round and sustained throughout systole, the rapid filling wave is prominent and the A wave has normal amplitude.

Systolic Time Intervals

The systolic time intervals are of no diagnostic value in patients with patent ductus arteriosus.

Vectorcardiogram

The vectorcardiographic features of patent ductus arteriosus with moderate or large left-to-right shunts are identical to the ones seen in patients with left and right ventricular hypertrophy.

Echocardiogram

Echocardiography can be a valuable tool in patients with patent ductus arteriosus. In these infants and children, one usually detects an increase in left atrial internal dimension, particularly if there is a large left-to-right shunt. If the diagnosis of patent ductus arteriosus is suspected, serial echocardiograms should be obtained. If the recordings demonstrate a progressive increase in left atrial size, this is usually indicative of a progressive increase in the left-to-right shunt through the ductus. However, caution must be exercised in the interpretation of these findings because an increase in left atrial diameter can also be seen in patients with respiratory distress syndrome. Spontaneous or surgical closure of the ductus will result in a decrease in left atrial size. The suprasternal approach should be used in all patients presenting with this abnormality because the left atrium may have more length than depth (Fig. 10.19). Because the echocardiographic findings are nonspecific for this particular lesion, it is important in studying the disease state that an increase in left atrial size be correlated with all of the previously described noninvasive techniques.

COARCTATION OF THE AORTA

The first heart sound is normal. The second heart sound may be single or split. Paradoxical splitting of the pulmonic component, which precedes the aortic component of the second heart sound, is seen in about 10% of patients with coarctation of the aorta and is due to delayed emptying of the left ventricle. The aortic component of the second heart sound is accentuated due to an increase in ascending aortic pressures (Fig. 10.20).

A systolic ejection murmur with maximal intensity in midsystole is often heard best at the level of the thoracic spine and the left upper chest at the sternal area. The murmur may extend through the aortic component of the second heart sound

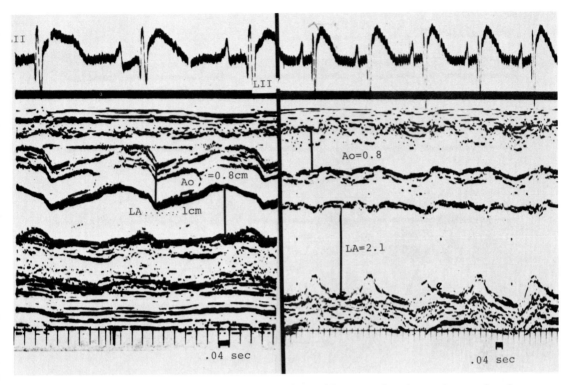

Figure 10.19. *Left:* Echocardiogram of a patient with patent ductus arteriosus using the sternal approach. On this recording the left atrium (LA) measures only 1 cm and the aortic root (AO), 0.8 cm. *Right:* The suprasternal approach with the left atrial size 2.1 cm as compared with sternal approach measurement of 1 cm. The aortic root size is still 0.8 cm. The suprasternal approach allowed for a more reliable measurement of left atrial size which is important in the diagnosis of patent ductus arteriosus.

terminating in early diastole. This murmur represents turbulent flow across the coarctation segments of the aorta (Fig. 10.20). Patients with severe coarctation and a marked degree of collateral circulation through the intercostal arteries may exhibit a continuous high frequency machinery type murmur with maximum intensity at the time of the second heart sound similar to the ones seen in patients with patent ductus arteriosus. This murmur is due to increased flow through dilated collateral circulation. Arterial diastolic murmurs of aortic insufficiency heard in approximately 35% of patients with coarctation of the aorta are related to the presence of an insufficient aortic valve, which may frequently have only two cusps instead of the normal three cusps.

Carotid Pulse Tracing

The carotid pulse tracing is not diagnostic in patients with coarctation of the aorta except to rule out the possibility of associated aortic valve disease. Recording of the peripheral arterial pulses, especially the femoral artery pulse as compared with the carotid pulse tracing, shows a delay in the upstroke time of the transcutaneous

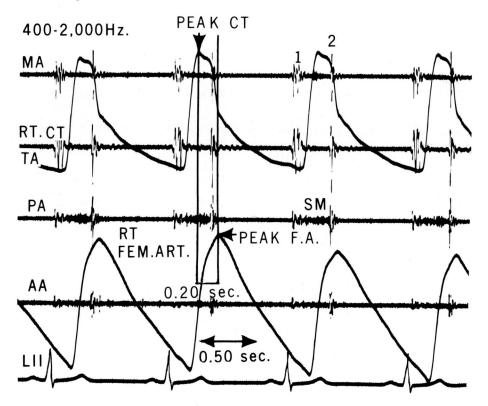

Figure 10.20. Simultaneously recorded phonocardiogram at the mitral (MA), tricuspid (TA), pulmonic (PA) and aortic areas (AA), right carotid pulse tracing (RT CT), right femoral artery pulse tracing (RT FEM ART), and lead II (LII) of the electrocardiogram in a patient with coarctation of the aorta. The first (1) heart sound is normal. The second (2) heart sound is accentuated. There is a high frequency, high amplitude systolic murmur (SM) that has a peak in mid-to-late systole. There are no diastolic murmurs. Note the difference in the time interval between the peaks of the carotid and femoral artery pulses (0.20 sec), which is markedly prolonged.

femoral pulse tracing, which exceeds the normal delay of 0.09 sec (Fig. 10.20). The contour of the femoral artery pulse tracing is essentially identical to the one described in patients with aortic valvular stenosis.

Jugular Venous Pulse Tracing

The jugular venous pulse tracing is nondiagnostic in this condition.

Apexcardiogram

The apexcardiogram frequently shows a prominent A wave, usually exceeding 15% of the total amplitude of the apexcardiogram (E through O amplitude). A sustained systolic wave representing left ventricular hypertrophy may be seen in patients with severe coarctation of the aorta.

Systolic Time Intervals

Systolic time intervals have no value in the diagnosis of coarctation of the aorta.

Vectorcardiogram

In patients with severe coarctation of the aorta, the vectorcardiogram shows signs of left ventricular hypertrophy.

Echocardiogram

No definite abnormalities have been described using echocardiography in patients with coarctation of the aorta unless the patient has an associated bicuspid aortic valve or aortic insufficiency, in which case the findings are identical to the ones seen in those conditions. Left ventricular thickness may be increased as seen in aortic stenosis.

PULMONARY VALVULAR STENOSIS

Heart Sounds and Murmurs

The first heart sound is normal and may be followed by a systolic ejection click. The time interval between the first high frequency vibration of the first heart sound and the systolic ejection click is a gross indicator of the severity of pulmonary stenosis. The shorter the first sound–click interval, the higher the gradient across the pulmonic valve. An ejection click is present in only 10 to 15% of patients with pulmonary infundibular stenosis, and this finding may be useful in differentiating valvular from infundibular stenosis (see tetralogy of Fallot). The second heart sound is important in assessing the degree of severity of pulmonary valvular stenosis. This sound is widely split and fixed; the pulmonic component is diminished in proportion to the degree of stenosis and may be absent in approximately 20% of patients with a pressure gradient across the pulmonic valve exceeding 80–100 mm Hg. The aortic valve closure sound is normal. The time between the aortic closure–pulmonary closure sound (A2–P2 interval), is also proportional to the gradient across the stenotic pulmonic valve. The longer the A2–P2 interval, the greater the gradient across the valve. Third heart sounds are rare.

The murmur of pulmonary valvular stenosis is characteristically a high frequency, noisy systolic ejection murmur having maximal intensity in mid- or late systole (Fig. 10.21). This murmur is best heard at the pulmonic and tricuspid areas. Timing of the peak of this murmur is grossly proportional to the gradient across the valve. With gradients exceeding 80 mm Hg, the murmur has late systolic accentuation continuing through the aortic valve closure sound and terminating with P2. This murmur, at times, is well transmitted to the carotid arteries. Diastolic murmurs are not heard in this condition.

Carotid Pulse Tracing

The carotid pulse contour is normal. However, recording of this pulse wave is useful as a reference tracing to identify the two components of splitting of the

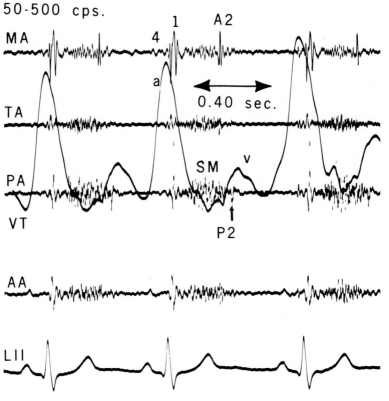

Figure 10.21. Simultaneously recorded phonocardiogram at the mitral (MA), tricuspid (TA), pulmonic (PA) and aortic areas (AA), jugular venous pulse tracing (VT), and lead II (LII) of the electrocardiogram in a 7-year-old patient with pulmonary valvular stenosis. The first (1) heart sound is normal. The aortic (A2) component of the second heart sound is normal. There is a wide splitting of the second heart sound (0.06 sec) and the pulmonic (P2) component is markedly diminished. There is a high frequency, high amplitude systolic ejection murmur (SM), reaching a maximal peak toward the end of systole. The jugular venous pulse shows a prominent A wave. There is also a fourth (4) heart sound that coincides with the peak of the A wave of the jugular venous pulse tracing.

second heart sound. The aortic component, which has normal amplitude, precedes the dicrotic notch and the pulmonic component follows it.

Jugular Venous Pulse Tracing

A good recording of the jugular venous pulse tracing is important in pulmonary stenosis. The A wave increases in amplitude in proportion to the increased pressures in the right ventricle. In very severe forms of pulmonary valvular stenosis, the A wave becomes extremely prominent with an A/V ratio exceeding 3 (normal, 1.5:1). In mild forms of pulmonary valvular stenosis, the jugular venous tracing may be normal.

Apexcardiogram

An apexcardiogram of the left ventricle is of no value in the diagnosis of pulmonary valvular stenosis. However, in many patients the right ventricular impulse can be recorded. In mild forms of pulmonary valvular stenosis, the right ventricular impulse recorded near the tricuspid area, or at the subxyphoid area, may show normal systolic retraction and a small A wave. However, in patients with severe pulmonary stenosis and associated right ventricular hypertrophy, the A wave of the right ventricular apexcardiogram becomes quite prominent, systolic retraction is absent, and there is a sustained systolic wave. The rapid filling wave becomes inconspicuous or may be absent.

Systolic Time Intervals

Systolic time intervals are of no value in the diagnosis of pulmonary valvular stenosis.

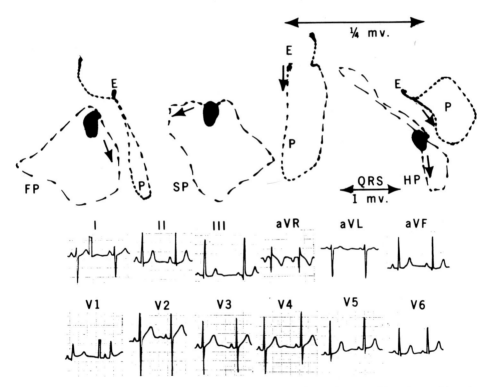

Figure 10.22. Vectorcardiogram and electrocardiogram in a 10-year-old patient with pulmonary valvular stenosis. Most of the forces seen in the horizontal (HP) plane are located posteriorly and to the right, which is indicative of right ventricular hypertrophy. The frontal plane (FP) vectorcardiogram shows clockwise rotation with most of the forces located inferiorly and to the right, indicating right ventricular hypertrophy. The P loop is in front of the E point, which is a typical feature for right atrial hypertrophy. The electrocardiogram shows sinus rhythm, prominent P waves in leads II, III, aVF, and V1, indicative of right atrial hypertrophy. There is also a tall R wave in V1 indicative of right ventricular hypertrophy.

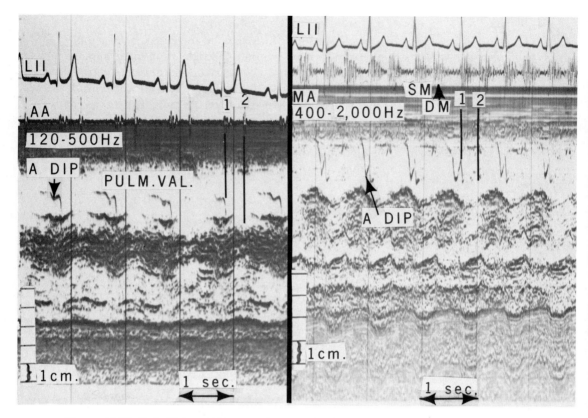

Figure 10.23. *Left:* Echocardiogram of a normal pulmonic valve (PULM VAL) showing a normal "a" dip. *Right:* Echocardiogram of the pulmonic valve in a patient with pulmonary stenosis showing a markedly exaggerated "a" dip. MA = mitral area phonocardiogram, LII = lead II of the electrocardiogram, SM = systolic murmur, DM = diastolic murmur, AA = aortic area phonocardiogram.

Maneuvers and Pharmacologic Agents

Inhalation of amyl nitrite usually causes an increase in amplitude of the systolic ejection murmur. This pharmacologic test is useful in differentiating pulmonary valvular stenosis from tetralogy of Fallot. Amplitude of the systolic murmur increases in patients with pulmonary valvular stenosis and decreases in patients with tetralogy of Fallot. The amplitude also decreases during the Valsalva maneuver in patients with pulmonary valvular stenosis.

Vectorcardiogram

The vectorcardiogram in pulmonary stenosis shows signs of right ventricular and right atrial hypertrophy. The QRS forces are oriented inferiorly, anteriorly, or posteriorly and to the right. The P loop is inscribed anterior to the O point (Fig. 10.22).

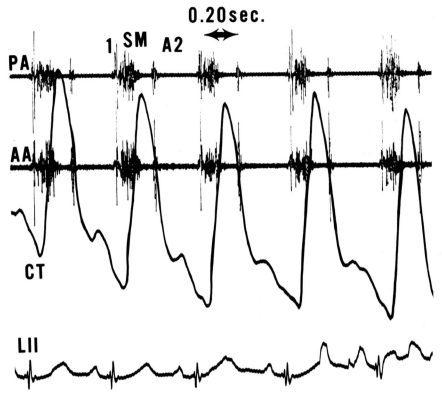

Figure 10.24. Simultaneously recorded phonocardiogram at the pulmonic (PA) and aortic areas (AA), carotid pulse tracing (CT), and lead II (LII) of the electrocardiogram in a six-year-old patient with tetralogy of Fallot. The first (1) heart sound is normal. The second (A2) heart sound is single and accentuated due to aortic valve closure. There is a high frequency, high amplitude systolic murmur (SM) that has a peak in early systole and terminates in midsystole. This is the typical murmur of patients with this disease state. The carotid pulse tracing is normal.

Echocardiogram

Echocardiography is valuable in the diagnosis of pulmonary valvular stenosis. Two of the three cusps of the pulmonic valve are usually recorded in infants but are sometimes difficult to record in children. Anatomical fusion of the pulmonic cusps results in a doming effect of the valve. The excursion of this valve during atrial contraction, which follows the P wave of the electrocardiogram, is called the "a" dip (Fig. 10.23). The more severe the stenosis, the greater the excursion of the "a" dip. Great caution should be exercised in interpreting this finding because some patients with moderately severe pulmonary stenosis may show normal excursion of the pulmonic valve and a normal "a" dip. The anterior wall of the right ventricle and/or interventricular septum should have increased thickness reflecting right ventricular hypertrophy.

PULMONARY ARTERY STENOSIS

In patients with peripheral pulmonary artery stenosis, the stenotic lesion may be single or multiple and may involve either the right or left pulmonary artery or both. The phonocardiographic and pulse wave abnormalities are somewhat similar to the ones described in patients with pulmonary valvular stenosis except that systolic ejection clicks are rare; the pulmonic component of the second heart sound is normal. Systolic ejection murmurs are best heard at the second or third intercostal space close to the anterior axillary line, either on the right or left depending upon the anatomical location of the stenosis. In pulmonary artery stenosis, the first heart sound is also normal. The carotid pulse tracing, apexcardiogram, and systolic time intervals are of no value in this condition. The jugular venous tracing may show an exaggerated A wave if right ventricular pressure is elevated.

Echocardiogram

No definite echocardiographic features have been described for this condition, although one might expect normal motion of the pulmonic valve instead of the abnormal features described for patients with pulmonary valvular stenosis.

TETRALOGY OF FALLOT

Heart Sounds and Murmurs

The first heart sound is normal. The second heart sound is single and accentuated due to aortic valve closure. The pulmonary valve closure sound is usually absent. Systolic ejection clicks are rare. Fourth heart sounds, part of the normal auscultatory findings, are of no diagnostic value in assessing the severity of the stenotic lesion. In tetralogy of Fallot, the obstructive disease is located in the infundibular tract of the right ventricle in about 85% of patients. Combinations of infundibular and pulmonary valvular stenosis may cause auscultatory findings similar to those described in patients with pulmonary valvular stenosis.

Systolic, high frequency ejection murmurs are heard best at the level of the third left intercostal space (Fig. 10.24). The murmur starts shortly after the first heart sound, has a maximal peak in early systole, and terminates in the last third of systole. The murmur is due to turbulent flow across the infundibular stenosis and not through the ventricular septal defect. Diastolic murmurs are not present unless the patient has prominent bronchial arterial collateral circulation causing a continuous murmur (see patent ductus arteriosus), which is heard at multiple areas over the precordium or unless the patient has been subjected to operative correction of this disease.

Carotid Pulse Tracing

The carotid pulse tracing is normal in patients with tetralogy of Fallot.

Jugular Venous Pulse Tracing

The jugular venous pulse usually shows a prominent A wave but not to the extent seen in patients with moderate-to-severe isolated pulmonary valvular stenosis.

Apexcardiogram

The apexcardiogram of the right ventricle may show a sustained systolic wave with a diminished rapid filling wave and a slightly prominent A wave due to right ventricular hypertrophy.

Vectorcardiogram

The vectorcardiographic findings in tetralogy of Fallot are signs of right ventricular hypertrophy and right atrial hypertrophy (Fig. 10.25).

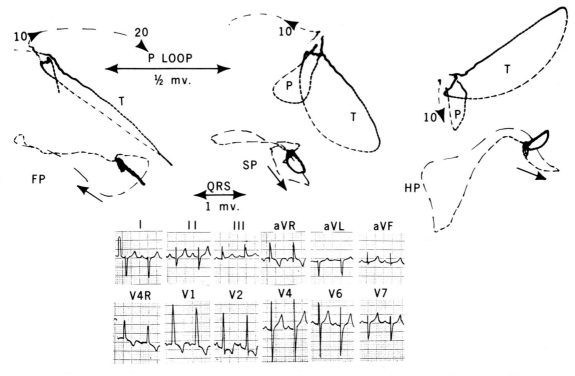

Figure 10.25. Vectorcardiogram and electrocardiogram in an eight-year-old patient with tetralogy of Fallot. The frontal plane (FP) vectorcardiogram shows most of the forces oriented inferiorly and to the right, indicating right ventricular hypertrophy. In the horizontal plane (HP), the QRS loop rotates counterclockwise, but most of the forces are located anteriorly and to the right in keeping with the diagnosis of right ventricular hypertrophy. Note that the entire P loop is anterior to the E point, indicative of right atrial hypertrophy. The electrocardiogram shows sinus rhythm with axis deviation and signs of right atrial and right ventricular hypertrophy based on the presence of prominent P waves in leads II, III, and aVF and tall R waves in V4R, V1, and V2. There is also right ventricular strain indicated by abnormalities of the T waves and ST segments in V1 and V2.

Echocardiogram

Echocardiographic features include demonstration of the anatomical discontinuity of the interventricular septum (Fig. 10.26) in relation to the anterior aortic wall. Anatomically, in this condition the aorta overrides the interventricular septum. There is continuity between the mitral annulus and the posterior aortic wall. Recording of the pulmonic valve is technically difficult. When obtained, it helps in the differential diagnosis between tetralogy of Fallot and truncus arteriosus.

Additional echocardiographic features in patients with tetralogy of Fallot include an enlarged aortic root, and possibly a thickened interventricular septum and right ventricular anterior wall and dilatation of the right ventricle. In severe forms of this condition with a marked decrease in size of the pulmonary artery, also called pseudo truncus, one may not identify the small segments of the pulmonic valve, which is almost atretic in this condition. These patients may also present with associated atrioventricular canal. They can be subjected to a number of operative procedures, including creation of a right subclavian–pulmonary artery anastomosis (Blalock procedure), aortic–pulmonary artery anastomosis (Potts procedure), or total correction of the lesion. The palliative shunt procedure at times can cause large left-to-right shunts and some of these patients may develop heart failure. Echocardiography is useful in detecting progressive enlargement of the left atrium in these patients, which is usually indicative of impending heart failure.

Congenital malformations such as tricuspid atresia, truncus arteriosus, transpositions of the great vessels and others were not included due to their complexity. For those interested in the use of noninvasive techniques in studying these conditions, other texts are available.

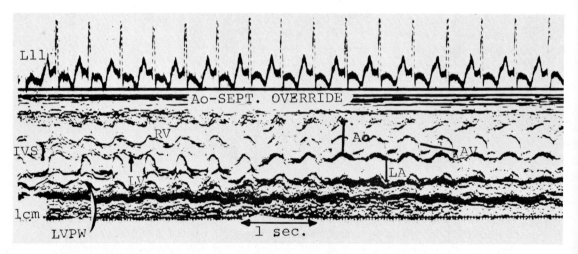

Figure 10.26. Echocardiogram of a patient with tetralogy of Fallot and pulmonary atresia. Note that the aorta (AO) overrides the interventricular septum (IVS). This is one of the characteristic features of patients with tetralogy of Fallot. LA = left atrium, AV = aortic valve, LV = left ventricle, RV = right ventricle, LVPW = left ventricular posterior wall.

BIBLIOGRAPHY

Abbasi, A.S., MacAlpin, R.N., Eber, L.M., and Pearce, M.L.:   Echocardiographic diagnosis of idiopathic hypertrophic cardiomyopathy without outflow obstruction. Circulation *46*:897, 1972.

Alderman, E.L., Rytand, D.A., Crow, R.S., Finegan, R.E., and Harrison, D.C.:   Normal and prosthetic atrioventricular valve motion in atrial flutter. Correlation of ultrasound, vectorcardiographic, and phonocardiographic findings. Circulation *45*:1206, 1972.

Allen, H.D., and Goldberg, S.J.:   Echocardiography in congenital heart disease. Ariz. Med. *31*:571, 1974.

Beller, B.M., and Dexter, L.:   Clinical and hemodynamic stability in a patient with a large atrial septal defect: a 17-year follow-up. J.A.M.A. *195*:588, 1966.

Benchimol, A., Barreto, E.C., and Gartlan, J.L.:   Right atrial flow velocity in patients with atrial septal defect. Am. J. Cardiol. *25*:381, 1970.

Benchimol, A., and Desser, K.B.:   Diagnostic value of arterial and venous wave forms. Cardiovasc. Clin. *6*:73, 1975.

Benchimol, A., and Dimond, E.G.:   Phonocardiography in ventricular septal defect. Correlation between hemodynamics and phonocardiographic findings. Am. J. Med. *28*:347, 1960.

Benchimol, A., and Lucena, E.G.:   Vectorcardiography in congenital heart disease with the use of the Frank system. Br. Heart J. *27*:236, 1965.

Benchimol, A., Wu, T.L., and Dimond, E.G.:   Apex cardiogram in the diagnosis of congenital heart disease. Am. J. Cardiol. *17*:63, 1966.

Benchimol, A., and Tippit, H.C.:   The clinical value of the jugular and hepatic pulses. Prog. Cardiovasc. Dis. *10*:159, 1967.

Benchimol, A., and Tippit, H.C.:   The clinical value of the jugular and hepatic pulses. In Physical diagnosis in cardiovascular diseases. Friedberg, C.K., (ed); New York: Grune & Stratton, 1969, chap. 3.

Betriu, A., Wigle, E.D., Felderhof, D.H., and McLoughlin, M.J.:   Prolapse of the posterior leaflet of the mitral valve associated with secundum atrial septal defect. Am. J. Cardiol. *33*:126, 1974.

Bialostozky, D., Horwitz, S., and Espino-Vela, J.:   Ebstein's malformation of the tricuspid valve. A review of 65 cases. Am. J. Cardiol. *29*:826, 1972.

Brammell, H.L., Vogel, J.H.K., Pryor, R., and Blount, S.G. Jr.:   The Eisenmenger syndrome. A clinical and physiologic reappraisal. Am. J. Cardiol. *28*:679, 1971.

Chang, J.H., and Burrington, J.D.:   Coarctation of the aorta in infants and children. J. Pediatr. Surg. *7*:127, 1972.

Chesler, E., Joffe, H.S., Beck, W., and Schrire, V.:   Echocardiography in the diagnosis of congenital heart disease. Pediatr. Clin. North Am. *18*:1163, 1971.

Chung, K.J., Alexson, C.G., Manning, J.A., and Gramiak, R.:   Echocardiography in truncus arteriosus: the value of pulmonic valve detection. Circulation *48*:281, 1973.

Colman, A.L.:   Clinical examination of the jugular venous pulse. Springfield, Ill.: Charles C. Thomas, 1966.

Craig, R.J., and Selzer, A.:   Natural history and prognosis of atrial septal defect. Circulation *37*:805, 1968.

Crews, T.L., Pridie, R.B., Benham, R., and Leatham, A.:   Auscultatory and phonocardiographic findings in Ebstein's anomaly. Correlation of first heart sound with ultrasonic records of tricuspid valve movement. Br. Heart J. *34*:681, 1972.

Davis, R.H., Feigenbaum, H., Chang, S., Konecke, L.L., and Dillon, J.C.:   Echocardiographic manifestations of discrete subaortic stenosis. Am. J. Cardiol. *33*:277, 1974.

DeMonchy, C.:   Phonocardiography and external pulsation tracings in infants with congenital heart disease. Cardiologia *52*:160, 1968.

Diamond, M.A., Dillon, J.C., Haine, C.L., Chang, S., and Feigenbaum, H.:   Echocardiographic features of atrial septal defect. Circulation *43*:129, 1971.

Dimond, E.G., and Benchimol, A.:   Phonocardiography in atrial septal defect: correlation between hemodynamics and phonocardiographic findings. Am. Heart J. *58*:343, 1959.

Dimond, E.G., and Benchimol, A.:   Phonocardiography in pulmonary stenosis: correlation between hemodynamics and phonocardiographic findings. Ann. Intern. Med. *52*:145, 1960.

Edler, I.:   The diagnostic use of ultrasound in heart disease. Acta. Med. Scand. *308*:32, 1955.

Eshaghpour, E., Turnoff, H.B., Kingsley, B., and Linhart, J.W.:   Echocardiographic features of endocardial cushion defect. Am. J. Cardiol. *33*:135, 1974.

Feigenbaum, H.:   Echocardiography. Philadelphia: Lea & Febiger, 1972.

Feigenbaum, H., Popp, R.L., Chip, J.N., and Haine, C.L.:   Left ventricular wall thickness measured by ultrasound. Arch. Intern. Med. *121*:391, 1968.

Feigenbaum, H., Popp, R.L., Wolfe, S.B., Troy, B.L., Pombo, J.F., Haine, C.L., and Dodge, H.T.:   Ultrasound measurements of the left ventricle. A correlative study with angiocardiography. Arch. Intern. Med. *129*:461, 1972.

Feigenbaum, H., Stone, J.M., Lee, D.A., Nasser, W.K., and Chang, S.:   Identification of ultrasound echoes from the left ventricle by use of intracardiac injections of indocyanine green. Circulation *51*:615, 1970.

Fisher, E., and Paul, M.H.:   Transposition of the great arteries: recognition and management. Cardiovasc. Clin. *2*:211, 1970.

Friedberg, C.K. (ed.):   Physical diagnosis in cardiovascular disease. New York: Grune & Stratton, 1969.

Friedman, S., Harris, T.N., Atac, M.S., and Peker, H.:   Some characteristics of diastolic flow murmurs in congenital and acquired heart disease. J. Pediatr. *71*:52, 1967.

Fyler, D.C., Gallaher, M.E., and Nadas, A.S.:   Auscultation in the evaluation of children with heart disease. Prog. Cardiovasc. Dis. *10*:363, 1968.

Genton, E., and Blount, S.G.:   The spectrum of Ebstein's anomaly. Am. Heart J. *73*:395, 1967.

Gibson, D.G., and Brown, D.:   Measurement of instantaneous left ventricular volumes and filling rate in man by echocardiography. Br. Heart J. *35*:559, 1973.

Glasser, S.P., Cheitlin, M.D., McCarty, R.J., Haas, J.H., Hall, R.J., and Mullins, C.E.:   Thirty-two cases of interventricular septal defect and aortic insufficiency. Am. J. Med. *53*:473, 1972.

Godman, M.J., Tham, P., and Kidd, B.S.L.:   Echocardiography in the evaluation of the cyanotic newborn infant. Br. Heart J. *36*:154, 1974.

Goldberg, B.B.:   Suprasternal ultrasonography. J.A.M.A. *15*:245, 1971.

Goldberg, S.J., Allen, H.D., and Sahn, D.J.:   Pediatric and adolescent echocardiography. Chicago: Year Book Medical Publishers, Inc., 1975.

Gramiak, R., Nanda, N.C., and Shah, P.M.:   Echocardiographic detection of the pulmonary valve. Radiology *102*:153, 1972.

Gramiak, R., and Shah, P.M.:   Echocardiography of the normal and diseased aortic valve. Radiology *96*:1, 1970.

Grossman, W., McLaurin, L.P., Moos, S.P., Stefadouros, M., and Young, D.T.: Wall thickness and diastolic properties of the left ventricle. Circulation 49:129, 1974.

Guller, B., and Bozie, C.: Right-to-left shunting through a patent ductus arteriosus in a newborn with myocardial infarction. Cardiology 57:348, 1972.

Henry, W.L., Clark, C.E., and Epstein, S.E.: Asymmetric septal hypertrophy. Echocardiographic identification of the pathognomonic anatomic abnormality of IHSS. Circulation 47:225, 1973.

Henry, W.L., Clark, C.E., and Epstein, S.E.: Asymmetric septal hypertrophy (ASH): the unifying link in the IHSS disease spectrum. Observations regarding its pathogenesis, pathophysiology, and course. Circulation 47:827, 1973.

Hipona, F.A., and Arthachinta, S.: Ebstein's anomaly of the tricuspid valve. A report of 16 cases and review of the literature. Prog. Cardiovasc. Dis. 7:434, 1965.

Hirata, T., Wolfe, S.B., Popp, R.L., Helmen, C.H., and Feigenbaum, H.: Estimation of left atrial size using ultrasound. Am. Heart J. 78:43, 1969.

Hirschfeld, S., Meyer, R.A., and Kaplan, S.: Non-invasive right and left systolic time intervals by echocardiography. Pediatr. Res. 8:350, 1974.

Hoffman, J.I.: Natural history of congenital heart disease. Problems in its assessment with special reference to ventricular septal defects. Circulation 37:97, 1968.

Johnson, S.L., Baker, D.W., Lute, R.A., and Murray, J.A.: Detection of mitral regurgitation by Doppler echocardiography. Am. J. Cardiol. 33:146, 1974.

Joyner, C.R., Hey, E.D., Johnson, J., and Reid, J.M.: Reflected ultrasound in the diagnosis of tricuspid stenosis. Am. J. Cardiol. 19:66, 1967.

Kamigaki, M., and Goldschlager, N.: Echocardiographic analysis of mitral valve motion in atrial septal defect. Am. J. Cardiol. 30:343, 1972.

Keith, J.D., Rowe, R.D., and Vlad, P.: Heart disease in infancy and childhood. New York: Macmillan, 1967.

King, D.L., Steeg, C.N., and Ellis, K.: Demonstrations of transposition of the great arteries by cardiac ultrasonography. Radiology 107:181, 1973.

King, D.L., Steeg, C., and Ellis, K.: Visualization of ventricular septal defects by cardiac ultrasonography. Circulation 48:1215, 1973.

Kloster, F.E., Roelandt, J., Cate, F.J.T., Bom, N., and Hugenholtz, P.G.: Multiscan echocardiography. II. Technique and initial clinical results. Circulation 48:1075, 1973.

Kotler, M.N.: Tricuspid valve in Ebstein's anomaly. Circulation 47:597, 1973.

Kraus, Y., Yahini, J.H., Shem-Tov, A., and Neufeld, H.N.: Precordial pulsations in corrected transposition of the great vessels. Diagnostic value of the electromechanical interval. Am. J. Cardiol. 23:684, 1969.

Lester, R.G., Osteen, R.T., and Robinson, A.E.: Infundibular obstruction secondary to pulmonary valvular stenosis. Am. J. Roentgen. 94:78, 1965.

Linhart, J.W., and Razi, B.: Late systolic murmur: a clue to the diagnosis of aneurysm of the membranous ventricular septum. Chest 60:283, 1971.

Luisada, A.A., and Feigen, L.P.: Technical progress in phonocardiography and pulse tracings. Acta. Cardiol. 28:392, 1972.

Lundstrom, N.R.: Echocardiography in the diagnosis of Ebstein's anomaly of the tricuspid valve. Circulation 47:597, 1973.

Lundstrom, N.R., and Edler, I.: Ultrasound cardiography in infants and children. Acta. Paediatr. Scand. 60:117, 1971.

Lundstrom, N.R., and Mortensson, W.: Clinical applications of echocardiography in infants and children. II. Estimation of aortic root diameter and left atrial size: a comparison between echocardiography and angiocardiography. Acta. Paediatr. Scand. *63*:33, 1974.

Macartney, F., Deverall, P., and Scott, O.: Significance of continuous murmurs in cyanotic congenital heart disease. Br. Heart J. *34*:205, 1972.

McDonald, I.G., Feigenbaum, H., and Chang, S.: Analysis of left ventricular wall motion by reflected ultrasound. Circulation *46*:14, 1972.

Meyer, R.A., and Kaplan, S.: Echocardiography in the diagnosis of hypoplasia of the left or right ventricles in the neonate. Circulation *46*:55, 1972.

Meyer, R.A., Schwartz, D.C., Benzing, G. III, and Kaplan, S.: Ventricular septum in right ventricular volume overload. An echocardiographic study. Am. J. Cardiol. *30*:349, 1972.

Moreyra, E., Klein, J.J., Shimada, H., and Segal, B.L.: Idiopathic hypertrophic subaortic stenosis diagnosed by reflected ultrasound. Am. J. Cardiol. *23*:32, 1969.

Moss, A.J., and Adams, F.H. (eds.): Heart disease in infants, children and adolescents. Baltimore: Williams & Wilkins, 1968.

Moss, A.J., Hutter, A.M. Jr., Lipchik, E.O., and Gallagher, R.E.: Congenital corrected transposition of the great vessels without cardiac anomalies. Am. J. Med. *47*:986, 1969.

Myler, R.K., and Sanders, C.A.: Normal splitting of the second heart sound in atrial septal defect. Am. J. Cardiol. *19*:874, 1967.

Nagle, R.E., and Tamara, F.A.: Left parasternal impulse in pulmonary stenosis and atrial septal defect. Br. Heart J. *29*:735, 1967.

Nanda, N.C., Gramiak, R., Manning, J., Mahoney, E.B., Lipchik, E.O., and DeWeese, J.A.: Echocardiographic recognition of the congenital bicuspid aortic valve. Circulation *49*:870, 1974.

Neufeld, H.N., Lucas, R.V. Jr., Lester, R.G., Adams, P. Jr., Anderson, R.C., and Edwards, J.E.: Origin of both great vessels from the right ventricle without pulmonary stenosis. Br. Heart J. *24*:393, 1962.

Perasalo, O., Halonen, P.I., and Siltanen, P.: Endocardial cushion defect. Clinical and surgical considerations. Acta. Chir. Scand. *128*:592, 1964.

Perloff, J.K.: Diagnostic inferences drawn from observation and palpation of the precordium with special reference to congenital heart disease. Advances Cardiopulm. Dis. *4*:13, 1969.

Perloff, J.K., Caulfield, W.H., and DeLeon, A.C.: Peripheral pulmonary artery murmur of atrial septal defect. Br. Heart J. *29*:411, 1967.

Pestana, C., Weidman, W.H., Swan, H.J.C., and McGoon, D.C.: Accuracy of preoperative diagnosis in congenital heart disease. Am. Heart J. *72*:446, 1966.

Popp, R.L., Brown, O.R., and Harrison, D.C.: Diagnostic accuracy of an ultrasonic multitransducer cardiac imaging system. Circulation *48*(Suppl IV):125, 1973.

Popp, R.L., Silverman, J.F., French, J.W., Stinson, E.B., and Harrison, D.C.: Echocardiographic findings in discrete subvalvular aortic stenosis. Circulation *49*:226, 1974.

Popp, R.L., Wolfe, S.B., Hirata, T., and Feigenbaum, H.: Estimation of right and left ventricular size by ultrasound. A study of the echoes from the interventricular septum. Am. J. Cardiol. *24*:523, 1969.

Pridie, R.B., and Oakley, C.M.: Mitral valve movement in hypertrophic obstructive cardiomyopathy. Br. Heart J. *31*:390, 1969.

Rao, B.N., and Edwards, J.E.: Conditions simulating the tetralogy of Fallot. Circulation *49*:173, 1974.

Rashkind, W.J.:   Transposition of the great arteries. Pediatr. Clin. North Am. *18*:1075, 1971.

Ravin, A., and Frame, F.K.:   International bibliography of cardiovascular auscultation and phonocardiography. New York: The American Heart Association, 1971.

Rossen, R.M., Goodman, D.J., Ingham, R.E., and Popp, R.L.:   Ventricular systolic septal thickening and excursion in idiopathic hypertrophic subaortic stenosis. N. Engl. J. Med. *291*:1317, 1974.

Sahn, D.J., Deely, W.J., Hagan, A.D., and Friedman, W.F.:   Echocardiographic assessment of left ventricular performance in normal newborns. Circulation *49*:232, 1974.

Sahn, D.J., Terry, R., O'Rourke, R., and Friedman, W.F.:   Multiple crystal cross-sectional echocardiography in the diagnosis of cyanotic congenital heart disease. Circulation *50*:230, 1974.

Sato, F.:   Symposium on limitation of diagnostic value of electrocardiography and phonocardiography. I. Electrocardiogram and phonocardiogram in relation to operative findings. Electrocardiogram of congenital heart disease in relation to their operative findings. Jap. Circ. J. *30*:1537, 1966.

Segal, B.L. (guest ed.):   Symposium on echocardiography. (Diagnostic ultrasound). Am. J. Cardiol. *19*:1, 1967.

Shah, P.M., Gramiak, R., Adelman, A.G., and Wigle, E.D.:   Role of echocardiography in diagnostic and hemodynamic assessment of hypertrophic subaortic stenosis. Circulation *44*:891, 1971.

Shepherd, R.L., Glancy, D.L., Jaffe, R.B., Perloff, J.K., and Epstein, S.E.:   Acquired subvalvular right ventricular outflow obstruction in patients with ventricular septal defect. Am. J. Med. *53*:446, 1972.

Solinger, R., Elbl, F., and Minhas, K.:   Echocardiography in congenital heart disease. Lancet *2*:1093, 1971.

Storstein, O., Rokseth, R., and Sorland, S.:   Congenital heart disease in a clinical material. An analysis of 1,000 consecutive cases. Acta. Med. Scand. *176*:195, 1964.

Tajik, A.J., Gau, G.T., Ritter, D.G., and Schattenberg, T.T.:   Echocardiogram in tetralogy of Fallot. Chest *64*:107, 1973.

Tajik, A.J., Gau, G.T., Ritter, D.G., and Schattenberg, T.T.:   Echocardiographic pattern of right ventricular diastolic volume overload in children. Circulation *46*:36, 1972.

Tatsuno, K., Konno, S., Ando, M., and Sakakibara, S.:   Pathogenetic mechanisms of prolapsing aortic valve and aortic regurgitation associated with ventricular septal defect. Anatomical, angiographic, and surgical considerations. Circulation *48*:1028, 1973.

Tavel, M.E.:   Phonocardiography and venous pulsations. The use of the jugular pulse in the diagnosis of atrial septal defect. Dis. Chest *54*:544, 1968.

Tavel, M.E., Baugh, D., Fisch, C., and Feigenbaum, H.:   Opening snap of the tricuspid valve in atrial septal defect. A phonocardiographic and reflected ultrasound study of sounds in relationship to movements of the tricuspid valve. Am. Heart J. *80*:550, 1970.

Troy, B.L., Pombo, J., and Rackley, C.E.:   Measurement of left ventricular wall thickness and mass by echocardiography. Circulation *45*:602, 1972.

Ultan, L.B., Segal, B.L., and Likoff, W.:   Echocardiography in congenital heart disease. Preliminary observations. Am. J. Cardiol. *19*:74, 1967.

Van Der Hauwaert, L.G.:   The effect of the Valsalva maneuver on the splitting of the second sound. Acta. Cardiol. *19*:518, 1964.

Van Praagh, R.:   What is the Taussing–Bing malformation? Circulation *38*:445, 1968.

Van Praagh, R., Corwin, R.D., Dahlquist, E.H., Freedom, R.M., Mattioli, L., and Nebesar, R.A.:   Tetralogy of Fallot with severe left ventricular outflow tract obstruction due to anomalous attachment of the mitral valve to the ventricular septum. Am. J. Cardiol. *26*:93, 1970.

Victoria, B.E., Gessner, I.H., and Schiebler, G.L.:   Phonocardiographic findings in persistent truncus arteriosus. Br. Heart J. *30*:812, 1968.

Wayne, H.H.:   Noninvasive technics in cardiology. The phonocardiogram, apexcardiogram, and systolic time intervals. Chicago: Year Book Medical Publishers, 1973.

Weyman, A.E., Dillon, J.C., Feigenbaum, H., and Chang, S.:   Echocardiographic patterns of pulmonic valve motion in pulmonic stenosis. Am. J. Cardiol. *33*:178, 1974.

Williams, R.G., and Rudd, M.:   Echocardiographic features of endocardial cushion defects. Circulation *49*:418, 1974.

Zoneraich, S. (ed.):   Non-invasive methods in cardiology. Springfield, Ill.: Charles C. Thomas, 1974.

Zuberbuhler, J.R., Bauersfeld, S.R., and Pontius, R.G.:   Paradoxic splitting of the second sound with transposition of the great vessels. Am. Heart J. *74*:816, 1967.

11
Myocardial Disease

Primary myocardial disease is a pathological state involving the heart muscle. Its etiology is unknown. Many names have been given to this disease, including diffuse myocardial disease, idiopathic cardiomyopathy, and others. Several etiologic factors have been implicated—viral, toxic, infectious, metabolic, congenital, etc. This disease is commonly classified as obstructive or nonobstructive. Obstructive disease, which is associated with abnormal hypertrophy of the myocardium, is seen in patients with idiopathic hypertrophic subaortic stenosis and is described in Chapter 6. In patients with obstructive disease there is usually a significant pressure gradient between the apex or inflow tract of the left ventricle and the outflow tract. In this chapter nonobstructive disease will be discussed.

Nonobstructive cardiomyopathies are classified as: (1) restrictive and (2) congestive. Restrictive disease is associated with marked restriction of ventricular filling. Its features are very similar to those seen in patients with constrictive pericarditis (see Chap. 12). Congestive cardiomyopathy is most frequently associated with early onset of congestive heart failure and cardiomegaly. The auscultatory, phonocardiographic, and pulse wave abnormalities seen in both types of disease have a few features in common.

Heart Sounds and Murmurs

The first heart sound is normal or diminished (Fig. 11.1). The second heart sound may be normal if pulmonary artery pressures are in the normal range. Most patients, especially the ones with congestive disease, have heart failure and pulmonary hypertension, and the combination of these findings causes the second heart sound to be single and accentuated due to increased intensity of the pulmonary component (Fig. 11.2). Conduction defects of the right and left bundle branches are a frequent finding. Wide and fixed splitting of the second heart sound is recorded if a right bundle branch block is present, or reversed splitting in the presence of left bundle branch block. A fourth heart sound is usually heard, particularly in patients with congestive myocardial disease, indicating decreased ventricular compliance and large left ventricular end-diastolic volume (Fig. 11.1). A third heart sound, which is almost always present in this condition, occurs 0.10 to 0.16 sec after the aortic valve closure sound (Fig. 11.1). In restrictive disease, this sound has the characteristics of an early, diastolic pericardial "knock," which is also heard in patients with constrictive pericarditis. Alternation of heart sounds is frequently observed in patients who also have pulsus alternans as demonstrated in the carotid pulse tracing (Fig. 11.2).

285

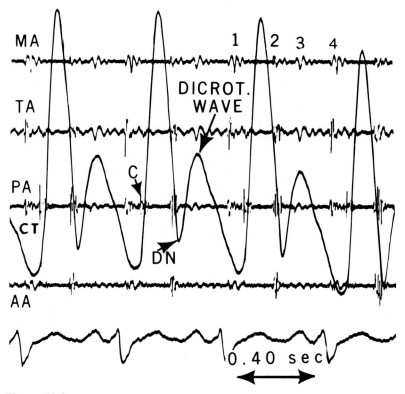

Figure 11.1.

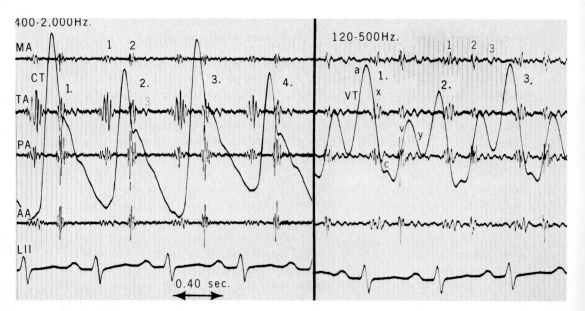

Figure 11.2.

286

Systolic ejection clicks may be heard if patients have pulmonary hypertension and dilated pulmonary arteries (Fig. 11.1).

Systolic murmurs due to mitral and/or tricuspid insufficiency are recorded frequently in congestive myocardial disease due to dilatation of the mitral or tricuspid annulus, and these patients have marked enlargement of the right and left ventricles. A soft, high frequency, systolic ejection murmur is present in both restrictive and constrictive disease due to turbulent blood flow across the pulmonic and aortic valves. Diastolic murmurs are not usually recorded in this condition.

Carotid Pulse Tracing

The carotid pulse tracing shows a rapid ascending limb with a rapid downward systolic wave, a dicrotic wave, and diminished ejection time (Fig. 11.1). Because most patients are in heart failure, pulsus alternans is a common finding (Fig. 11.2). It may occur in the left or right heart circulation, or simultaneously in both. If pulsus alternans is not present at rest, a mild degree of stress exercise will precipitate the appearance of this abnormality. It may also be induced by cardiac arrhythmias. The presence of pulsus alternans implies a poor prognosis since it is usually seen in the end stage of cardiomyopathies.

Jugular Venous Pulse Tracing

The jugular venous pulse tracing shows a conspicuous A wave, a normal C wave, and a normal or sustained systolic X descent (Figs.11.2 through 11.5). The V wave is large, with a rapid Y descent followed by a quick rise in early diastole. On the

---

Figure 11.1. Simultaneously recorded phonocardiogram at the mitral (MA), tricuspid (TA), pulmonic (PA) and aortic areas (AA), carotid pulse tracing (CT), and electrocardiogram in a 38-year-old patient with myocardial disease. Note the diminished first heart sound. The second heart sound is slightly accentuated. There are prominent third and fourth heart sounds. A systolic ejection click is recorded best at the pulmonic area. This patient had elevated pulmonary artery pressure during cardiac catheterization. The carotid pulse tracing has an abnormal contour. It shows diminished ejection time, a low placed dicrotic notch (DN), and a prominent dicrotic wave (DICROT. WAVE).

Figure 11.2. *Left:* Simultaneously recorded phonocardiogram at the mitral (MA), tricuspid (TA), pulmonic (PA) and aortic areas (AA), carotid pulse tracing (CT), and lead II (LII) of the electrocardiogram in a 55-year-old patient with a severe degree of congestive cardiomyopathy. Note the presence of alternans on the phonocardiogram and carotid pulse. The large beats (1 and 3) are usually associated with strong contractions of the heart. The small beats (2 and 4) usually indicate that the left ventricle is ejecting less blood into the aorta. The prominent third heart sound on the phonocardiogram indicates alternation in the left ventricle. *Right:* Simultaneously recorded phonocardiogram at the mitral, tricuspid, pulmonic and aortic areas, jugular venous tracing (VT), and lead II of the electrocardiogram. Note alternation in the jugular venous tracing. Beats 1 and 3 are strong. Beat 2 is weak. The presence of pulsus alternans on the jugular venous tracing indicates that the patient also has a severe degree of right ventricular disease. The phonocardiogram shows a third heart sound and a diminished first heart sound.

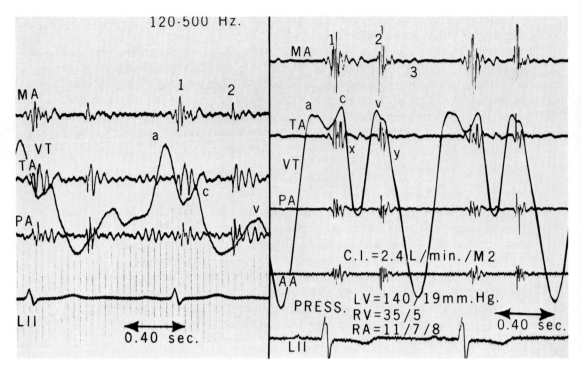

Figure 11.3.

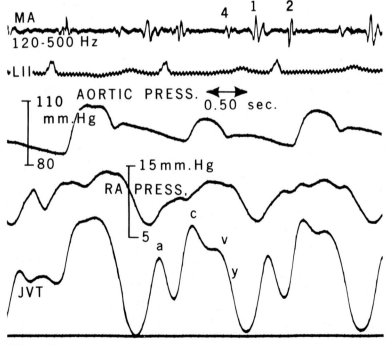

Figure 11.4.

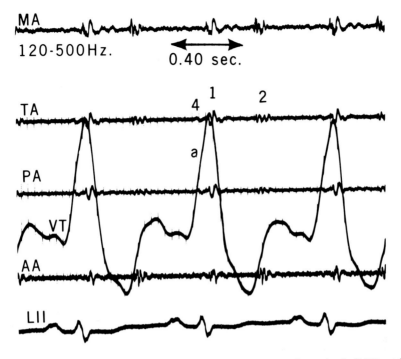

Figure 11.5. Simultaneously recorded phonocardiogram at the mitral (MA), tricuspid (TA), pulmonic (PA) and aortic areas (AA), jugular venous tracing (VT), and lead, II (LII) of the electrocardiogram in a 48-year-old patient with idiopathic pulmonary hypertension and myocardial disease involving the right ventricle. There is a faint fourth heart sound on the phonocardiogram. The first and second heart sounds are normal. The jugular venous tracing shows a markedly increased A wave. The V wave is normal.

Figure 11.3. *Left:* Simultaneously recorded phonocardiogram at the mitral (MA), tricuspid (TA) and pulmonic areas (PA), jugular venous tracing (VT), and lead II (LII) of the electrocardiogram in a normal subject to illustrate the normal configuration of the jugular venous pulse. Compare this panel with the right panel. *Right:* Simultaneously recorded phonocardiogram at the mitral, tricuspid, pulmonic and aortic areas, jugular venous tracing, and lead II of the electrocardiogram in a patient with restrictive pericarditis. There are prominent C and V waves with a rapid Y descent. The cardiac index on this patient was 2.4 L/min/M², which was within the normal limits. The left ventricular end-diastolic pressure was elevated to 140/19 mm Hg. Right ventricular pressure of 35/5 was within normal limits. The right atrial pressure of 11 for the A wave, 7 for the V wave, and 8 for the mean was within the normal range.

Figure 11.4. Simultaneously recorded phonocardiogram at the mitral area (MA), lead II (LII) of the electrocardiogram, aortic pressure (AORTIC PRESS.), right atrial pressure (RA PRESS.), and jugular venous tracing (JVT) in a 37-year-old patient with idiopathic restrictive primary myocardial disease. Note the presence of a prominent fourth heart sound on the phonocardiogram. The aortic pressure is normal. Note the similarity in contours of the right atrial pressure and the jugular venous pulse. Both are abnormal showing a prominent A wave, sustained systolic wave (from C to V), and a rapid Y descent.

289

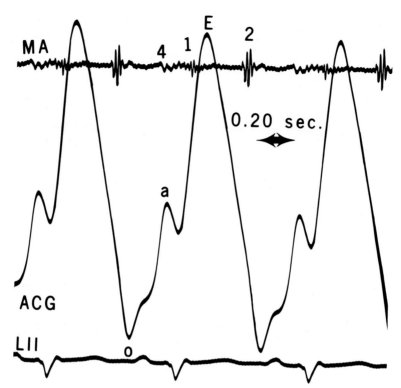

Figure 11.6.

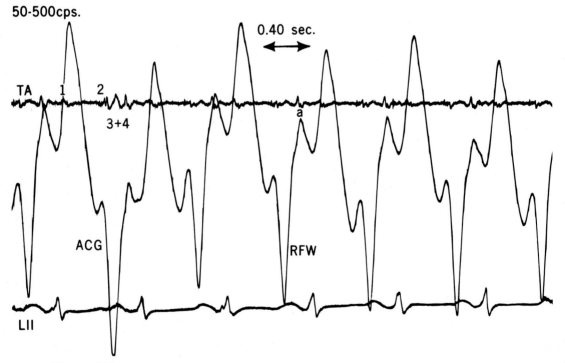

Figure 11.7.

jugular venous tracing, it may be difficult to differentiate between cardiomyopathy and constrictive pericarditis. Alternation of the jugular venous pulse indicates the presence of associated severe right ventricular disease (Fig. 11.2).

Apexcardiogram

The apexcardiogram shows a large A wave and a sustained systolic contraction (Fig. 11.6). Late systolic bulges are common and indicate left ventricular dyskinesis. The rapid filling wave is prominent. Pulsus alternans can also be seen on the apexcardiogram as shown in Figure 11.7.

Systolic Time Intervals

Ejection time (ET) is short and the pre-ejection period (PEP) is prolonged. Several reports have indicated that the ratio of PEP/ET is a good indicator of abnormal left ventricular function, which is almost always present in primary myocardial disease. This ratio is above the normal value of 0.40 and seems to correlate well with abnormal cardiovascular functions.

Vectorcardiogram

The vectorcardiogram is valuable in studying patients with myocardial disease. Most patients with primary myocardial disease due to viral or bacterial infections, or secondary to any systemic disease will present with either left ventricular enlargement or hypertrophy (Fig. 11.8). In addition, many patients will have a significant degree of fibrosis of the left ventricular myocardium. In this particular disease, recording without filtering is critically important because fibrosis of the myocardium results in an abnormal pattern of depolarization of the heart. Therefore, one may record what is called a "bite." A "bite" is a sudden change of direction and inscription of the QRS loop in any plane and the QRS loops look as if something were missing. The "bite" usually indicates the presence of scattered fibrosis around various areas of the myocardium. In addition, because of the loss

---

Figure 11.6. Simultaneously recorded phonocardiogram at the mitral area (MA), apexcardiogram (ACG), and lead II (LII) of the electrocardiogram in a 15-year-old patient with congestive primary myocardial disease. The phonocardiogram shows a diminished first heart sound, a fourth heart sound, and a normal second heart sound. There are no murmurs. The apexcardiogram shows a markedly prominent A wave. (From A. Benchimol: Non-Invasive Diagnostic Techniques in Cardiology. Copyright 1977 by the Williams & Wilkins Company, Baltimore. Used by permission.)

Figure 11.7. Simultaneously recorded phonocardiogram at the tricuspid area (TA), apexcardiogram (ACG), and lead II (LII) of the electrocardiogram in a 41-year-old patient with congestive cardiomyopathy and pulsus alternans on the left ventricular apexcardiogram. Note that each tall beat is followed by a small beat. On the tall beats, there are prominent A and rapid filling waves (RFW). Due to the rapid heart rate, both the rapid filling and A waves appear almost at the same time, causing a summation gallop as seen in the first heart beat at the left of the illustration.

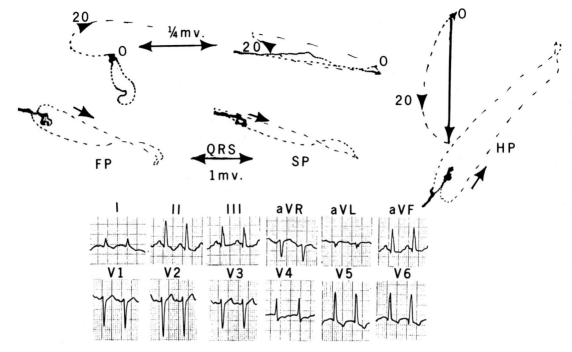

Figure 11.8.

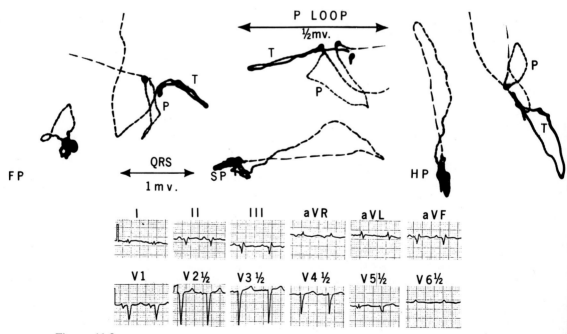

Figure 11.9.

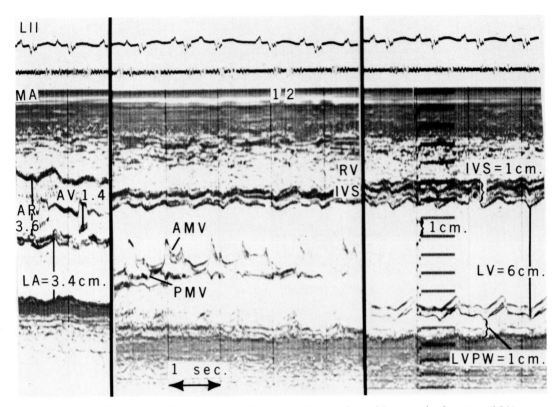

Figure 11.10. Echocardiogram recorded simultaneously with a mitral area (MA) phonocardiogram and lead II (LII) of the electrocardiogram in a 74-year-old patient with myocardial disease. Note an increase in the left ventricular (LV) internal dimension, 6 cm. The left atrium (LA) and aortic valve (AV) are within the normal limits. The middle panel shows the mitral valve floating in the left ventricle. AR = aortic root, AMV = anterior mitral valve, PMV = posterior mitral valve, IVS = interventricular septum, LVPW = left ventricular posterior wall.

Figure 11.8. Vectorcardiogram and electrocardiogram in a 16-year-old patient with cardiomyopathy and a marked degree of septal hypertrophy. The vectorcardiogram shows increased forces in the horizontal plane (HP) to the front of the O point, which is seen in patients with septal hypertrophy. There is also an increase in the total length of the QRS loop in the horizontal and frontal plane (FP), indicative of left ventricular hypertrophy. The electrocardiogram shows sinus rhythm and signs of left ventricular hypertrophy. The precordial leads were recorded at half standard. There are also some abnormalities of the T waves and ST segments, which are quite common in patients with cardiomyopathy.

Figure 11.9. Vectorcardiogram and electrocardiogram in a 15-year-old patient with primary myocardial disease. In the frontal plane (FP), the vectorcardiogram shows that all forces are above the O point, indicating some kind of conduction defect, and also simulating myocardial infarction. This is also seen in the horizontal plane (HP) where there are no forces in front of the P loop, indicating the presence of an anteroseptal myocardial infarction, which is seen frequently in patients with cardiomyopathy. The electrocardiogram is also abnormal showing signs of an inferior wall and anteroseptal myocardial infarction, as well as left ventricular hypertrophy.

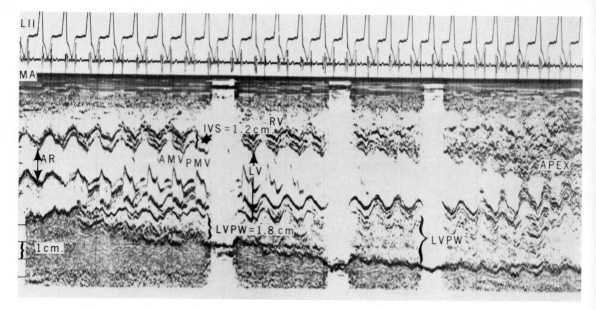

Figure 11.11.

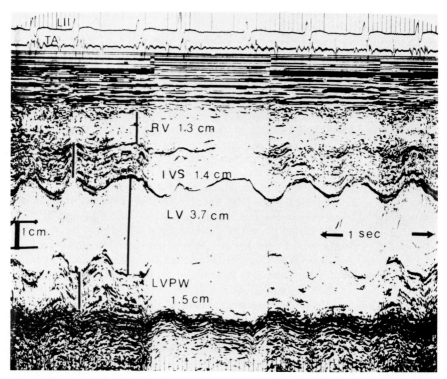

Figure 11.12.

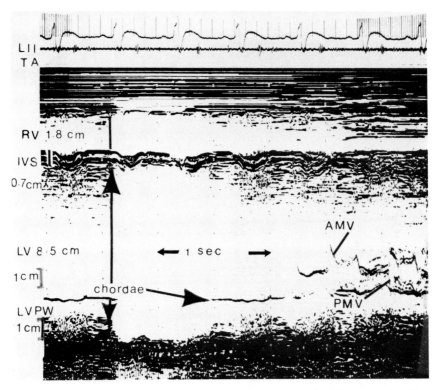

Figure 11.13. Simultaneously recorded echocardiogram, phonocardiogram at the tricuspid area (TA), and lead II (LII) of the electrocardiogram in a 41-year-old patient with cardiomyopathy. Note marked enlargement of the left ventricle, 8.5 cm. The right ventricular size and interventricular septal size are within the normal limits. The left ventricular posterior wall has poor motion.

Figure 11.11. Echocardiographic scan from the aorta to the apex recorded simultaneously with lead II (LII) of the electrocardiogram and a mitral area (MA) phonocardiogram in a 17-year-old patient with hypertrophic cardiomyopathy. Note an increase in left ventricular posterior wall (LVPW) thickness to 1.8 cm. Thickness of the interventricular septum (IVS), 1.2 cm is at the upper limits of normal. AR = aortic root, AMV = anterior mitral valve, PMV = posterior mitral valve.

Figure 11.12. Echocardiogram in a 22-year-old patient with primary myocardial disease, recorded with a tricuspid area (TA) phonocardiogram and lead II (LII) of the electrocardiogram. Note a significant increase in thickness of the interventricular septum (IVS), 1.4 cm, and the left ventricular posterior wall (LVPW), 1.5 cm, indicating concentric left ventricular hypertrophy. The left ventricular (LV) internal dimension is normal (3.7 cm). RV = right ventricle.

of a large mass of myocardial tissue in patients with primary myocardial disease, they may exhibit patterns that simulate vectorcardiographic findings of myocardial infarction (coronary artery disease) (Fig. 11.9) or a decrease in voltage of the QRS forces. Signs of left atrial enlargement can be detected on the vectorcardiogram by an enlarged P loop. In the late stage of this disease, there is an increase in the pulmonary artery pressure and the patient exhibits signs of right ventricular hypertrophy that can be detected on the vectorcardiogram.

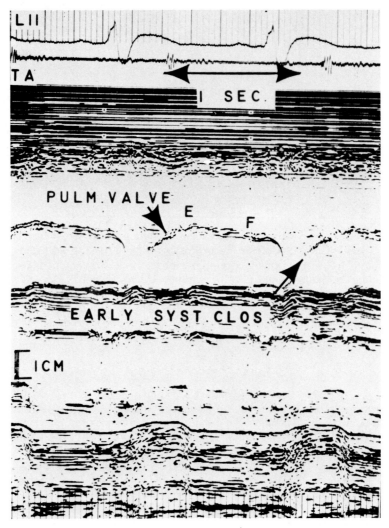

Figure 11.14. Echocardiogram in a patient with congestive cardiomyopathy and severe pulmonary hypertension recorded with a phonocardiogram at the tricuspid area (TA) and lead II (LII) of the electrocardiogram. The pulmonic valve has a reduced e–f slope, a minimal "a" dip, and appears to close early, which are the signs usually present in patients with severe pulmonary hypertension secondary to congestive heart failure.

Echocardiogram

In patients with primary myocardial disease, diminished excursion of the interventricular septum and posterior wall of the left ventricle (Fig. 11.10) are seen. True paradoxical motion of the interventricular septum is rare. In patients with idiopathic hypertrophic cardiomyopathy, there is an increase in the thickness of the interventricular septum and/or the posterior wall of the left ventricle (Fig. 11.11, 11.12). When right and/or left ventricular end-diastolic pressures are elevated, abnormal motion of the mitral and/or tricuspid valve is frequently seen, especially at the time of atrial contraction (tall A wave) or in addition, the A–C interval is prolonged and the P–R interval minus the A–C interval is less than 0.06 sec. The mitral valve usually demonstrates a double diamond appearance where the posterior leaflet has a diastolic excursion equal to or greater than the anterior leaflet. The valve also may appear to float in the middle of the left ventricle (Fig. 11.10). The aortic valve excursion is small, reflecting diminished cardiac output and stroke volume. Abnormalities of the pulmonic valve (flat motion without a dip) may also be seen, indicating the presence of pulmonary hypertension (Fig. 11.13). Measurements of intracavitary diameters almost always demonstrate increased left atrial and left ventricular (Fig. 11.14) and/or right ventricular diameters.

BIBLIOGRAPHY

Abbasi, A.S., MacAlpin, R.N., Eber, L.M., and Pearce, M.L.:   Echocardiographic diagnosis of idiopathic hypertrophic cardiomyopathy without outflow obstruction. Circulation *46*:897, 1972.

Anger, L.E.:   Mitral and aortic valve incompetence in endocardial fibroelastosis. Diagnostic and hemodynamic significance. Am. J. Cardiol. *28*:309, 1971.

Cheng, T.O.:   Prompt squatting and systolic murmurs. Am. Heart J. 77:433, 1969.

Epstein, E.J., Coulshed, N., Brown, A.K., and Doukas, N.G.:   The "A" wave of the apex cardiogram in aortic valve disease and cardiomyopathy. Br. Heart J. *30*:591, 1968.

Feigenbaum, H.:   Newer aspects of echocardiography. Circulation *47*:833, 1973.

Goodwin, J.F., and Oakley, C.M.:   The cardiomyopathies. Br. Heart J. *34*:545, 1972.

Gould, L., and Lyon, A.F.:   Pulsus alternans. An early manifestation of left ventricular dysfunction. Angiology *19*:103, 1968.

Hanby, R.I.:   Primary myocardial disease. A prospective clinical and hemodynamic evaluation in 100 patients. Medicine (Balt) *49*:55, 1970.

Harvey, W.P., Segal, J.P., and Gurel, T.:   The clinical spectrum of primary myocardial disease. Progr. Cardiov. Dis. 7:17, 1964.

Hill, C.A., Harle, T.S., and Gaston, W.:   Cardiomyopathy: A review of 59 patients with emphasis on the plain chest roentgenogram. Am. J. Roentgen. *104*:433, 1968.

Karatzas, N.B., Hamill, J., and Sleight, P.:   Hypertrophic cardiomyopathy. Br. Heart J. *30*:826, 1968.

Lundstrom, N.R., and Edler, I.:   Ultrasound cardiography in infants and children. Acta. Paediatr. Scand. *60*:117, 1971.

McDonald, I.G., and Hobson, E.R.:   A comparison of the relative value of noninvasive techniques—echocardiography, systolic time intervals, and apexcardiography—in the diagnosis of primary myocardial disease. Am. Heart J. *88*:454, 1974.

Morrow, A.G., Fisher, R.D., and Fogarty, T.J.:   Isolated hypertrophic obstruction to right ventricular outflow. Clinical, hemodynamic and angiographic findings before and after operative treatment. Am. Heart J. *77*:814, 1969.

Nagle, R.E., Boicourt, O.W., Gillam, P.M., and Mounsey, J.P.D.:   Cardiac impulse in hypertrophic obstructive cardiomyopathy. Br. Heart J. *28*:419, 1966.

Shah, P.M., Gramiak, R., Kramer, D.H., and Yu, P.N.:   Determinants of atrial (S$_4$) and ventricular (S$_3$) gallop sounds in primary myocardial disease. New Engl. J. Med. *278*:753, 1968.

12
Pericardial Disease

Diseases of the pericardium (the membrane surrounding the heart) are classified as acute or chronic pericarditis with or without constriction. The disease may be due to primary infection of the pericardial membrane. Rarely, it may be secondary to a chronic or recurrent systemic disease process, such as recurrent viral, fungal, or bacterial pericarditis, or involvement of the pericardium primary or secondary to malignancy. It is usually secondary to involvement of the pericardium. Pericarditis following open heart surgery is fairly common but in most cases it does not have any major clinical significance.

PERICARDITIS

Heart Sounds, Friction Rubs, and Murmurs

The first and second heart sounds are normal in acute pericarditis without significant effusion. The most characteristic feature of acute or chronic pericarditis without constriction is the presence of a pericardial friction rub that has three major components (Figs. 12.1, 12.2). The first occurs during mid- or late systole, the second during early or mid-diastole at the time of rapid filling of the ventricles or shortly thereafter, and the third during atrial contraction (Figs. 12.1, 12.2). If the patient's rhythm is atrial fibrillation, the third component is absent because of the lack of coordinated atrial contraction. The triphasic rub consists of high frequency vibrations of variable amplitude (Figs. 12.1, 12.2). It is best recorded at the tricuspid and/or mitral areas. The friction rub varies with respiration, being loudest during expiration and when the patient is in the left lateral decubitus position. Mid- or late systolic clicks are uncommon but may be found in 10 to 15% of patients with this disease state.

PERICARDIAL EFFUSION

Pericardial effusion may result from a multitude of pathological conditions involving the pericardium as the primary site, or it may be secondary to a systemic disease process. Abnormalities in cardiac function resulting from pericardial effusion are present when the amount of fluid exceeds 200 cc, which causes significant impairment of ventricular filling.

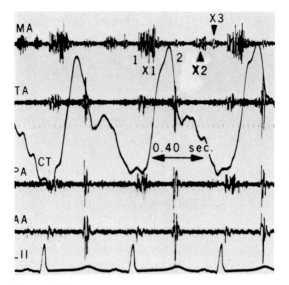

Figure 12.1.

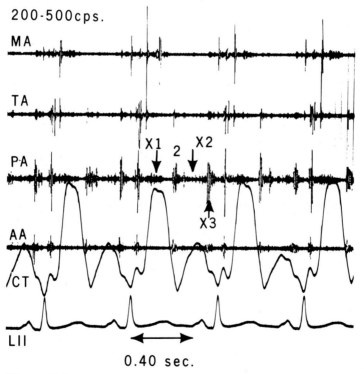

Figure 12.2.

Heart Sounds and Murmurs

The first heart sound has diminished amplitude because late ventricular filling is decreased at the time of atrial contraction and the atrioventricular valves are in a semiclosed position. As a result, the rate of excursion of these valves is short. Amplitude of the second heart sound is also diminished because stroke volume (blood volume ejected per heart beat), and pulmonary artery and aortic pressures are low. Third and fourth heart sounds are rarely present, particularly in younger patients. High frequency, low amplitude systolic regurgitant murmurs due to mitral and/or tricuspid insufficiencies are present in approximately 5 to 10% of patients.

Carotid Pulse Tracing

The carotid pulse tracing has a normal contour or may show rapid upstroke time and a short ejection time corresponding to the diminished stroke volume. Respiratory variations may occur and changes in the amplitude of the carotid pulse tracing correspond to so-called "pulsus paradoxicus" (inspiratory fall in systolic arterial pressure below 10 to 15 mmHg). A great deal of care should be exercised in the clinical evaluation of pulsus paradoxicus, since it may be present in patients without significant pericardial effusion. However, it is of clinical value if the auscultatory, phonocardiographic, and pulse wave abnormalities are present. Pulsus alternans (see Chap. 11) may be seen, particularly in patients with a large effusion, and is usually indicative of major impairment of left ventricular function.

Jugular Venous Pulse Tracing

The jugular venous pulse tracing may be normal when the amount of pericardial fluid is less than 150 to 300 cc. In the presence of significant right ventricular restriction, the jugular venous pulse tracing shows a prominent A wave, sustained

---

Figure 12.1. Simultaneously recorded phonocardiogram at the mitral (MA), tricuspid (TA), pulmonic (PA) and aortic areas (AA), carotid pulse tracing (CT), and lead II (LII) of the electrocardiogram in a 17-year-old patient with pericarditis. The phonocardiogram was recorded at a setting of 500–2000 Hz. The first (1) and second (2) heart sounds have normal amplitude. Note the characteristic triphasic pericardial friction rub. The first component (X1) of the rub occurs during midsystole. The second component (X2) is present during mid-, or early diastole. The third component (X3) occurs during atrial contraction following the P wave of the electrocardiogram. These vibrations of the rub have different characteristics from beat to beat. The carotid pulse tracing is normal. (From A. Benchimol: Non-Invasive Diagnostic Techniques in Cardiology. Copyright 1977 by The Williams & Wilkins Company, Baltimore. Used by permission.)

Figure 12.2. Simultaneously recorded phonocardiogram at the mitral (MA), tricuspid (TA), pulmonic (PA) and aortic areas (AA), carotid pulse tracing (CT), and lead II (LII) of the electrocardiogram in a 23-year-old patient who developed pericarditis following mitral valvulotomy. Again, note the three components of the pericardial friction rub, X1 during systole, X2 in mid-diastole, and X3 during atrial contraction, with marked variation in the amplitude of these noisy vibrations especially at the pulmonic area.

systolic wave, and rapid Y descent followed by a rapid early diastolic rise. The tracing is identical to that of patients with constrictive pericarditis and resembles the square root symbol ($\sqrt{}$).

Apexcardiogram

The precordial pulsations are diminished and a technically satisfactory apexcardiogram is rarely recorded. However, if a good recording is obtained, it may show a marked retraction during systole.

Systolic Time Intervals

Ejection time is normal or diminished and varies with respiration. This is probably secondary to decreased stroke volume and decreased aortic pressure during respiration. These changes occur, however, only in patients with large effusions exceeding 500 cc.

Vectorcardiogram

The vectorcardiogram is not used to evaluate patients with pericardial effusion or constrictive pericarditis. However, if pericardial effusion is of clinical importance, it usually shows the same findings seen on the electrocardiogram, i.e., a decrease in the magnitude of the QRS vectors in all three planes.

Echocardiogram

One of the first clinical applications of echocardiography was evaluation of patients with pericardial effusion. It gave great impetus to this diagnostic technique. The echocardiogram detects the presence of pericardial effusion and grossly quantitates the amount of pericardial fluid in the anterior and/or posterior aspects of the heart. Pericardial fluid is recognized by an "echo free" space separating the epicardial surface of the heart from the pericardium (Figs. 12.3 through 12.5). Tracings should be recorded at multiple damping settings. Additional findings on the echocardiogram include the presence of flat or paradoxical motion of the interventricular septum and an increase in thickness of the parietal pericardium. With significant effusion, abnormal valve motion can be seen, such as prolapse of the mitral and tricuspid valves. The prolapse should not be considered a true finding but a result of the pericardial effusion itself. A small effusion is approximately 1 cm anterior and/or posterior, medium effusion 1.5 to 2 cm, and a large effusion is over 2 cm anterior and/or posterior. In massive effusions, the whole heart swings in the pericardium and the structures are almost unidentifiable (Fig. 12.3).

A careful scan from the aorta to the left ventricle is essential to follow the pericardium beneath the left atrium to the left ventricle. Good slow damping is important to delineate clearly the pericardium from the epicardium (Fig. 12.6). In the presence of a moderate to large pericardial effusion, structure motion cannot be determined with any accuracy. If a pleural effusion is present, a pericardial effusion may be easier to quantitate by placing the patient in a left lateral position (Figs. 12.4, 12.5).

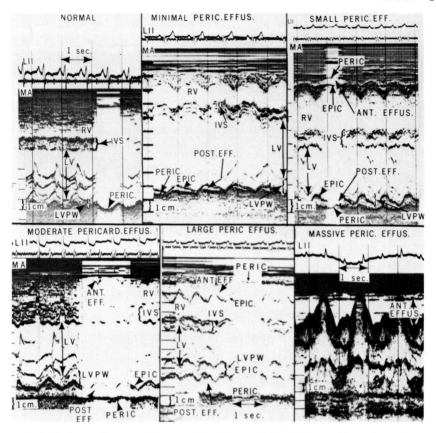

Figure 12.3. Echocardiogram of a normal patient and in subjects with various degrees of pericardial effusion. *Top Left:* A normal left ventricle and pericardium without pericardial effusion. *Top Middle:* A tracing of a patient with a minimal amount of pericardial fluid. The epicardium is well seen. The posterior effusion is indicated by an arrow. *Top Right:* In the patient with a small pericardial effusion, there is an echo free space located anteriorly and posteriorly. *Bottom Left:* Recording of a patient with a moderate pericardial effusion. There is an echo free space located anteriorly and posteriorly. Damping is quite important to delineate clearly the epicardium. *Bottom Middle:* A large echo free space located in the anterior and posterior aspects of the pericardium is seen in a patient with a large pericardial effusion. *Bottom Right:* Massive pericardial effusion. Note the large echo free space located anteriorly. The structures are impossible to visualize due to the swinging motion of the heart.

CONSTRICTIVE PERICARDITIS

Constriction is defined as impairment of ventricular filling because the cardiac chambers cannot expand as much as the normal heart. Constrictive pericarditis (Pick's disease) is due to marked fibrosis with or without calcification of the pericardium around the epicardial surface of the heart. Constriction is usually present on the surface of the left ventricle but it may involve multiple cardiac chambers.

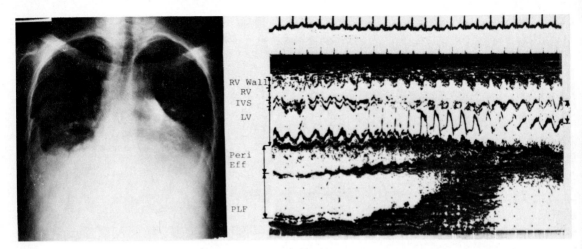

Figure 12.4. Echocardiographic scan from the aorta to the mitral valve on a patient with pericardial and pleural effusion. The chest X-ray shows a moderate enlargement of the cardiac silhouette. On the scan, one can clearly appreciate an echo free space behind the pericardium, which is a large pericardial effusion, and another echo free space located posteriorly representing a large pleural effusion.

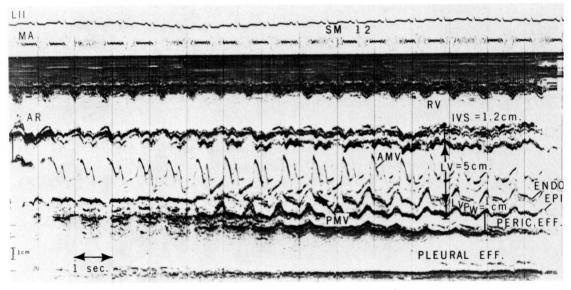

Figure 12.5. Echocardiographic scan from the aorta to the left ventricle recorded simultaneously with a mitral area (MA) phonocardiogram and lead II (LII) of the electrocardiogram in a 37-year-old patient who developed pericardial and pleural effusion following aortic valve replacement for aortic stenosis. The echo free space behind the pericardium represents pleural effusion. If one follows the pericardium beneath the left atrium to the left ventricle, an echo free space is noted between the epicardium and pericardium representing a small to moderate effusion.

304

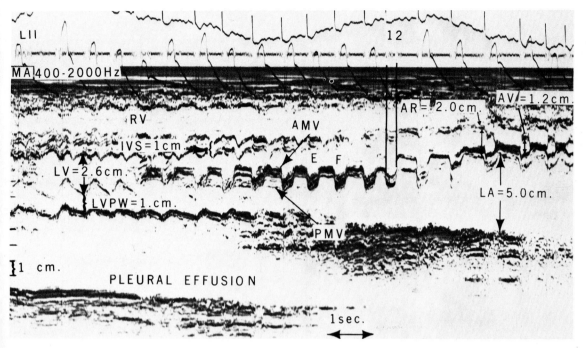

Figure 12.6. Echocardiogram simultaneously recorded with a mitral area (MA) phonocardiogram and lead II (LII) of the electrocardiogram in a 55-year-old patient with severe mitral stenosis and a large isolated pleural effusion. This illustration demonstrates the importance of clear damping in order to observe the pericardium so that pericardial effusion is not confused with pleural effusion. The mitral valve motion is characteristic of patients with mitral stenosis. The left atrium (LA) is enlarged to 5.0 cm. RV = right ventricle, LV = left ventricle, LVPW = left ventricular posterior wall, AMV = anterior mitral valve, AR = aortic root, AV = aortic valve, IVS = interventricular septum.

Heart Sounds and Murmurs

The first heart sound is normal. The second heart sound is usually widely split with marked variations during respiration. One of the most striking features in patients with constrictive pericarditis is the presence of an early diastolic sound called a "pericardial knock" (Figs. 12.7 through 12.9). This "early third heart sound" occurs within the range of 0.04 to 0.12 sec after the aortic valve closure sound and has high amplitude and high or low frequency characteristics. In many situations, this sound may be difficult to differentiate from a split second heart sound or opening snap of the mitral valve. However, with simultaneous recording of a phonocardiogram and apexcardiogram, this early diastolic sound should coincide with the peak of the rapid filling wave on the apexcardiogram, and if there is a split second sound both components should precede the O point of the apexcardiogram. The production mechanism for "pericardial knock" is not well known but it is probably related to increased rapid filling of the nondistensible ventricles in the early diastolic phase of the cardiac cycle. This sound is best heard at the mitral and tricuspid areas. Prominent fourth heart sounds are frequently recorded in patients with constrictive pericarditis due to forceful atrial contraction

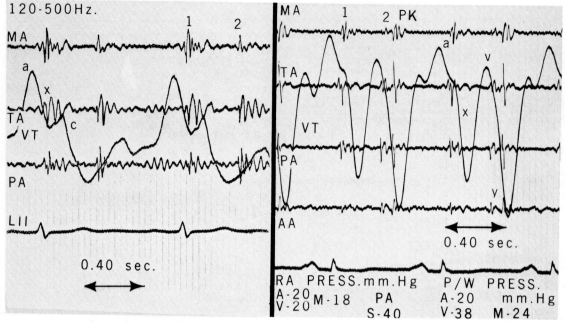

Figure 12.7. *Left:* Simultaneously recorded phonocardiogram at the mitral (MA), tricuspid (TA) and pulmonic areas (PA), jugular venous tracing (VT), and lead II (LII) of the electrocardiogram in a normal subject. Note the normal contour of the jugular venous pulse. *Right:* Simultaneously recorded phonocardiogram at the mitral (MA), tricuspid (TA), pulmonic (PA), and aortic areas (AA), jugular venous tracing (VT), and lead II (LII) of the electrocardiogram in a patient with constrictive pericarditis. The tracings were recorded at a filter setting of 50–500 Hz. The first (1) and second (2) heart sounds are normal. The extremely prominent vibration following the second heart sound is the third heart sound, which is also called a pericardial knock (PK). The jugular venous pulse shows prominent A and V waves that resemble the square root sign ($\sqrt{}$). At cardiac catheterization, right atrial (RA) pressures were markedly elevated, A wave 29 and V wave 20 with a mean of 18. The pulmonary artery (PA) pressure was 40, systolic. The pulmonary "wedge" (P/W) pressures were markedly elevated, A wave 20 and V wave 38 with a mean of 24 mm Hg.

against a nondistensible ventricle, which also has poor compliance during the late diastolic phase of the cardiac cycle.

No definite characteristic murmurs can be detected. Low frequency atrioventricular diastolic murmurs resembling mitral and/or tricuspid stenosis have been described, but are rare. They may be the result of constriction around the atrioventricular valve rings causing a decrease in size of the mitral and/or tricuspid orifices, thus simulating mitral and/or tricuspid stenosis (see Chaps. 5 and 7).

Carotid Pulse Tracing

The carotid pulse tracing has normal contour.

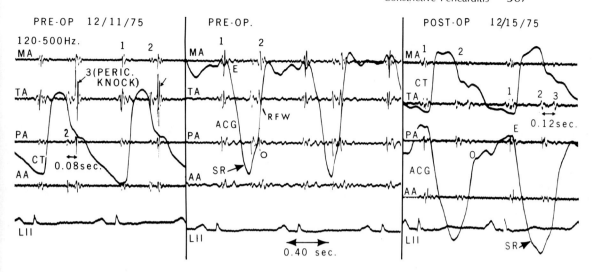

Figure 12.8. *Left:* Phonocardiogram at the mitral (MA), tricuspid (TA), pulmonic (PA), and aortic areas (AA), carotid pulse tracing (CT), and lead II (LII) of the electrocardiogram in a patient with constrictive pericarditis simultaneously recorded prior to surgery. The first (1) and second (2) heart sounds are normal. Note the presence of a very prominent vibration following the second heart sound, which is called pericardial knock (PERIC. KNOCK). *Middle:* Left ventricular apexcardiogram on the same patient, which shows the typical midsystolic retraction (SR) after the E point. Following the O point, there is a rapid filling wave that coincides with the pericardial knock. *Right:* This tracing was recorded after a pericardectomy. Note that the pericardial sound has much less amplitude and has a low frequency characteristic. On the preoperative tracing the interval from the second sound to the pericardial knock was 0.08 sec, and following surgery it was 0.12 sec. The carotid pulse tracing was normal. The apexcardiogram continues to show a midsystolic retraction following surgery.

Jugular Venous Pulse Tracing

Inspection of the jugular venous pulsations should make the observer suspect the presence of constrictive pericarditis. It will show a large A wave, small X descent, sustained systolic, and large V and H waves (Fig. 12.7). The tracing resembles the square root symbol ($\sqrt{}$) and reflects abnormalities of right ventricular function.

Apexcardiogram

In constrictive pericarditis, the apexcardiogram shows a large A wave representing forceful atrial contraction against a nondistensible left ventricle during late diastole. The E point is sharp. During systole, there is a systolic retraction followed by a late systolic wave indicating the presence of left ventricular dyskinesis (Figs. 12.8, 12.9). A prominent and sharp rapid filling wave is present because most of left ventricular filling occurs during the early phase of diastole. The peak of the rapid filling wave coincides with the prominent "early third heart sound."

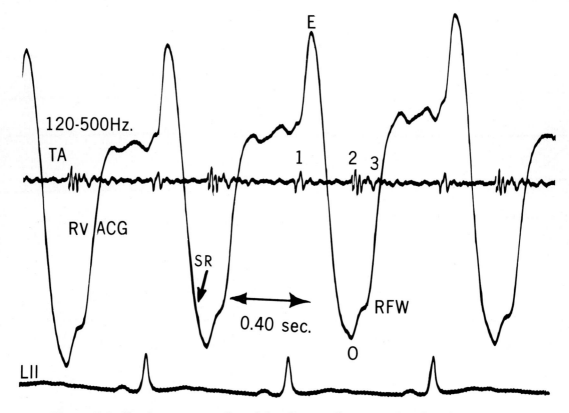

Figure 12.9. Simultaneous recording of the phonocardiogram at the tricuspid area (TA), right ventricular apexcardiogram (RV ACG), and lead II (LII) of the electrocardiogram in a patient with constrictive pericarditis. The first and second heart sounds have diminished amplitude. A very prominent third heart sound is inscribed close to the second heart sound. The second sound–third sound interval measures approximately 0.08 sec., which is abnormal. This is a typical pericardial knock seen in patients with constrictive pericarditis. There are no murmurs. The apexcardiogram is abnormal. Following the E point, there is a rapid systolic retraction terminating with the O point, which is inscribed very early. The rapid systolic retraction is one of the characteristic features on the apexcardiogram in patients with constrictive pericarditis. After the O point, the tracing moves upward and the rapid filling wave (RFW) is identified. Near the peak of the rapid filling wave, the third heart sound is recorded.

Systolic Time Intervals

Ejection time is usually diminished, corresponding to decreased stroke volume, ejection fraction, and aortic pulse pressures.

Echocardiogram

No definite patterns have been described outlining the use of echocardiography in patients with constrictive pericarditis. However, one may find decreased diastolic motion of the posterior left ventricular wall. A rapid E–F slope of the anterior mitral valve may be present, probably representing an increased rapid rate of flow in the left ventricle during early diastole. The interventricular septum may show paradoxical motion. These findings should be interpreted with caution because they may also be seen in patients with primary myocardial disease.

BIBLIOGRAPHY

Abbasi, A.S., Ellis, N., and Flynn, J.J.:   Echocardiographic M-scan technique in the diagnosis of pericardial effusion. J. Clin. Ultrasound *1*:300, 1973.

Boicourt, O.W., Nagle, R.E., and Mounsey, J.P.:   The clinical significance of systolic retraction of the apical impulse. Br. Heart J. *27*:379, 1965.

Braunwald, E., and Ross, J. Jr.:   Hemodynamic alterations in pericardial diseases. Nat. Conf. Cardiov. Dis. *2*:508, 1964.

Clauss, R.H.:   Pericardial disease. Cardiovasc. Clin. *3*:45, 1971.

Durant, T.M.:   Pericardial disease: diagnostic procedures. Nat. Conf. Cardiovasc. Dis. *2*:506, 1964.

Ellis, K., and King, D.L.:   Pericarditis and pericardial effusion. Radiologic and echocardiographic diagnosis. Radiol. Clin. North Am. *11*:393, 1973.

el-Sherif, A., and el-Said, G.:   Jugular, hepatic, and praecordial pulsations in constrictive pericarditis. Br. Heart J. *33*:305, 1971.

Feigenbaum, H.:   Echocardiographic diagnosis of pericardial effusion. Am. J. Cardiol. *26*:475, 1970.

Glaser, J.:   Echocardiographic diagnosis of septic pericarditis in infancy. J. Pediatr. *83*:697, 1973.

Goldberg, B.B., Ostrum, B.J., and Isard, H.J.:   Ultrasonic determination of pericardial effusion. J.A.M.A. *202*:927, 1967.

Holmes, J.C., and Fowler, N.O.:   Diagnosis of pericarditis. Postgrad. Med. *44*:92, 1968.

Holt, J.P.:   The normal pericardium. Am. J. Cardiol. *26*:455, 1970.

Horowitz, M.S., Schultz, C.S., Stinson, E.B., Harrison, D.C., and Popp, R.L.:   Sensitivity and specificity of echocardiographic diagnosis of pericardial effusion. Circulation *50*:239, 1974.

Idriss, F.S., Hisashi, N., and Muster, A.J.:   Constrictive pericarditis simulating liver disease in children. Arch. Surg. *109*:223, 1974.

Kay, C.F., Joyner, C.R., Helwig, J. Jr., and Raymond, T.F.:   The "late systolic heartbeat" of pericardial effusion. Am. Heart J. *72*:7, 1966.

Kahn, A.M., Nejat, M., and Bloomfield, D.A.:   The measurement of pericardial effusion volume. Chest *63*:762, 1973.

Lange, R.L., Botticelli, J.T., Tsagaris, T.J., Walker, J.A., Gani, M., and Bustamante, R.A.:   Diagnostic signs in compressive cardiac disorders. Constrictive pericarditis, pericardial effusion, and tamponade. Circulation *33*:763, 1966.

Lundstrom, N.R., and Edler, I.:   Ultrasoundcardiography in infants and children. Acta. Paediatr. Scan. *60*:117, 1971.

Madaras, J.S. Jr., Taber, R.E., and Lam, C.R.:   Constrictive pericarditis: diagnosis and operative management. Dis. Chest *52*:746, 1967.

Moreyra, E., Knibbe, P., and Segal, B.L.:   Constrictive pericarditis masquerading as mitral stenosis. Chest *57*:245, 1970.

Moscovitz, H.L.:   Pericardial constriction versus cardiac tamponade. Am. J. Cardiol. 26:546, 1970.

Moss, A.J., and Bruhn, F.:   The echocardiogram. An ultrasound technic for the detection of pericardial effusion. New Engl. J. Med. 274:380, 1966.

Potter, D.J., and Cohen, A.I.:   Diagnosis and management of uremic constrictive pericarditis. Ariz. Med. 28:302, 1971.

Pridie, R.B., and Turnbull, T.A.:   Diagnosis of pericardial effusion by ultrasound. Br. Med. J. 3:356, 1968.

Ramsey, H.W., Sbar, S., Elliott, L.P., and Eliot, R.S.:   The differential diagnosis of restrictive myocardiopathy and chronic constrictive pericarditis without calcification. Value of coronary arteriography. Am. J. Cardiol. 25:635, 1970.

Ratshin, R.A., Smith, M., and Hood, W.P. Jr.:   Possible false–positive diagnosis of pericardial effusion by echocardiography in presence of large left atrium. Chest 65:112, 1974.

Shabetai, R., Fowler, N.O., and Fenton, J.C.:   Restrictive cardiac disease. Pericarditis and the myocardiopathies. Am. Heart J. 69:271, 1965.

Shapiro, E., and Salick, A.I.:   A clarification of the paradoxic pulse. Adolf Kussmaul's original description. (Kussmaul, A.) Am. J. Cardiol. 16:426, 1965.

Simcha, A., and Taylor, J.F.N.:   Constrictive pericarditis in childhood. Arch. Dis. Child. 46:515, 1971.

Spodick, D.H.:   Acoustic phenomena in pericardial disease. Am. Heart J. 81:114, 1971.

Spodick, D.H.:   Pericardial friction. Characteristics of pericardial rubs in fifty consecutive, prospectively studied patients. New Engl. J. Med. 278:1204, 1968.

Weiss, A., and Luisada, A.A.:   The friction rubs of pericarditis. Chest 60:491, 1971.

Index